Do It Yourself
Pure Plant Skin Care

Do It Yourself
Pure Plant Skin Care

second edition

Carolyn Stubbin

Black Pepper Creative

First published in 1999 by
The International Centre of Holistic Aromatherapy
PO Box 273, Zillmere QLD 4034
Australia
ISBN: 0 646 38318 3

Second edition published in 2022 by
Black Pepper Creative Pty Ltd
PO Box 273, Zillmere QLD 4034
ISBN: 978-0-6482606-9-1

Note to the reader
To the fullest extent of the law, neither the author nor the publisher, contributor or editor assumes any liability for any injury and/or damage to persons or property as a matter of product liability, negligence or otherwise, or from any use or operation of any methods, products, instructions or ideas contained in this book.

A catalogue record for this book is available from the National Library of Australia
ISBN: 9780648260691

Edited by Kyoko Mizoguchi
Proofreading by Gail Cartwright
Cover design by Bill Adrisurya
Text design by Bill Adrisurya
Illustrations by Romana Gruber-Hallam
Photography by Carolyn Stubbin
Models — Gemma Edwards and Kiki Fung
Typeset by Watson Ferguson and Company, Brisbane
Printed and bound in China by Everbest Printing Investment Ltd

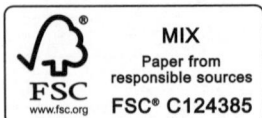

MIX
Paper from responsible sources
FSC® C124385
FSC
www.fsc.org

Acknowledgements

I acknowledge the Traditional Custodians of Country, the Aboriginal and Torres Strait Islander peoples, throughout Australia and recognise their continuing connection to land, waters and community. I pay my respects to them and their cultures, and to Elders both past and present.

I would like to thank Ugarapul Elders Uncle Burragun John Long and Auntie Teenie Wilton and their families for their friendship and for regularly taking the time to share their Dreaming with me. I grew up on their country in the Scenic Rim and they have taught me a deep appreciation of all their country holds. They have shown me the healing it provides them, and all of us, and how we must continue to care for this sacred land.

There are many other people I would like to thank for their encouragement, support and inspiration — especially my husband, Salvatore Battaglia, for his love and support. I would like to thank my parents, Beverly and Robert Stubbin, for always making natural therapies a central part of my life as I was growing up.

Thank you to all my students, colleagues at Perfect Potion and customers who have been a constant source of information and questions, and who inspire me to seek knowledge and understanding. Keep asking and keep telling me of your successes too.

I am also indebted to all the medicine people, herbalists and aromatherapists who have gone before me. The knowledge you have imparted has been truly invaluable.

About the author

Carolyn Stubbin was born in 1967 in Boonah, a country town on Ugarapul country in south-east Queensland, where she grew up and lived with her family on a farm. From a very young age, Carolyn knew she wanted to be a herbalist and work with plant medicines. Carolyn holds qualifications in herbal medicine, aromatherapy and cosmetic science. Most recently she completed a Master of Arts in Visual Arts.

Carolyn and her partner, Salvatore Battaglia, founded Perfect Potion and have developed a range of pure aromatherapy products. Carolyn currently works as the creative director of Perfect Potion.

Foreword

This book is for those of you who find joy in nature and respect the innate wisdom it holds. It provides a repository of restorative and healing elements for both body and spirit.

In this book, you will learn how to make luscious creams to moisturise your skin, gorgeous soaps to lather up with, relaxing bath soaks to calm the spirit, healing ointments to repair and protect your skin and much more, using the purest plant and natural ingredients.

The ingredients recommended in this book have been chosen both for their therapeutic properties as well as their availability. Do not limit your preparations to the ingredients recommended in this book. You may find that your knowledge of local indigenous plants and herbs or having access to rarer ingredients will allow you to substitute them into many of the recipes. Once you have mastered the basics, the possibilities are infinite.

As well as containing pure plant and natural ingredients, your preparations will contain lots of love — a truly special ingredient. I wish you joy in making your own preparations from this book.

In this second edition of *Do It Yourself Pure Plant Skin Care*, you will find many new recipes and be introduced to a range of new ingredients, including Australian ingredients. There are over 300 recipes, and among them you will find powders and pastes for cleaning your teeth, simple colour cosmetics such as blush, face powder and eye colours, as well as shampoo and conditioner bars.

The new Clean & Minimal section features a range of 'clean', simple and effective skin care recipes. They are made with minimal ingredients, in a minimum amount of time, with minimal effort, and are all preservative-free. In the new Home section, you will learn how to make recipes to clean and care for your home and discover essential oil blends to use in your aromatherapy diffuser to create a home sanctuary.

Please note

All ingredients must be selected and used with care and respect to ensure compatibility with your skin. The best quality certified organic ingredients available should always be selected where possible.

Product outcomes or skin reactions may vary due to a variety of factors such as:

- **Light** — botanical colourants can alter if exposed to UV light and will change over time.

- **Temperature** — products such as balms will be softer in warmer temperatures and harder in cooler temperatures. A warmer temperature may also reduce product preservation and stability.

- **Humidity** — products such as bath bombs can absorb moisture from the air. This affects their ability to fizz and remain compacted.

- **Ingredient quality and processing** — ingredients may have been processed differently. For example, granules may be smaller or larger, affecting their feel on the skin. Herbs may be cut into smaller pieces or left whole. Castile soap made by one supplier may differ from that made by another supplier due to different ratios of starting material used and the addition of other ingredients.

- **Common names** — the common name for an ingredient may vary from supplier to supplier or from one location to another. Botanical names are listed in the ingredients section of this book and should be referred to when sourcing ingredients.

- **Storage conditions** — exposure to air, moisture, heat or light may affect the quality of ingredients. Ingredients may become too old to use.

- **Skin and health conditions** — if you have skin concerns or health conditions that may be exacerbated by ingredients that you have never used or you are not familiar with, please consult with your health practitioner.

While many of the recipes in this book may form starting points for commercial products, it is important to note that rigorous testing must be carried out before releasing a product to market. This includes product efficacy testing, preservative efficacy testing, stability testing, packaging testing and skin sensitisation testing. Compliance with regulatory requirements and insurance must also be undertaken. These matters are beyond the scope of this book.

The recipes given in this book are not to be used as substitutes for professional health or medical advice.

Contents

Acknowledgements   v
About the Author   vi
Foreword   vii
Please Note   viii

Essentials
Basics   1
Raw Ingredients   7
Base Products   32
Aromatherapy   35
Herbal Extracts and Preparations   49
Ointments and Balms   59
Gels   65
Emulsions   69

Clean & Minimal
Beauty Infusions   91
Beauty Powders and Pastes   93
Beauty Sugar and Salt Scrubs   99
Beauty Washes   101
Beauty Oils and Elixirs   103
Beauty Vinegars   108
Beauty Balms   111

Face
Skin Types and Conditions   117
Cleansers   121
Toners   129
Moisturisers   133
Facial Treatment Oils   139
Lip Balms and Scrubs   141
Facial Compresses   145
Eye Creams and Gels   147
Masks   149
Scrubs and Exfoliants   155
Teeth Powders and Pastes   159
Colour Cosmetics   161

Soap
Introduction to Soap Making   167
Basic Soap Making   168
Soap Balls   177

Body
Body Washes   181
Body Scrubs   183
Body Masks   187
Body Moisturisers   189
Body Massage Preparations   191
Deodorants   197
Insect Repellents   202
Hair Removal   205
Sun Care   208
Body Powders   210
Hand Care   211
Foot Care   215
Baths   221
Mother and Baby Care   236

Perfumes
Fragrant Harmony   241
Creating Perfumes   244

Hair
Hair and Scalp Care Ingredients   251
Shampoos   255
Conditioners   261
Hair and Scalp Treatments   265
Styling   269
Colours   273

Home
Basic Cleaning Ingredients   279
Green Cleaners   280
Home Fragrance   282

Useful Information
Guide to Herbs and Essential Oils for Skin Care   288
Guide to Herbs and Essential Oils for Hair Care   291
Ingredient Suppliers   292
Guide to Green Terms   293
Glossary   300
Bibliography and Further Reading   304

Index   307

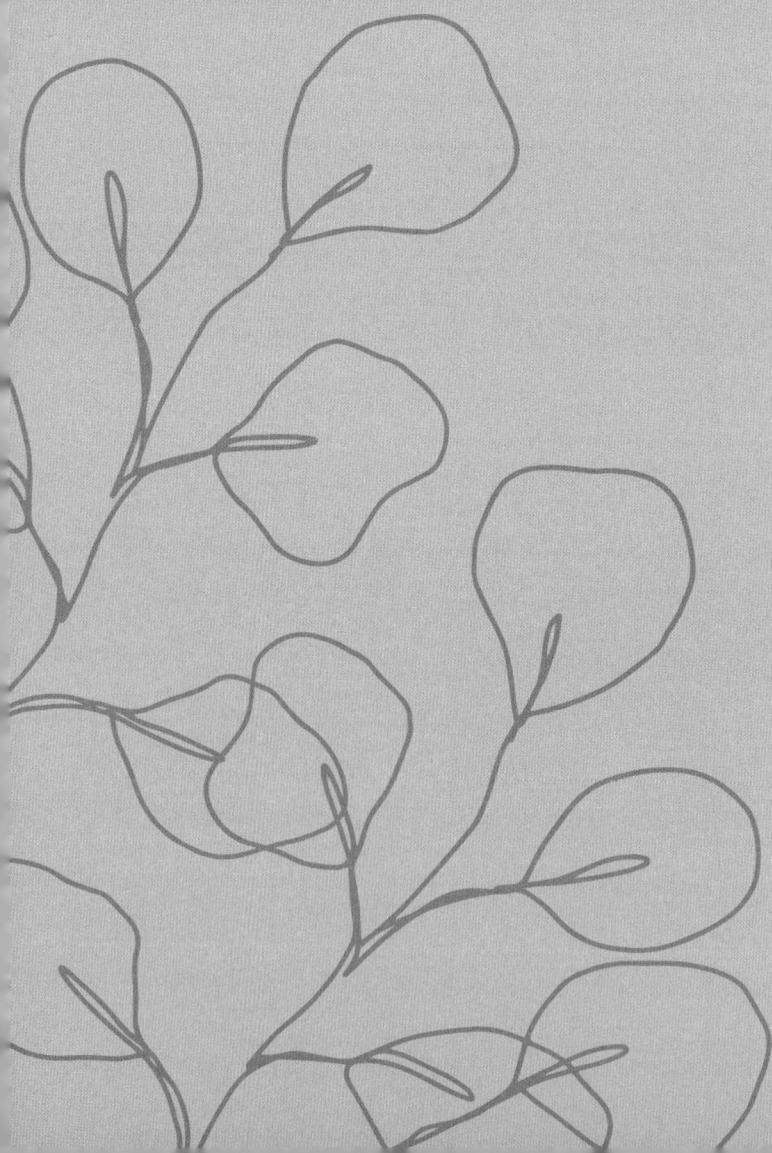

Essentials

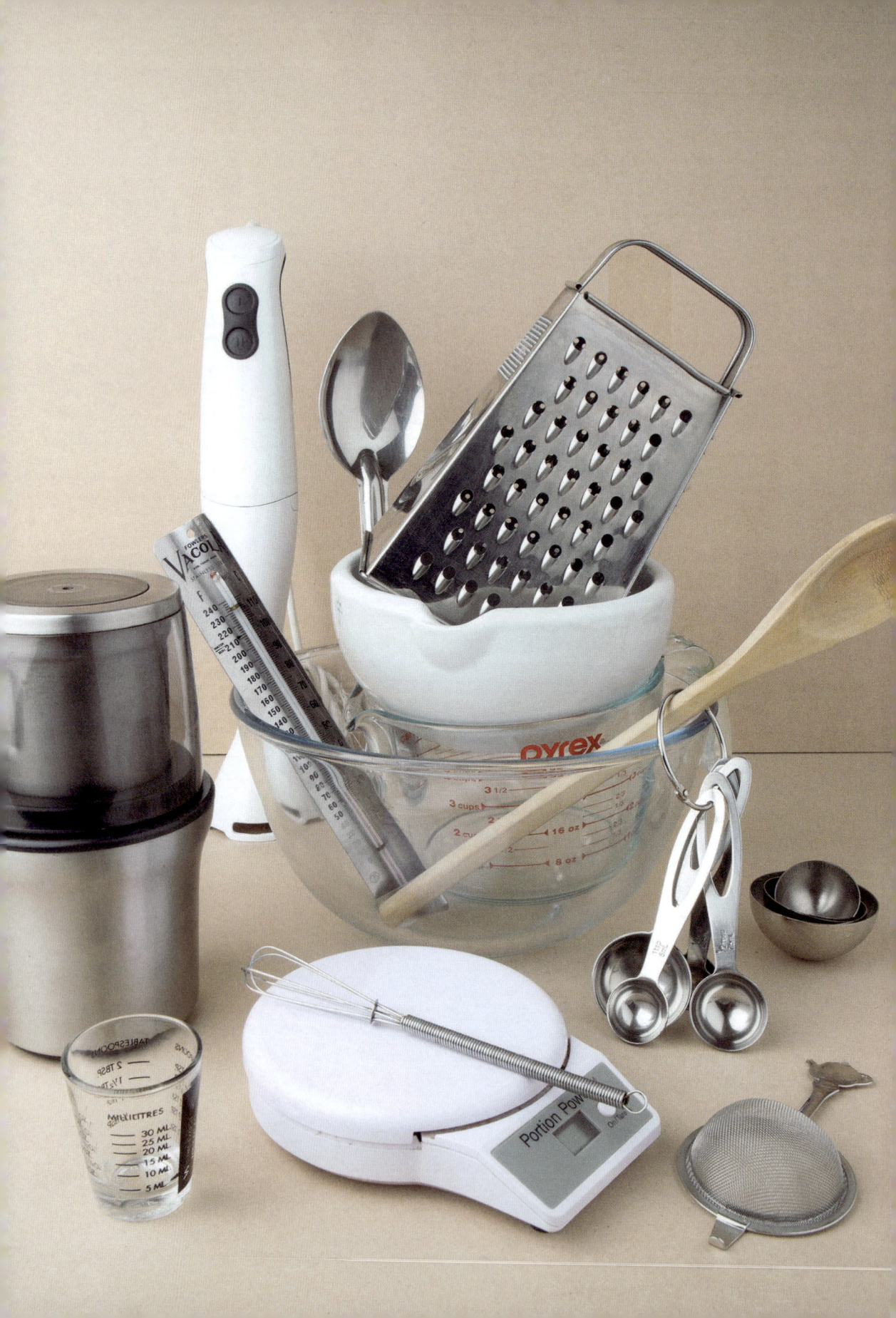

Basics

Equipment and Utensils

To make your natural and organic preparations, you will require a variety of basic equipment and utensils. Most of the utensils you need can be found in your kitchen. If not, you will be able to obtain them from kitchen shops, supermarkets, department stores, hardware stores, laboratory suppliers or online. The list below summarises the range of utensils that you may require.

- Scales — digital kitchen scales (with minimum weighing capacity of 1 g for larger ingredient quantities) and laboratory scales (with minimum weighing capacity of 0.01 g for smaller ingredient quantities)
- Cooking thermometers — two are often required, with a temperature range from 0°C to 100°C or higher
- Electric stick mixer
- pH meter or pH strips
- Heat-resistant glass mixing bowls
- Mixing bowls — stainless steel, ceramic or glass
- Stainless steel spoons of various sizes
- Measuring glass, cups, spoons
- Sharp knife
- Stainless steel saucepans
- Cutting board
- Strainer/sieve
- Kettle
- Teapot
- Funnel

- Cheesecloth/muslin
- Coffee or laboratory filter paper
- Grater
- Egg whisk
- Mortar and pestle
- Electric coffee grinder
- Latex gloves
- Oven gloves
- Apron
- Protective eyewear
- Dust mask
- Moulds — soap, bath bomb, chocolate, candle, muffin tins
- Pipettes/eyedroppers
- Glass bottles/jars
- Glass spray bottles/pump bottles
- Glass dropper bottles/rollerball bottles
- Labels
- Marking pens
- Notebook and pen
- Scissors
- Calculator

Abbreviations

Throughout this book, these abbreviations will be used regularly:

tbsp = tablespoon

tsp = teaspoon

qs = quantum sufficit, which means only as much as required

EO = essential oil

Weights and Measures

The recipes in this book are intended to be easy and fun to make. For that reason, I have included measurements such as spoons and cups where minor variations do not affect the outcome of the recipe.

As tiny amounts of essential oil are used in many recipes, their measurements are given in drops where 20 drops of essential oil approximates 1 g. However, it is worth noting that this can only be an approximation due to variations in dripolator size and viscosity of essential oils. This variability is acceptable for the recipes in this book. However, for accuracy and consistency from batch to batch, it is important to weigh ingredients and convert all measurements to grams.

For the most part, recipes are given as bases into which a range of essential oils may be added. Most recipes are given in increments of 100 g, with the essential oils given as an addition to this. This means if the base is 100 g and a 1% dilution of essential oils is recommended, 1 g of essential oil is added to the 100 g with the entire recipe adding

up to 101 g. This has been done for ease of measurement. This means the actual dilution of essential oil will be less than 1%. In this case, it will be 0.9%. For the most part, this lower dilution is acceptable. However, for accuracy and consistency from batch to batch, it is important that the formula adds up to 100%. If the essential oils are 1% of the formula, the base should be converted to 99% of the formula, with the entire formula adding up to 100%.

Australian measuring standards have been used throughout this book, where 1 cup is 250 mL, 1 tbsp is 20 mL and 1 tsp is 5 mL.

Hygiene and Sanitisation

It is important to consider hygiene and sanitisation for two reasons. Firstly, contamination with bacteria, yeast and mould will cause your beautiful preparations to deteriorate quickly, and secondly, the application of preparations containing bacteria, yeast and mould can be harmful, especially if applied to broken or weakened skin.

Therefore, the following points need to be addressed when making your preparations.

- Wash your hands.
- Make sure the utensils you use are clean.
- Ensure that your containers are clean.
- When removing your preparations from jars, use a clean spoon or spatula rather than your fingers, which are naturally covered in bacteria and other contaminants. Alternatively, pouring or pumping from a container can reduce contamination.

Sanitising Containers and Equipment

Sanitising containers is important if they have not been stored in clean conditions after manufacturing, especially when the recipe contains water or moisture. Equipment should be sanitised to reduce contamination of your preparations.

To sanitise your containers and equipment, follow these steps:

- Begin by washing your containers or equipment with hot soapy water and rinsing them well.
- Spray them with a 70% ethanol (or isopropyl alcohol) and 30% water solution. Wipe over with clean paper towel or leave to dry.

Labelling and Storage

Labelling

When you make your preparations, include a label with the name of the product and the date it was made. This way you can tell what it is and how fresh it is and can refer back to your recipe if you need to.

Storage

Your preparations, if not being used immediately, should be stored in sealed containers in a cool, dark, dry environment. In warm climates, the refrigerator is often the best place. Preparations such as infusions and decoctions and any made with fresh fruit or vegetable matter should be used in a matter of days.

Opaque, amber or dark glass containers are preferable, where possible, to prevent light fading and oxidising the contents. Otherwise, apply an opaque label which covers as much of the container as possible.

Adverse Reactions

Many people are under the impression that natural ingredients will not cause adverse reactions, such as inflammation and irritation. While careful selection of natural ingredients means they are less likely to, there is no guarantee that an adverse reaction will not happen. Some people are generally more sensitive than others or may have unique individual sensitivities.

Immediately wash the substance from your skin if an adverse reaction occurs.

Sometimes it may take several applications of a substance before a reaction occurs. This is known as sensitisation.

If the reaction appears to be due to your preparation, it may be easier to identify the irritant or allergen. Performing a patch test may assist with identification. Apply one of the ingredients to a band-aid and attach it firmly to the soft skin just inside your elbow. Leave it on for 24 hours and check for any reaction. You may want to test two substances on each elbow at the same time. Just make sure they are far enough away from each other to be able to distinguish between each substance.

A reaction may also occur if the dilution of an active ingredient is too high. Remember that essential oils are very concentrated substances and that lowering the concentration used in your preparations may be helpful if a reaction occurs. Some essential oils are more likely to be skin irritants than others. Check whether or not your chosen essential oils are suitable for use in the skin care preparation you are making and that they are not skin irritants.

Sometimes stress, heat, cold, change in humidity, change in diet, hormonal changes, illness or medication can make you more prone to an adverse reaction than you otherwise might be. If you are unable to identify a particular ingredient in your preparation, it may be some other agent with which you have come into contact, such as an animal, plant or cleaning agent.

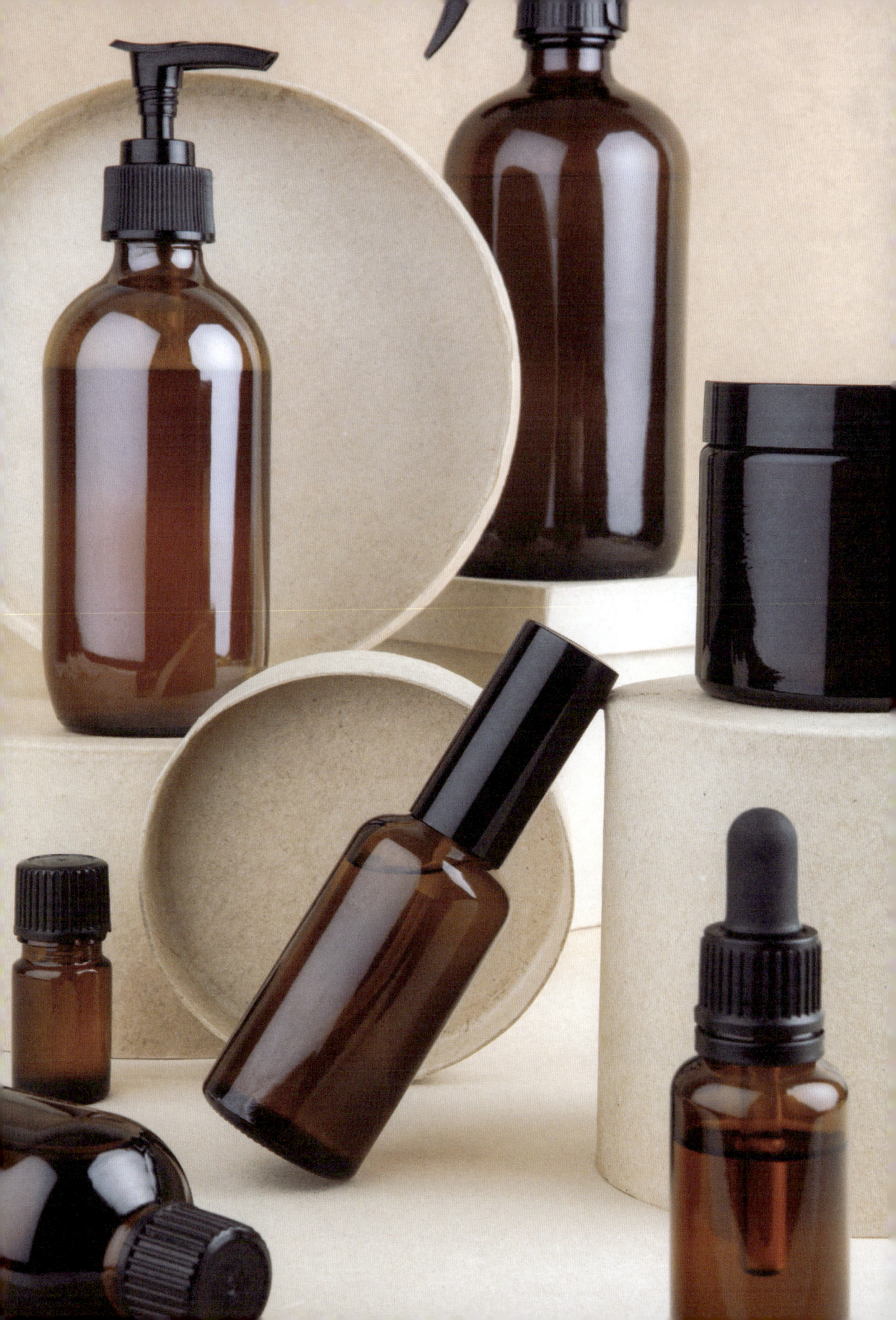

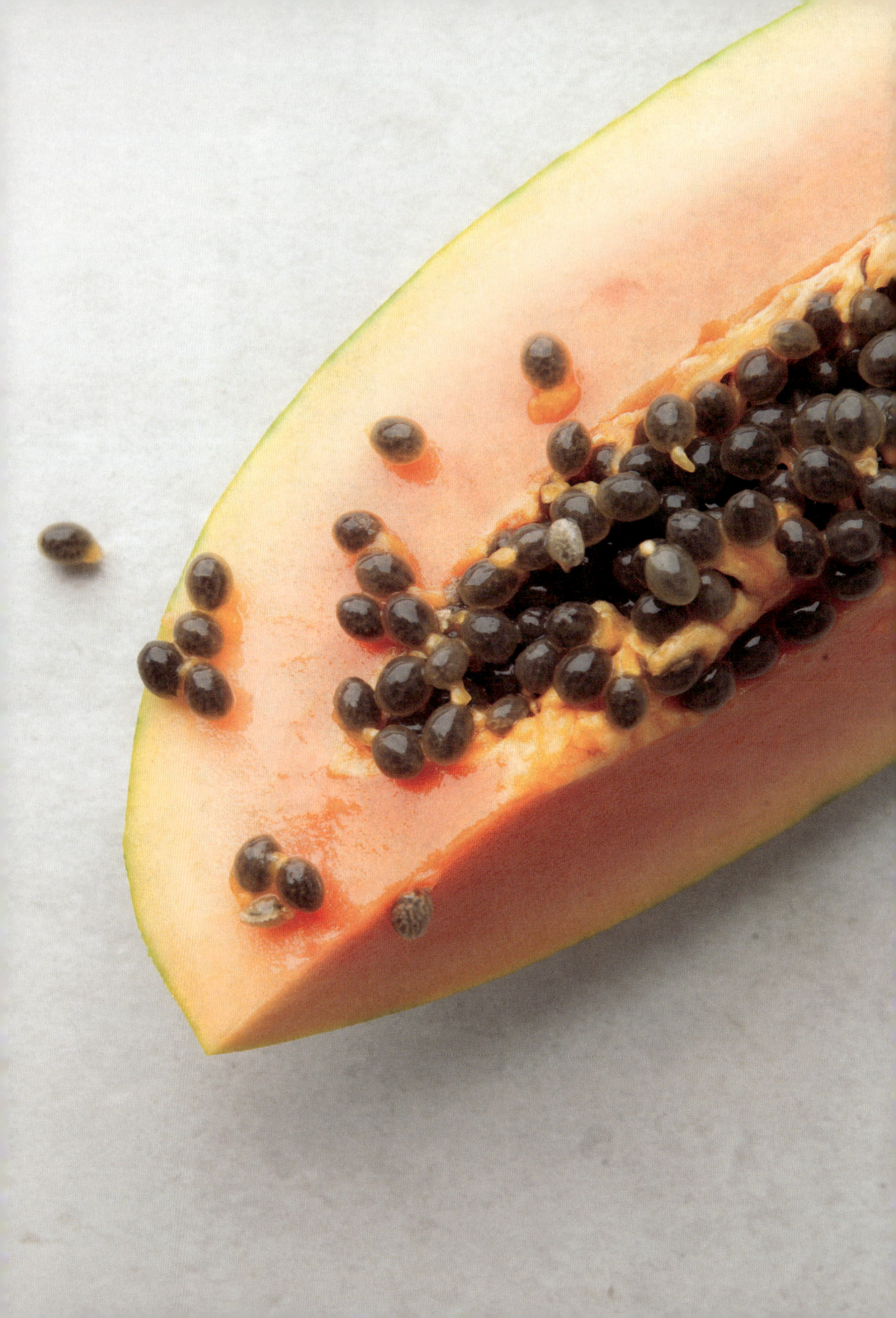

Raw Ingredients

Fruits and Vegetables

Mashed, juiced, grated or sliced, fresh fruits and vegetables are incredibly beneficial to the skin. They are complex blends of natural chemical substances that make available to you such things as fruit acids, enzymes, sugars, proteins, fats, vitamins, minerals and water, all of which can be beneficial to your skin.

Fresh fruits and vegetables are best used in treatment masks or cold poultices. They can be mashed, juiced, grated or sliced depending on the fruit or vegetable and the type of preparation being made. Fruits and vegetables may also be incorporated into your skin-exfoliating preparations.

Remember to wash your fruits and vegetables before use to remove any soil, microbes and spray residues. Using organically grown produce ensures there will be no concern over pesticide or herbicide residues.

Dehydrated and powdered fruits and vegetables may be mixed with other dry ingredients, which are then rehydrated at the time of use, especially in face and body masks.

Apple *Malus domestica*

Grated apple is very soothing and smoothing to dry skin. It contains malic and tartaric acids, which gently exfoliate the skin.

Avocado *Persea Americana*

Mashed avocado flesh is very soothing, softening and emollient to dry skin. It is rich in natural oils.

Banana *Musa × paradisiaca*

Mashed banana is used in skin care preparations for its soothing and skin softening properties. It contains mucopolysaccharides, which improve skin hydration. Also available as banana flour, which can be rehydrated to create masks.

Beetroot *Beta vulgaris*

Beetroot powder can be used to colour preparations such as bath bombs.

Blueberry *Vaccinium corymbosum*

Blueberries are rich in antioxidants. Fresh blueberries or blueberry juice powder can be added to face masks or exfoliants to refresh and smooth the skin.

Coconut *Cocos nucifera*

The versatile coconut offers up oil (page 12), flour, milk, cream, sugar and water, which can be used to make natural skin care preparations. Coconut water is high in electrolytes and natural sugars, making it hydrating to the skin and hair. Coconut sugar is made from the sap collected from incisions made in the coconut flowers and can be used in natural exfoliants.

Cucumber *Cucumis sativus*

Cucumber slices and juice are very soothing and anti-inflammatory, hydrating and mildly astringent to the skin.

Grapes *Vitus species*

Crushed grapes are very soothing, cooling and toning to the skin.

Kakadu plum *Terminalia ferdinandiana*

Kakadu plum is a unique fruit endemic to northern Australia. It has the highest known level of vitamin C content of any fruit in the world, along with a range of other antioxidants. Freeze dried Kakadu plum powder can be incorporated into face masks, helping to improve skin smoothness, suppleness and brightness.

Lemon *Citrus limon*

Lemon juice is acidic and is used diluted in hair and skin preparations to counteract the alkalinity of soaps and shampoos, thus reducing any product build up and irritation that may result from their use. It is also antibacterial and astringent, and contains citric acid, making it useful for treating oily and blemished skin. Do not use undiluted. Dry, powdered lemon peel can be added to face masks in small quantities to encourage skin exfoliation, revealing fresh healthy skin.

Lettuce *Lactuca sativa*

Lettuce juice is soothing to the skin and promotes the healing of blemishes.

Lime *Citrus aurantifolia*

Dry, powdered lime peel can be added to face masks in small quantities to encourage skin exfoliation, revealing fresh healthy skin.

Oats *Avena sativa*

Oat preparations are very soothing to the skin, relieving irritation, inflammation and itching. They are used in bath preparations, cleansing preparations, face masks, face and body scrubs, and soaps. Oatmeal, oat bran and oat flour can be used in these skin care preparations.

Orange *Citrus sinensis*

Dry, powdered orange peel can be added to face masks in small quantities to encourage skin exfoliation, revealing fresh healthy skin. Dried orange slices can be used for decoration of bath salts and soaps.

Passionfruit *Passiflora incarnata*

Passionfruit pulp is hydrating, softening and refreshing to the skin.

Paw paw or papaya *Carica papaya*

Paw paw flesh is used in face and body masks as a very gentle exfoliant. It contains the enzyme papain, which has the ability to dissolve keratin and hence our dead surface skin cells. Green paw paw contains more of this enzyme.

Peach *Prunus persica*

Peach slices, juice or pulp can be used to soothe, soften and hydrate dry skin.

Pear *Pyrus communis*

Pear slices, juice or pulp can be used to soothe, soften and hydrate dry skin.

Pineapple *Ananas comosus*

Pineapple flesh or juice is used in face and body masks as an exfoliant. It contains the enzyme bromelain, which has the ability to dissolve keratin and hence our dead surface skin cells.

Pomegranate *Punica granatum*

Pomegranate juice can be used in face masks to hydrate, soothe and refresh the skin. Dry, powdered pomegranate juice can be used in face masks and rehydrated before applying to the skin.

Potato *Solanum tuberosum*

Potato juice or grated potato is soothing and anti-inflammatory. It reduces bruising and calms puffy eyes.

Quandong *Santalum acuminatum*

Quandong is a fruit native to the deserts of Australia. It is high in Vitamin C, antioxidants and protein. Freeze dried quandong powder can be incorporated into face masks and exfoliants, helping to exfoliate, smooth and soothe the skin.

Rockmelon or cantaloupe
Cucumis melo cantalupensis

Rockmelon slices, pulp or juice are used to hydrate and soothe dry and inflamed skin.

Seaweed

Seaweeds are macroscopic algae. There are many varieties including bladderwrack (*Fucus vesiculosus*) and kelp (*Ascophyllum nodosum*), which are used in *thalassotherapy*. Thalassotherapy is a term applied to treatments using ingredients from the sea. It is derived from the Greek word, *thalassa* meaning ocean.

Seaweed is used in skin care for its ability to attract and retain moisture and for its cell regenerative properties. It is soothing, hydrating and healing to the skin. It has been used as a traditional skin healing remedy by many cultures to heal burns, rashes, wounds, bruises and swelling.

Strawberry *Fragaria vesca*

Strawberries can be mashed and juiced to make skin care preparations that are soothing, toning and mildly bleaching. Dry, powdered strawberry juice can be used in face masks and rehydrated before applying to the skin.

Strawberry leaves can be made into an infusion and used on an oily skin to help balance overactive sebaceous glands.

Tomato *Lycopersicum esculentum*

Tomato slices or pulp are used in skin care preparations. It has astringent properties, which make it useful for the treatment of oily skin.

Watermelon *Citrullus lanatus*

Watermelon slices are very soothing, hydrating and toning to the skin.

Nuts, Seeds, Grains and Pulses

Ground and polished nuts, seeds, grains and pulses make superb granules for your skin-exfoliating preparations. The following granules are suitable for this purpose:

- almond meal
- bran
- ground adzuki beans
- ground lentils
- ground wattle seeds
- hemp flour
- oat flakes
- oatmeal
- rice flour
- semolina.

The finer, softer granules are more suitable for facial preparations, and the harder, larger granules are more suitable for places where the skin is hardest and toughest, such as on the feet.

Starches and flours can be combined with clays, essential oils and herbs to make luxurious fragrant body powders, as well as soothing powders for baby's bottom. Their absorbent properties make them suitable for deodorising powders for the body and feet. They can also be used to make absorbent hair powders/dry shampoos. They can be combined with active ingredients to create masks and exfoliants. Choose from:

- arrowroot powder/starch/flour
- chickpea (besan) flour
- corn starch
- potato starch
- rice starch
- tapioca starch/flour.

An electric coffee grinder is useful for creating granules and powders from dried herbs, fruits, vegetables, seeds and grains.

Vegetable Oils, Fats and Waxes

Skin softening and smoothing describe the emollient properties of pure vegetable oils, fats and waxes. Even though they are often referred to as vegetable oils, fats and waxes, they are mostly extracted from the seeds, nuts and kernels of the plant, except for avocado, which is pressed from the flesh.

Vegetable oils are used as 'base' or 'carrier' oils for essential oils to create aromatherapy face, body and massage oils. They are also referred to as 'fixed' oils.

Vegetable oils, fats and waxes are used in moisturising preparations such as creams and lotions to protect and soften the skin and prevent moisture evaporating from the skin. They supply the skin with essential fatty acids and vitamins and also make effective hair conditioning treatments.

Vegetable oils, fats and waxes may be combined for different purposes, depending on what they do for the skin, and their consistency, skin-feel and odour.

It is important to use cold-pressed vegetable oils unless otherwise specified as they have been exposed to the least heat and processing, and hence contain many unaffected and useful nutrients.

The following vegetable oils, fats and waxes are commonly used in face, body and hair care preparations.

Almond oil, sweet
Prunus amygdalis var. *dulcis*
Sweet almond oil is an excellent, all-purpose emollient suitable for most skin types. Composed of oleic and linoleic acids, it can be used on the body and face, as a massage oil base, and in cleansers, creams, lotions and balms.

Apricot kernel oil *Prunus armeniaca*
Apricot kernel oil has very similar constituents to sweet almond oil and is used for similar purposes. If a person has nut allergies, they may prefer to use apricot kernel oil in recipes rather than sweet almond oil. It has a slightly richer texture than sweet almond oil, which makes it good for drier skin.

Argan oil *Sideroxylon spinosum*

Argan oil is extracted from the kernels of the fruit of the argan tree, which is indigenous to Morocco. It is rich in carotene and tocopherol, omega-6 fatty acids and linoleic acid. It softens, smooths, protects and soothes the skin, encourages skin repair and elasticity and reduces dryness. It also makes an excellent hair and scalp conditioning oil. It can be used on your face or body and is suitable for all skin types. It is absorbed readily and is non-greasy.

Avocado oil *Persea americana*

Avocado oil consists mostly of oleic, linoleic and linolenic acids. Other constituents include palmitic and palmitoleic acids, lecithin, phytosterol, carotenoids, and a high concentration of vitamins A, D and E. Unlike other oils, this oil is not obtained from the seed or nut, but is obtained from pressing the ripe avocado flesh. It has a rich consistency and has a beautiful deep green colour. Dry and mature skin benefits most from this oil. It also acts as a mild sun filter.

Candelilla wax *Euphorbia cerifera*

Candelilla wax comes from the leaves of a shrub indigenous to Mexico and the south-west of the US. The plant is immersed in boiling acidified water and the resultant floating wax that is released from the leaves is then collected. This wax is a stiffening and hardening agent and is often used to make balms and various stick and solid products. It assists in reducing moisture loss from the skin.

Carnauba wax *Copernicia prunifera*

Carnauba wax comes from the leaves of the carnauba palm, which is grown in north-eastern Brazil. The leaves are dried and the wax beaten from them. This wax is a stiffening and hardening agent and is often used to make balms and various stick and solid products. It assists in reducing moisture loss from the skin and provides a glossy finish.

Castor oil *Ricinus communis*

Castor oil is pressed from the seeds of the castor oil plant. This thick, viscous oil is used in balms to create a barrier, protect and soften dry, cracked skin, and reduce skin dehydration. For this reason, it is often used in lip balms, hand balms and baby bottom balms.

Cocoa butter *Theobroma cacao*

Cocoa butter smells like chocolate and is actually used to make chocolate. It is pressed from roasted cacao beans. It makes a wonderful emollient and lubricant, softening and protecting dry skin. Cocoa butter is useful in creams, lotions, ointments and balms. It is especially good in balms as it is solid until it warms to body temperature, when it will melt and spread easily over the skin.

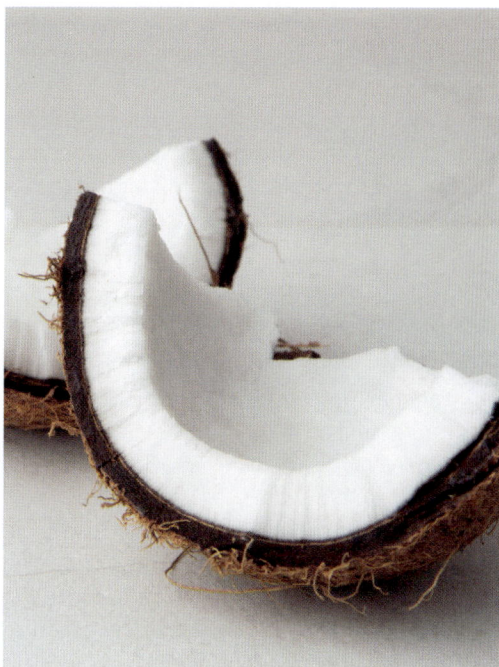

Coconut oil *Cocos nucifera*

Coconut oil is an opaque white solid or a clear liquid depending on the temperature. It liquefies readily in warm temperatures and solidifies at lower temperatures. It remains relatively stable when exposed to the air as it is highly saturated. It is extracted from copra, the white flesh of the coconut. Unrefined coconut oil has the benefit of smelling and tasting like coconuts.

Coconut oil is used as hair and body oils and in creams, ointments and balms. It is often chemically treated to make foaming agents for shampoos, bubble baths and other foaming products. It is, along with palm oil, often used as a major component in vegetable soaps, making them hard and giving them very good lathering properties.

Fractionated coconut oil, also known as caprylic/capric triglycerides or medium chain triglyceride (MCT) oil, is a fraction of coconut oil created by refining the coconut oil. Coconut oil is heated and as it cools, the longer chain fatty acids, which solidify first, are removed. Nutrients are also lost during this process. Medium chain saturated fatty acids remain. This version of the oil does not solidify, is very stable, feels light and is easily absorbed by the skin.

Evening primrose oil
Oenothera biennis

Evening primrose oil contains high levels of gamma linoleic acid, which is one of the essential fatty acids vital for the maintenance of healthy epidermal cells. It improves the skin's ability to develop normal barrier functions. It is used in the treatment of dry, flaky, sensitive skin conditions such as eczema and psoriasis. As evening primrose oil is rich in essential fatty acids, it is important not to expose it to high temperatures as it will oxidise rapidly, becoming rancid.

Hemp seed oil *Cannabis sativa*

Hemp seed oil is obtained by pressing hemp seeds. It contains omega-3 and omega-6 essential fatty acids. As it is rich in essential fatty acids, it is important not to expose it to high temperatures as it will oxidise rapidly, becoming rancid. It is suitable for soothing, softening and protecting most skin types.

Jojoba oil *Simmondsia chinensis*

Jojoba oil is made up primarily of unsaturated wax esters and is relatively resistant to rancidity. It has a very fine consistency and skin-feel and is absorbed readily by the skin. It makes an excellent facial oil and can be used in light, non-greasy moisturising preparations. It is also used as a hair conditioning oil. It was traditionally used by the First Peoples of the Sonora Desert for its beneficial properties. Jojoba oil is often used as the base of natural perfume oils due to its resistance to rancidity.

Macadamia oil *Macadamia integrifolia*

The macadamia tree is indigenous to Australia. The oil, pressed from the nuts, is rich in monounsaturated fats, making it relatively stable. Its high omega-7 content makes it especially protective and emollient, improving the condition of dry, chapped and mature skin.

Olive oil *Olea europaea*

Olive oil is a monounsaturated oil, rich in oleic acid. It is expressed from the olive flesh. The best grade comes from the first pressing and is known as extra virgin olive oil. It has a deep green colour and a distinctive odour, and is rich in consistency. It is often used in balms, soaps and hair conditioning preparations. Olive oil is traditionally used in Mediterranean countries.

Rosehip oil *Rosa rubiginosa*

Rosehip oil is high in both linoleic and linolenic fatty acids, beta-carotene and tretinoin, which are believed to be responsible for its ability to encourage regeneration and repair of skin tissue. It is used in the treatment of damaged skin tissue including scars and burns. It improves the texture of dry and wrinkled skin. It has a very fine consistency and makes a wonderful facial oil, and can be incorporated into creams. It is extracted from the seeds of a rose bush that grows wild in the southern Andes and other cool parts of the world. As rosehip oil is high in essential fatty acids, it is important not to expose it to high temperatures as it will oxidise rapidly, becoming rancid.

Shea butter *Butyrospermum parkii*

Karite nut butter, better known as shea butter, is a vegetable fat extracted from the fruit of a tree that grows in Africa. It protects the skin, improves its suppleness and elasticity, and promotes skin healing. It makes an excellent ingredient in skin creams and balms, especially for dry, damaged, irritated and sensitive skins.

Soyabean oil *Glycine max*

Soyabean oil is rich in vitamin E and contains more lecithin than any other vegetable oil. It is also high in unsaturated fatty acids. It makes a superb body and massage oil for normal to dry skin.

Wheatgerm oil *Triticum durum*

Wheatgerm oil has a very high vitamin E content. This makes it useful in healing preparations for damaged or scarred skin. It has a distinctive, nutty odour and is rich in

consistency. It can be used as a body oil or incorporated into creams. Especially good for dry skin.

Along with the vegetable oils discussed above, there are many more vegetable oils pressed from seeds and nuts that can be included in your formulations for their benefits to the skin and hair, including:

acai, apple seed, babchi, baobab, black currant, borage, Brazil nut, broccoli seed, camellia, canola, cherry kernel, corn, cottonseed, cucumber, grapeseed, guava, hazelnut, kiwi fruit, kukui nut, linseed (flaxseed), marula, meadowfoam, moringa, neem, papaya seed, passionfruit, peach kernel, pine nut, pistachio, pomegranate, poppy seed, prickly pear, pumpkin, raspberry, rice bran, safflower, sandalwood nut, sea buckthorn, sesame (black), sesame (white), sunflower, tamanu, walnut and watermelon.

Choosing a vegetable oil

The vegetable oils on page 14 have been listed in order of lightest and finest through to heaviest and thickest. It is useful to consider these properties when choosing an oil for a specific skin type or condition. For example, a fine and readily absorbed oil such as jojoba will be more suitable for combination skin, whereas dry, flaky skin will benefit from a rich, thick oil such as coconut, which will remain on the surface of the skin longer and is more protective. This list is a guide only, as the amount of processing that an oil undergoes, such as filtering, can influence its properties and skin-feel.

'Comedogenic' is a term that is often applied to ingredients such as vegetable oils and fats. It refers to the likelihood of an ingredient causing the skin to clog and develop pimples. Generally, heavier, thicker oils will be more comedogenic than finer lightweight oils, and a higher concentration of vegetable oils and fats in a product will have the potential to clog more than a water-based lotion with a low oil content.

Cold-pressed vegetable oils can be combined in order to make use of a range of benefits and to vary a preparation's texture and feel on the skin.

Argan oil

Hemp seed oil

Jojoba oil

Evening primrose oil

Rosehip oil

Apricot kernel oil

Sweet almond oil

Soyabean oil

Avocado oil

Wheatgerm oil

Olive oil

Macadamia oil

Coconut oil

Castor oil

LIGHTEST/FINEST/ MOST READILY ABSORBED

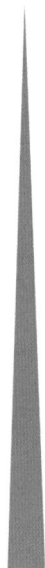

HEAVIEST/THICKEST

Drying, semi-drying, non-drying oils

The terms drying, semi-drying and non-drying do not refer to the effect vegetable oils have on the skin. Rather, they refer to what happens to the vegetable oils on exposure to air. Drying oils tend to feel finer and are absorbed faster by the skin, semi-drying oils remain on the skin longer and feel more emollient, while non-drying oils feel thicker and richer and remain on the skin surface a lot longer.

Herbs and Spices

Herbal preparations for your skin and hair can be made from the herbs in your garden or from herbs purchased from suppliers specialising in high quality dried herbs. Alternatively, herbal extracts can be purchased for use in skin and hair care preparations.

Herbs contain many active constituents that can be utilised in the treatment and care of your skin and hair.

Aloe vera *Aloe vera*

Aloe vera gel is obtained from the plant's succulent leaves. It is an effective healing agent for burns, injuries and acne. The gel is cooling, soothing and hydrating, and stimulates the growth of new cells and tissue. It can be incorporated into moisturising preparations or applied directly to the skin. If you have an aloe vera plant, a leaf can be cut off. The outer skin can then be removed by thinly slicing off the top, bottom and sides of the leaf to reveal the inner clear, firm gel. This inner gel can be laid directly on to the skin to soothe inflamed or burned skin. Alternatively, the gel can be blended into a liquid and smoothed over the skin. If you have prepared too much to use immediately, freeze it in an ice cube tray, and use the cubes as needed.

Aloe vera is also available as a dried powder and can be rehydrated with the addition of water. For example, if the aloe vera plant has been dehydrated to a 1:200 powder, 1 g can be rehydrated in 200 g of water to the equivalent of the original juice.

Calendula *Calendula officinalis*

Infusions or tinctures made from the petals of the calendula flower are antiseptic, healing,

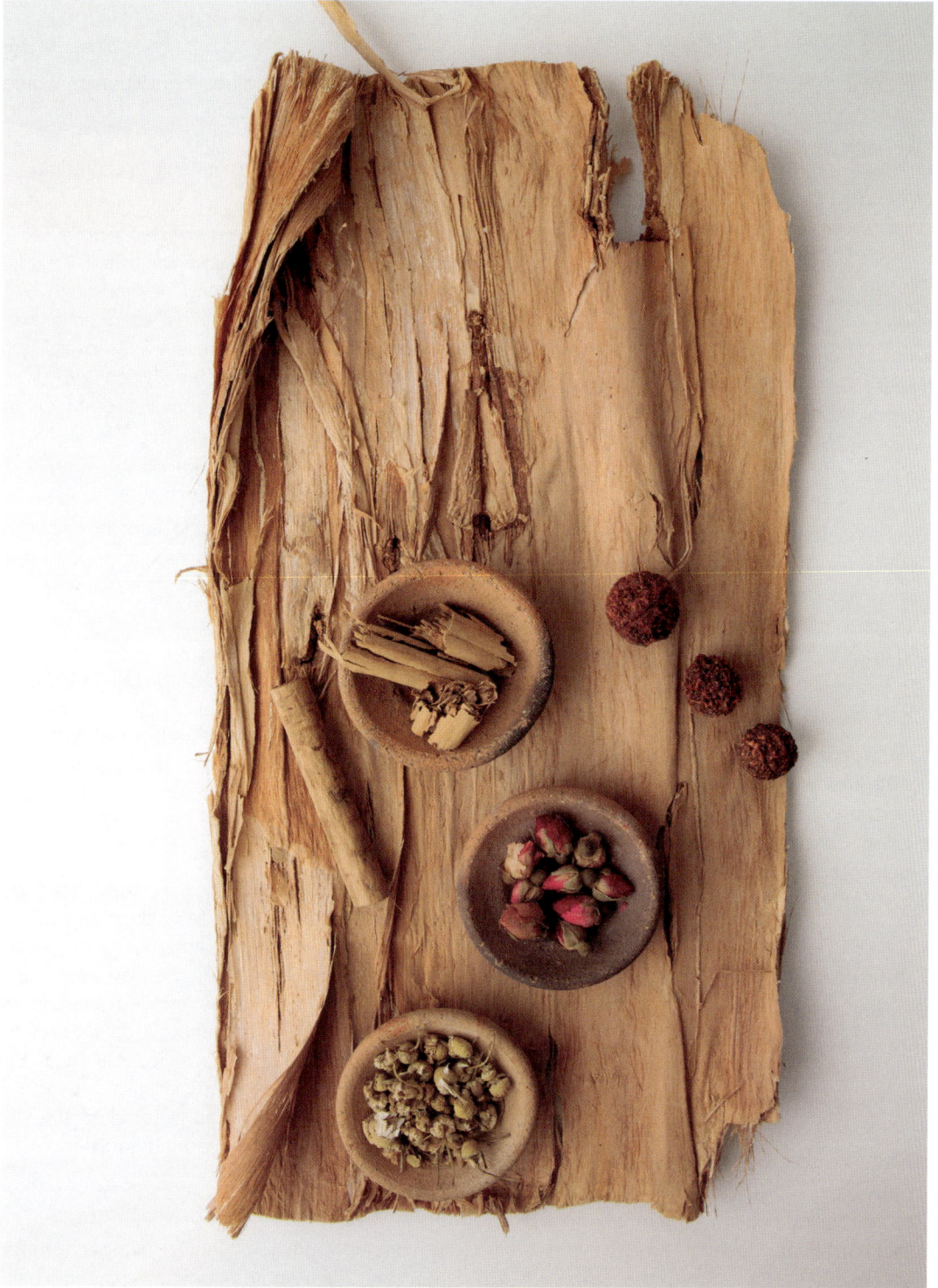

soothing and anti-inflammatory. Calendula may be used to treat wounds and burns and sensitive, inflamed skin conditions. It is also used in hair rinses to impart golden highlights to fair hair. Calendula flowers can be used in many preparations including oils, ointments, creams, infusions, poultices and compresses. See page 28 for infused oil.

Chamomile *Matricaria chamomilla*

German chamomile is most often used in skin and hair care preparations. Chamomile flowers can be made into an infusion and used as a compress to soothe the skin and eyes, reducing inflammation and irritation. An infused oil can also be made from the flowers and is particularly soothing to the skin. Chamomile preparations also improve wound healing. Infusions can be used as hair rinses for fair hair as they contain a substance called apigenin, which brightens and adds subtle golden highlights to the hair.

Chickweed *Stellaria media*

Chickweed has traditionally been used to soothe irritated and dry skin conditions such as eczema, and to heal minor wounds. An infused oil can be made from chickweed, which can then be made into a balm or added to a cream.

Cinnamon *Cinnamomum zeylanicum*

Cinnamon powder has a sweet, spicy aroma. It is often used in exfoliating preparations and masks. It has antibacterial properties and gently improves circulation, making it useful for pimples and acne. When added to soaps, cinnamon powder gives a speckled texture. Avoid using cassia (*cassia cinnamomum*), commonly found in supermarkets and labelled as cinnamon, as it is a skin irritant.

Comfrey *Symphytum officinale*

Comfrey leaves contain allantoin and mucilage, among other constituents, which give them their excellent skin healing and soothing properties. They can be used in infusions, poultices, ointments and creams.

Elderflowers *Sambucus nigra*

Elderflowers are used for their mildly astringent and soothing properties. An elderflower infusion can be used as a skin toner and to make an eye compress for irritated eyes. In the nineteenth century, it was recommended for clearing the complexion of freckles.

Fennel *Foeniculum vulgare*

Fennel seeds can be made into an infusion, which can then be used as a compress for inflamed eyes and eyelids.

Ginseng *Panax ginseng*

Ginseng aids in increasing skin elasticity, and revitalising and reactivating epidermal cell production. Extracts such as infusions or tinctures of the root can be incorporated into moisturisers.

Gotu kola *Centella asiatica*

Gotu kola has traditionally been used to improve dilated surface capillaries. It is healing and soothing, and used to relieve irritation. The leaves can be used to make an infusion that can be applied directly to the skin, used in a compress or added to a moisturiser. A cool poultice can also be made and applied to the skin. An infused oil made from gotu kola can be applied directly to the skin or incorporated into moisturisers.

Lavender *Lavandula officinalis*

Lavender infusion and vinegar make fragrant, calming additions to body and bath preparations. In addition, the dried purple flowers make bath soaks look attractive.

Lemon balm *Melissa officinalis*

Lemon balm is antiseptic, astringent, soothing and healing. It is used to treat sensitive, blemished skin. The infusion or diluted tincture can be used for this purpose. It can be made into a skin toner and wiped over the skin after cleansing.

Lemongrass *Cymbopogon citratus*

Lemongrass is used on oily skins to help normalise excessive sebaceous secretions. The infusion or diluted tincture can be used for this purpose. It can be made into a skin toner and wiped over the skin after cleansing.

Lemon myrtle *Backhousia citriodora*

Dried lemon myrtle leaves can be crushed or powdered and added to body care products such as exfoliants and soaps for texture, and bath salts to add a subtle fragrance.

Liquorice *Glycyrrhiza glabra*

Liquorice root preparations are very soothing to the skin and can be used in the treatment of skin inflammations such as eczema.

Marshmallow *Althaea officinalis*

Marshmallow root is prepared as a cold infusion. The chopped root is left to steep in water overnight to allow for the extraction of mucilage. Heat causes the mucilage to solidify. Mucilage gives marshmallow root its anti-inflammatory and soothing properties. The infusion may be applied to the skin directly or incorporated into moisturisers.

Myrrh *Commiphora myrrha*

Myrrh resin is used as a natural incense and in perfumes. It releases a warm, rich, earthy aroma. It has astringent and healing properties, with myrrh powder and tincture used in dental products to strengthen and improve gum health.

Nettle *Urtica dioica*

Stinging nettles sting when they are fresh. However, the dried herb is safe to touch. It encourages circulation and is particularly useful in hair preparations to improve the condition of the hair and scalp.

Neem *Azadirachta indica*

Neem leaves are used in skin and hair care preparations for their antibacterial, anti-inflammatory and antifungal properties. Neem oil, which is pressed from the seeds, is used as an insect repellent and to treat lice. It can be blended with other vegetable oils to improve dry skin conditions.

Parsley *Petroselinum crispum*

Fresh parsley can be used in masks to help reduce oiliness, calm inflammation and improve the healing of acne. It is rich in vitamin C and other antioxidants.

Peppermint *Mentha piperita*

An infusion made from peppermint leaves relieves skin irritation, inflammation and itching. It has a refreshing and cooling effect which is due to the constriction of capillaries. It is also used in hair care preparations to relieve dandruff.

Rose *Rosa centifolia*

An infusion made from fresh or dried rose petals can be used as a toner to sooth and refresh the skin. Powdered dried rose petals can be blended into face masks to help tone the skin. Finely powdered red rose petals also work well as a natural blush. Dried rose buds and petals added to bath soaks make them look attractive.

Rosemary *Rosmarinus officinalis*

Rosemary has antiseptic, astringent, deodorant and healing properties. It improves blood circulation and is helpful for devitalised skin. As rosemary stimulates circulation in the scalp and therefore the hair follicles, it is used in preparations to help encourage healthy hair growth. It also helps improve the condition of the scalp, including dandruff.

Sage *Salvia officinalis*

Sage leaves are used for their astringent, antibacterial, antiseptic and healing properties. Sage can be used in baths, in compresses, as a healing skin toner, in hair rinses and in deodorant preparations. Used over a period of time, sage infusion will begin to darken the hair. It also helps improve dandruff conditions and oily skin with pimples.

Slippery elm *Ulmus rubra*

Powdered slippery elm bark is very soothing, healing and hydrating to the skin. When mixed with water it swells and forms a thick gel-like substance due to its high content of mucilage. It can be used as a poultice or in face masks.

Soapwort *Saponaria officinalis*

Soapwort root is used as a mild cleansing agent for skin and hair. It soothes the skin and relieves itching. It can be used as a cleanser for sensitive and inflamed skin and as a mild cleanser for sensitive and inflamed scalps and fragile hair. Soapwort root produces a mild lather due to its saponin content.

Tea, green *Camellia sinensis*

Green tea is rich in potent antioxidants called catechins, and may provide anti-aging benefits if used with regularity. It also calms sensitive skin and has mild astringent properties. Matcha powder (finely powdered green tea) is easily incorporated into face masks and exfoliants.

Thyme *Thymus vulgaris*

Thyme leaves are used for their antiseptic, astringent and healing properties. Thyme can be made into an infusion, tincture, herbal vinegar or herbal oil. It can be used in deodorants, shampoos and hair rinses for dandruff and oily hair, aftershaves, skin toners for oily and blemished skin, and bath preparations.

Turmeric *Curcuma longa*

Turmeric powder is used in masks to reduce inflammation, encourage skin healing and treat acne. It is effective in small quantities. This means concerns over staining the skin yellow are minimised. Turmeric powder can be used as a natural colourant in soaps and cosmetics.

Yarrow *Achillea millefolium*

Yarrow flowers and leaves are used for their anti-inflammatory, antiseptic, astringent and healing properties. They are used to heal wounds, stop bleeding, and treat oily and blemished skin and greasy hair. They are used in poultices, compresses, infusions for the skin and hair rinses.

Clay

Clay is a naturally occurring geomaterial comprised mostly of fine-grained clay minerals (hydrous phyllosilicates), with varying amounts of associated minerals (silicates, such as quartz; carbonates; oxides and hydrated oxides of iron and aluminium), organic and inorganic matter. Clay forms as

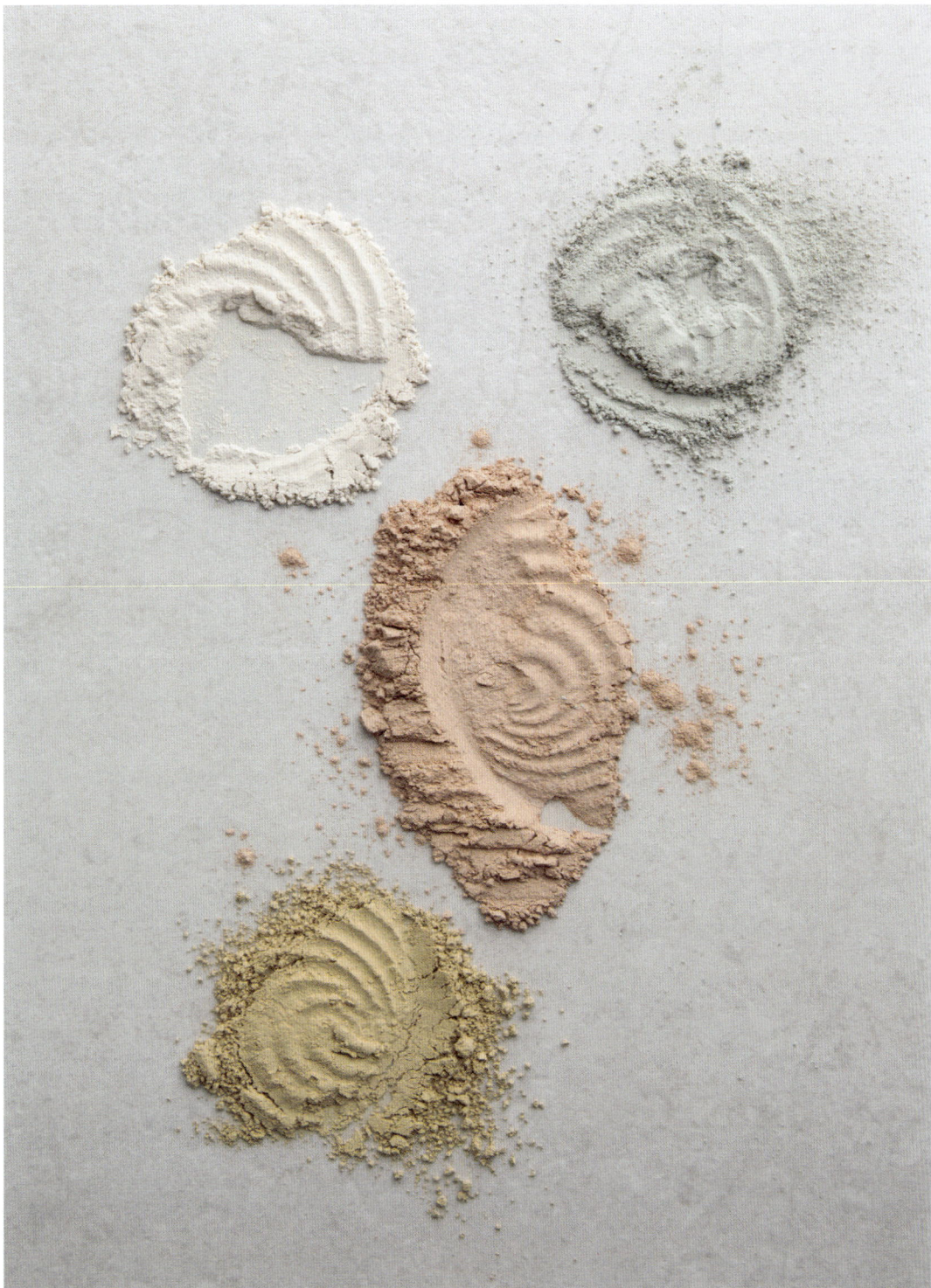

a result of the weathering of silicate-bearing rocks over long periods of time.

The clay mineral families most often used in skin care preparations are kaolin minerals (such as kaolinite and halloysite), smectites (such as montmorillonite) and illites. Smectites have the capacity to swell when mixed with water, while kaolin minerals and illites do not expand on absorption of water.

The properties of clay on the skin can be attributed largely to their varying adsorption, absorption and ionic exchange capabilities.

Clays are cleansing, healing and soothing, stimulate the circulation in the skin, and are most commonly applied in face and body masks. The use of clay in preparations to heal the skin is known as 'pelotherapy'. Clays come in a range of colours and are employed in colour cosmetics. They are used to add natural colour to soaps and bath soaks. They make great absorbent deodorising powders and are used in dry shampoos to adsorb excess oil and other impurities.

Clays vary in their proportion of mineral families as well as other components depending on where they are mined. Therefore, it is important not to attribute the same properties of one clay to another clay based on their colour.

Argiletz clays

Argile means 'clay' in French. Argiletz is a family business in France that was established in 1953, with the mother of the founder having treated wounded resistance fighters during World War II with green illite clay.

The Argiletz clays have a high mineral content, which gives them active properties on the skin such as cleansing, detoxifying, drawing, exfoliating, healing, soothing and toning. They are mined at specific depths in areas free from contamination, mainly from French

Making a Simple Clay Mask

To make a simple clay mask, mix the clay powder with water — approximately 2 teaspoons of clay with 1–2 teaspoons of water and mix into a smooth paste. As the amount of water needed to create a smooth paste may vary from clay to clay, add the water carefully, otherwise you may need to add more clay if you have added too much water. For example, while 2 teaspoons of the French Argiletz clays mix into a smooth paste with 1 teaspoon of water, 7 teaspoons of kaolin clay mix into a smooth paste with 1 teaspoon of water.

To use a clay mask, first cleanse and exfoliate the skin. Then while the skin is still damp, apply the clay mask with your fingers or a brush. The mask can be applied in layers to allow for a thick application of clay. For oily and acne skin, leave the mask on for approximately 10 minutes and allow the mask to dry but not completely dry out. For dry, dehydrated and sensitive skin, leave the mask on for 5 minutes, ensuring the mask remains damp. The mask can be misted with water or floral water while it is on to ensure it does not dehydrate the skin.

Remove the clay mask by dampening it well with a wet face cloth or sponge, then removing it well and flushing the skin with water, for example, while showering. Inspect the skin carefully to ensure it has all been removed. Follow with a toner and moisturiser. Use clay masks once or twice a week.

quarries, and are sun-dried in order to retain and enhance their healing properties.

Argiletz clays can be used in masks, poultices, absorbent powders and scalp treatments, and to colour soaps, bath soaks and other skin care preparations.

The Argiletz clays are generally available in the following colours, which are due to their various mineral contents. This gives each clay its unique healing properties.

Green

Green Argiletz clay is an illite clay. It is used in preparations such as face masks to adsorb excess sebum, draw out toxins, help with tissue repair and calm inflammation. It is especially useful in the treatment of acne and oily skin.

Yellow

Yellow Argiletz clay is an illite clay. It is cleansing and toning to normal and combination skin. It stimulates epidermal cellular regeneration.

Red

Red Argiletz clay is an illite clay rich in iron oxide. It is cleansing, softening and decongesting and revives dull, sallow skin, improving skin radiance.

Pink

Pink Argiletz clay is a mixture of white Argiletz clay and red Argiletz clay. It is gently cleansing and is suitable for use on sensitive and mature skin. It is softening, soothing and toning.

White

White Argiletz clay is kaolin. It gently cleanses the skin and is suitable for all skin types, including sensitive and mature.

Green clay is the most cleansing of the Argiletz clays, while pink and white clays are the gentlest of the clays.

Australian clays

Clays and ochres have long been an integral part of Aboriginal culture and trade, with uses including ceremonial, decorative, sun protection and healing.

Australian ivory clay

Australian ivory clay's main components are kaolin and quartz. It gently cleanses the skin and is suitable for use on sensitive skin.

Australian kaolin white clay

Australian kaolin white clay is available as a white powder and is used in cleansing masks. It is suitable for most skin types including sensitive. It may also be used to make body deodorants and foot powders. It can be mixed with red clay to produce pink clay.

Australian olive green clay

Australian olive green clay's main components are kaolin and quartz. It is used in preparations such as face masks to help with tissue repair, drawing out of toxins and calming inflammation. It is especially useful in the treatment of acne and oily skin.

Australian yellow clay

Australian yellow clay's main components are montmorillonite, quartz and anatase. It improves skin tone and gently cleanses and exfoliates the skin.

Bentonite clay

Sodium bentonite is a smectite clay, generally high in montmorillonite. It has the capacity to swell when mixed with water, which increases its surface area. It is used in face masks to combine and suspend active ingredients and cleanse the skin. It can also be used in dry shampoo powders and deodorant powders.

Brazilian clays

A range of mineral-rich Brazilian clays are available for use in masks, scrubs and dry shampoos, and as natural colourants in colour cosmetics, soaps and bath soaks. Colours include green, pink, red, purple, yellow, brown, white, grey and black.

French green montmorillonite clay

Montmorillonite clay is a smectite clay and has the capacity to swell when mixed with water. This increases its surface area. It is especially good at cleansing and exfoliating oily, clogged and acne skin.

Kaolin

Kaolin is also known as china clay and white clay. It is an aluminium silicate and is mined in many locations around the world. It is mostly available as a white powder and is used in cleansing masks. It may be used on all skin types as it has a gentle action. It is also used to make face, body and foot powders. It can be found with iron oxide, which can colour it with red, pink, orange or yellow tinges, depending on the concentration.

Mediterranean clays

This range of clays from the Mediterranean region includes caramel, chocolate, dusky rose, red and slate. They can be used in masks, scrubs and dry shampoos, and as natural colourants in colour cosmetics, soaps and bath soaks.

Rhassoul clay

Rhassoul clay is also known as ghassoul clay and Moroccan lava clay. It is a smectite clay and comes from the Atlas Mountains of Morocco, where it has traditionally been used to make skin and hair cleansing masks, and in body treatments in hammams. It contains a range of minerals and is an especially magnesium-rich phyllosilicate. It may also be used as a simple face and body cleanser by mixing the powdered clay with water into a liquid paste and massaging it over the body and face before rinsing. It can be used as an alternative to liquid shampoo. Massage a mixture of clay and water into the scalp and through the hair and leave on for 20–30 seconds before rinsing. Do not leave to dry. It can be used in face masks for normal to oily skin to cleanse clogged pores, and remove dead skin cells and excess oil.

Other Ingredients

Alcohol

The term alcohol applies to substances that have a hydroxyl (−OH) group in their chemical structure.

Alcohols exist in nature and in natural cosmetic ingredients in several forms, including volatile liquids, fragrance molecules and hard waxes. They each have a different function and can be very useful when chosen carefully and used in appropriate formulations.

Ethanol

The kind of alcohol which springs to mind immediately for most people is ethanol, or ethyl alcohol, which is manufactured from natural sources via the fermentation of starch, grains, sugar and other carbohydrates. It may also be derived from petrochemical sources. Methanol and isopropyl alcohol are other commonly available alcohols, but are not suitable for use in natural cosmetic preparations.

Ethanol has antiseptic and preservative properties and is a good solvent. Its solvent properties make it useful in making concentrated herbal extracts. It is also used to solubilise essential oils in perfumes and sprays. It is astringent and has a cooling effect on the skin. It has also been used in skin toners and aftershaves. It can be drying and irritating to the skin in high concentrations. This can be counteracted in skin care preparations by the incorporation of humectants such as glycerin and emollient oils and butters if, for example, alcoholic herbal extracts are used in creams and lotions.

Vodka is suitable for making homemade herbal extracts. A natural perfume base is available from some aromatherapy suppliers and is made from high-grade perfume ethanol that has been denatured (making it undrinkable and in compliance with sale of alcohol laws). This base is ideal for making perfumes, deodorants and body sprays.

Fatty alcohols

Fatty alcohols, such as cetyl alcohol and cetearyl alcohol, are actually wax-like substances and have a completely different function on the skin and in cosmetic preparations to ethanol. They act as co-emulsifiers and emollients in creams and lotions. If they are of plant origin, they are usually obtained from coconut or palm oil. Otherwise, they are petrochemically derived.

Aromatic alcohols

Aromatic alcohols are constituents in essential oils. For example, linalool is a monoterpene alcohol found in lavender oil. Aromatic alcohols often contribute to the antiseptic properties of essential oils.

Arrowroot *Maranta arundinacea*

Arrowroot powder, starch or flour is made from the dried rhizome of the plant. It makes an excellent absorbent body powder, can be used as a thickener in face masks, and may be added to balms (up to 2%) to reduce their greasy feeling. It is often used interchangeably with tapioca flour. Kudzu powder is also used for similar purposes.

Beeswax

Beeswax is one of the oldest raw ingredients used in cosmetic preparations. It serves as a base and stiffener in creams, balms, ointments, lipsticks and pomades, and helps regulate a formulation's consistency. When applied to the skin's surface in a balm, it acts as a barrier by forming a network rather than a totally occlusive film. White beeswax has been bleached, whereas unbleached beeswax can be various shades of brown and yellow.

Behentrimonium methosulphate & cetearyl alcohol

Behentrimonium methosulphate is a quaternary ammonium compound made using canola oil as a starting material, and is a cationic hair conditioning agent. It smooths the hair cuticle along the hair shaft via a positive charge. BTMS 25 combines 25% behentrimonium methosulphate with 75% cetearyl alcohol. It is available as a solid wax and is used in both liquid conditioners and hair conditioning bars.

Benzoin tincture

Tincture of benzoin is an alcoholic extract of benzoin gum, which comes from the *Styrax benzoin* tree. It grows mainly in Indonesia and Thailand. It has antibacterial and antioxidant properties. This makes it useful in helping to preserve creams, lotions and other herbal preparations. It also helps heal broken or cracked skin.

Borax

Borax, sodium borate, is an alkaline salt that was originally collected from a sea or lake bed after the evaporation of water, but is now mined. It is used with beeswax to form a soap-like emulsifier for water-in-oil emulsions. The more borax used, the stiffer an emulsion will become.

Brewer's yeast

Yeast is a type of fungus, with brewer's yeast often used in skin care. Incorporated into face masks, it is stimulating and gives the skin a healthy glow.

Cacao and cocoa powder
Theobroma cacao

Cacao powder has a delicious chocolatey aroma. After the fat has been removed from the cacao beans, the remaining dried component is ground into powder to produce cacao powder. It is high in antioxidants, improves blood flow to the skin and reduces inflammation. This makes it useful in face masks. It is used to give a chocolatey brown colour to soaps and can be added to bath bombs, bath salts and exfoliants to give them a range of brown colours depending on the amount added. Cocoa powder is a little different to cacao powder in that the beans have been roasted and subjected to high temperatures. For this reason, cocoa powder would only be used as a colouring agent in preparations such as soaps, bath bombs and bath salts.

Castile soap

Castile soap is available as a hard bar of soap or as a liquid soap. It is named after a region called Castile in Spain where olive oil is produced. Originally Castile soap contained 40–50% olive oil. Now, Castile soap is being sold with concentrations of 20% olive oil blended with other vegetable oils. Castile liquid soap is made by saponifying olive oil and potassium hydroxide. It is a very mild soap that can be used to wash the face and body. It is especially suitable for sensitive skin.

Caustic soda/caustic potash

Sodium hydroxide/potassium hydroxide is also known as lye and is used for making soap. See *Lye* on page 26.

Champagne/beer

Leftover flat champagne or beer can be used as a hair rinse. After shampooing, pour the beer or champagne through your hair, leave on for a few minutes and then rinse out. It leaves your hair feeling soft and shiny and gives it body.

Charcoal, activated

Charcoal is produced by burning carbon-based materials. Activated charcoal is made by exposing charcoal to high heat in the presence of a gas. This produces many tiny pores and increases its surface area, giving it adsorptive properties. It is often used in masks to adsorb oil, making it useful for oily and acne-prone skin. It has mild exfoliating properties and can be used in exfoliants and toothpastes. It is also used to colour soaps, bath bombs, bath salts and body scrubs. It will colour them grey through to black depending on the amount added. Choose activated charcoal made from coconut shells and husks that has been steam activated and is food, medicinal or cosmetic grade.

Citric acid

Originally derived from citrus fruits, citric acid is now more commonly manufactured via a process involving fermentation of the

Aspergillus niger mould with sugars. It is used for its antioxidant and preservative properties and to balance the pH of a product. It can be combined with sodium bicarbonate to create fizzy bath powders or bath bombs when added to the bathwater.

Cocamidopropyl betaine

Cocamidopropyl betaine is a liquid surfactant that creates foam and cleanses the hair and body in shampoos and body washes. It is made using coconut oil or palm oil and dimethylaminopropylamine as starting materials.

Coffee

Dried, used coffee grounds make a great body scrub. The granules encourage circulation and exfoliate the skin.

Cream

Cream can be used in face masks to soften and soothe dry skin. It is rich in butterfat and contains lecithin. It can also be used as a simple facial massage medium. Rinse after massage.

Emulsifying waxes

Emulsifying waxes are emulsifying agents used in creams and lotions to bind the water and oil ingredients. There are various types available, including ones derived from treated coconut and palm oils, animal fats, petroleum by-products and combinations of these. They are usually very efficient in ensuring emulsions remain stable.

Epsom salt

Epsom salt, magnesium sulphate, is a compound of magnesium, sulphur and oxygen. It is used for making bath salts to relax and relieve sore and aching muscles. Epsom salt can be used in drawing poultices.

The salt granules can also be mixed with oil to create a salt body scrub.

Essential oil solubiliser

Essential oil solubiliser is a common term that refers to a range of surfactants that disperse essential oils throughout water, including bathwater and aromatherapy face and body sprays. Solubilisers that are certified natural and produced using vegetable oil as the starting material are available. These include solubilisers such as caprylyl/capryl glucoside, or this ingredient in combination with other surfactants, for example, caprylyl/capryl glucoside, polyglyceryl-4 caprate, polyglyceryl-6 laurate, pentylene glycol and sodium dilauramidoglutamide lysine. When the combination is used, less solubiliser is required to create a clear, stable solution. Follow the instructions supplied by the manufacturer or supplier for using a solubiliser.

Glycerin

Glycerin, also known as glycerine or glycerol, is a clear syrupy liquid. It is obtained from vegetable oils or animal fats that have been heated under pressure or mixed with a strong alkali.

It is a humectant used in moisturisers due to its water-binding capabilities, which allow it to draw and absorb moisture from the air. However, its use has been cautioned in aggressive climatic conditions such as excessive wind, sun and low humidity, as it has been found to absorb moisture from the skin as well. Your preparation should contain no more than 20% glycerin.

Guar gum *Cyamopis tetragonoloba*

Guar gum is extracted from the beans of the guar plant. It is composed of galactomannans (complex carbohydrates), which form a gel when mixed with water. It acts as a thickener, stabiliser and gelling agent.

Honey

Honey has antiseptic, hygroscopic and healing properties. It can be incorporated into face masks, healing ointments and balms, and can be applied directly to help heal sores. Ensure that you use unprocessed honey if you wish to maintain a higher nutrient, enzyme and pollen content.

Lanolin

Lanolin is the fat found on sheep's wool. It is secreted by the sheep's sebaceous (oil) glands. It is used in creams for its rich, emollient properties. It is mainly used in preparations for dry skin. Anhydrous (water-free) lanolin is commonly available. It may sensitise irritated or sensitive skins; however, it seems to have no negative effect on normal skin.

L-ascorbic acid

L-ascorbic acid is a form of vitamin C synthesised from sorbitol which has been produced from wheat or corn. It exfoliates and brightens the skin. Use in low concentrations or in combination with other ingredients to buffer its low pH as it may irritate the skin.

Lecithin

Lecithin, also known as phospholipids, is generally obtained from eggs or soya beans and is available as a thick syrupy substance or in granule form. The phosphoric component is hydrophilic, while the lipid group is lipophilic. This enables it to be used as an emulsifier and skin-conditioning emollient.

Linseeds *Linum usitatissimum*

Also known as flax seeds, linseeds contain an oil high in essential fatty acids, which makes them highly nutritive. Linseeds are also high in mucilage and, when they are soaked in water, they form a soothing gel. Wonderful for soothing and moisturising inflamed, irritated skin.

Loofah *Luffa cylindrica*

A loofah is the dried, fibrous skeleton of a gourd. It looks like a giant cucumber or zucchini and grows on a vine. Use a loofah in a shower as a body sponge. It is used to exfoliate the skin and to stimulate the circulation in the skin.

Lye

Sodium hydroxide and potassium hydroxide are commonly called caustic soda and potash respectively. Lye is made by mixing either of these two ingredients with water to create a strong alkaline solution that reacts with oils and fats to form soap.

Milk

Full cream milk or powdered milk may be used when bathing to soften and soothe the skin.

Panthenol

Panthenol, also referred to as provitamin B5, is a humectant used in skin and hair care products to improve moisturisation. D-panthenol is available as a viscous liquid whereas DL-panthenol is available as a white, crystalline powder.

Pumice

Pumice stones are volcanic in origin and they are often seen washed up on beaches. They float on water. Pumice can be ground and used in exfoliating preparations, or the stones can be used whole and massaged over your feet to remove dry rough skin.

Red wine

Red wine contains tartaric acid and can be used on rough skin to smooth and soften it. It can be incorporated into face masks.

Salt

Sodium chloride, in combination with various other minerals, may be extracted from seawater, saline lake water and rock salt mines. Salt crystals are often used as exfoliants in body scrubs. They are also included in bath soak mixtures, which may help improve skin conditions. However, salt can be irritating to broken skin.

Sandalwood powder

This naturally fragrant, finely powdered wood can be incorporated into face and body masks and scrubs and blended into bath salts.

Sodium bicarbonate

Sodium bicarbonate is also known as bicarbonate of soda. It is used in baths to soothe itchy skin and can be combined with citric acid to create fun fizzy baths. It is used in hair rinses to remove residue build-up. Sodium bicarbonate can be used in deodorants. Its alkaline pH creates an environment in which odour causing bacteria find it difficult to live. Armpits are especially sensitive areas of skin and some people can be or become sensitised to sodium bicarbonate when used in deodorants.

Sodium cocoyl isethionate

Sodium cocoyl isethionate is an extremely gentle anionic surfactant made using either coconut or palm oil as starting materials. It is available in powder or flake form and is used in shampoos or body cleansing products. It is a popular ingredient in shampoo bars.

Spirulina *Arthrospira platensis*

Spirulina is a type of blue-green algae rich in chlorophyll and a range of other nutrients. In powdered form, it can be added to face masks to soothe and hydrate the skin. Its green colour makes powdered spirulina a natural way to colour bath soaks and other products.

Sugar *Saccharum officinarum*

Granulated sugar, including cane and coconut sugar, is used as an exfoliant in face and body scrubs. It is also the main ingredient in 'sugaring', a toffee-like mixture, which is used as an alternative to wax for hair removal.

Vinegar

Apple cider vinegar and white vinegar are both useful in making your own DIY preparations. Apple cider vinegar is made via the fermentation of apples, whereas white vinegar is made via the fermentation of grain. As they are both acidic, it is important that they are used diluted with water to avoid irritation.

Apple cider vinegar

Apple cider vinegar that still contains the 'mother' — a combination of beneficial yeast and bacteria, along with acetic acid, citric acid, vitamins, minerals and other micronutrients — is potentially more suitable for skin preparations. You will see the mother as the cloudy part that sits at the bottom of a bottle or floats around in it.

Apple cider vinegar helps restore the pH of the skin, is antibacterial and can act as a mild exfoliant. It balances oily skin and softens and reduces flakiness in dry skin. It must be well diluted before being applied to the skin.

It can be used to make herbal extracts, which are then used to make fragrant and healing baths, hair rinses and deodorants.

White vinegar

White vinegar is suitable for cleaning windows and glass. It is not recommended for cleaning all surfaces as it can etch into stone, varnishes and other coatings. Once again, it should be used diluted with water.

Xanthan gum

Xanthan gum is also known as corn sugar gum. It is produced through the fermentation of bacteria (*Xanthomonas campestris*) with a carbohydrate. It is used as a thickener, emulsion stabiliser and gelling agent.

Yoghurt

Yoghurt is made by the fermentation of certain types of beneficial bacteria with milk. It is very soothing, cooling and hydrating to the skin. Yoghurt makes an excellent base for face and body masks, especially for inflamed, irritated skin, and can be used on all skin types.

Zinc oxide

Zinc oxide is mainly produced by heating and vaporising zinc metal, with the vapour reacting with oxygen to produce zinc oxide.

It is available as a white powder in a range of particle sizes, and is added to products such as ointments and balms for its soothing, astringent and protective properties. For this reason, it is often used in nappy rash preparations. Zinc oxide is used in sunscreens as it offers physical protection from ultraviolet (UV) rays. It is also used as a colouring agent and provides skin coverage in colour cosmetics.

Infused Oils

Infused oils are made by macerating plant material in a vegetable oil over time to allow the active constituents of the plant to pass into the fixed oil. In some cases, the fixed oil and plant matter are heated to speed up the process. The plant material is then strained and filtered out of the preparation. The resulting infused oil can then be used directly on the skin or incorporated into creams, ointments or treatment oil blends.

Arnica infused oil *Arnica montana*

Arnica flowers are used to make arnica infused oil. It is dark green in colour and is used in the treatment of bruises, swelling and sprains.

Calendula infused oil
Calendula officinalis

Calendula flowers are used to make calendula infused oil. It is a beautiful orange colour and is healing and soothing to the skin. Calendula infused oil can be used in preparations for rashes and inflamed skin conditions such as eczema and dermatitis, for wound healing and to reduce scarring.

Carrot infused oil *Daucus carota*

Carrot roots are used to make carrot infused oil. Carrot infused oil has a beautiful deep orange colour and is rich in beta-carotene, an antioxidant and precursor to Vitamin A. Carrot infused oil is used to rejuvenate dry and mature skin conditions. It introduces a yellow to orange colour to products depending on the amount added.

Hypericum infused oil
Hypericum perforatum

Hypericum is also commonly known as St John's wort. The aerial parts of the herb are used to make this infused oil. It is deep red in colour due to its hypericin content. Hypericum oil is used in the treatment of inflamed, irritated skin conditions, for burns and bruises, and for wound healing. Do not apply this oil to areas of the skin that will be exposed to the sun as it may photosensitise the skin and cause the skin to burn more quickly.

Make your own infused oil by following the methods for making infused oils on page 52.

Floral Waters and Aromatic Hydrosols

Authentic floral waters are also known as waters of distillation, aromatic hydrosols and hydrolats. They are the by-product of essential oil distillation.

Once the distilled essential oil has been removed from the water, we are left with traces of water-soluble essential oil constituents in the remaining water. These constituents generally have anti-inflammatory and antiseptic properties. This makes floral waters suitable for use in soothing, healing compresses for inflamed skin and eyes. A teaspoon of floral water can be added to a teaspoon or so of clay to create a face mask.

They also make excellent skin toners and fresheners and can be incorporated into moisturising preparations. They have a subtle fragrance reminiscent of the essential oil. Pour a floral water into a spray bottle and use it to refresh and hydrate your skin throughout the day.

It is important to be aware that there are floral waters, such as rosewater or neroli water, that have been made by blending food or fragrance essences into water. They are not a by-product of distillation and do not contain the water-soluble components of the essential oil and yet are still called pure floral waters. They are usually sold for flavouring food and are generally inexpensive. These floral waters are not suitable for making skin care preparations. Furthermore, essential oils dispersed into water have also been labelled as floral waters. When purchasing floral waters, ensure that you are receiving the water of plant distillation.

As floral waters are mostly water, they are easily contaminated with microbes and provide a medium in which they can thrive. Unless you are using a floral water that has been freshly distilled or stored in sterile conditions, it will have a preservative added to it. This is important to guard against contaminating your preparations and causing skin or eye infections.

Many fragrant plants are suitable for distillation. The following floral waters are commonly used in skin care.

Chamomile water *Matricaria recutita*

Chamomile water is very soothing. It is suitable for use on sensitive and inflamed eyes and skin.

Lavender water *Lavandula angustifolia*

Lavender water is soothing and antiseptic. It helps soothe and heal blemished skin.

Neroli water
Citrus aurantium var. *amara*

Neroli water is also known as orange flower water. It has soothing and slightly astringent

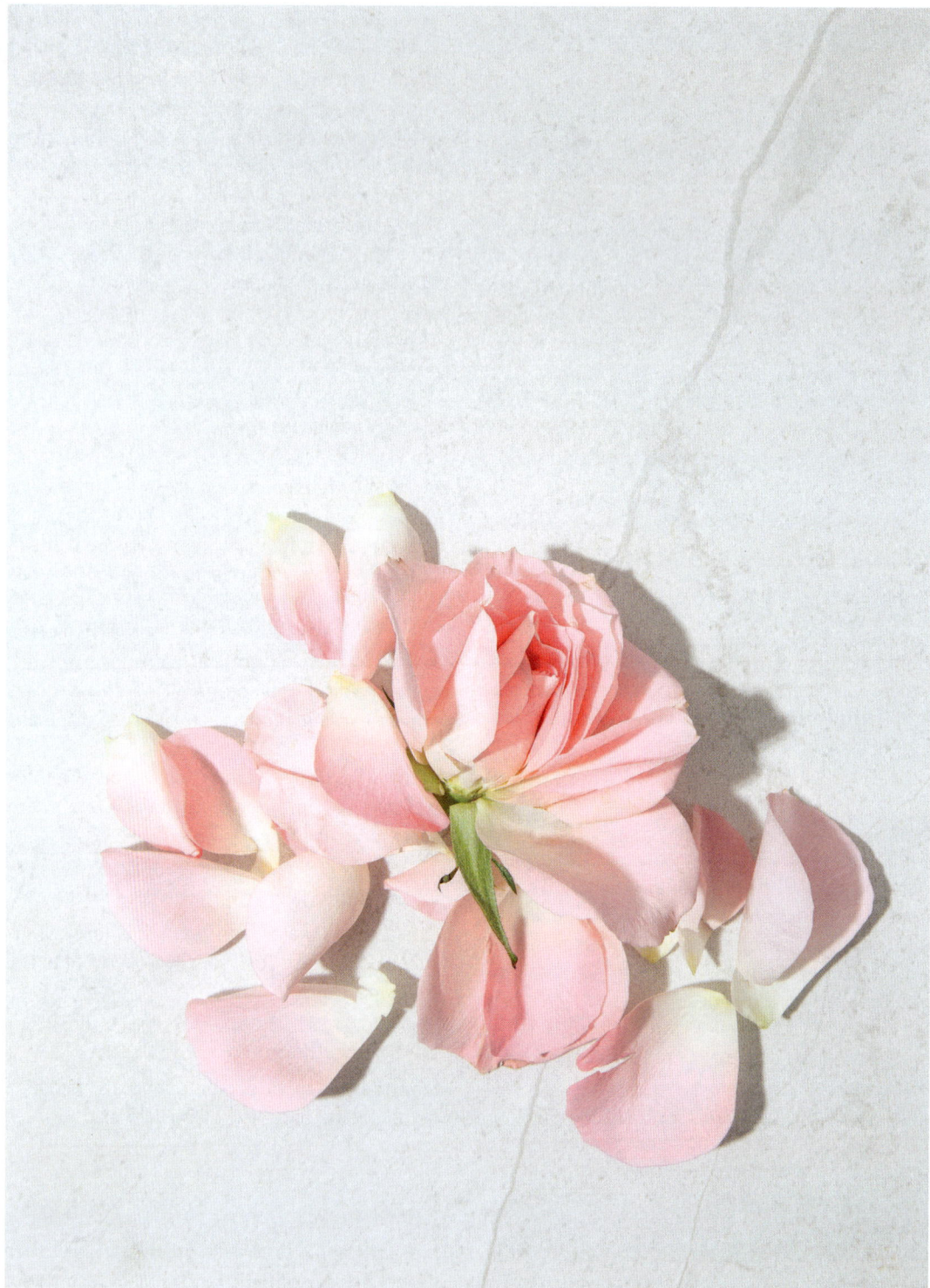

properties and is suitable for combination and sensitive skin.

Rosewater *Rosa damascena*

Rosewater is soothing and cooling to the skin. It can be used on all skin types, especially dry and sensitive skin. Rosewater applied to cotton pads can be placed over the eyes to soothe irritation.

Witch hazel water *Hamamelis virginiana*

Witch hazel water, which has been distilled, is mild on the skin and can be used to refresh, cool and calm. On the other hand, witch hazel extract is made using alcohol and is astringent and antiseptic due to its tannin content. It is especially useful on bites, stings, rashes and haemorrhoids.

Base Products

Base products are pre-made preparations into which herbal extracts and essential oils may be added. They are simple preparations and do not contain fragrances, colouring agents, essential oils, herbal extracts or the addition of any other active ingredients. This allows you to customise a preparation for a particular purpose very easily and quickly. The following suggested quantities of ingredients to be added to the base products are given as a guideline. You may want to check with your supplier for any variations. Due to the range in concentrations of herbal extracts, the following quantities are a guide only.

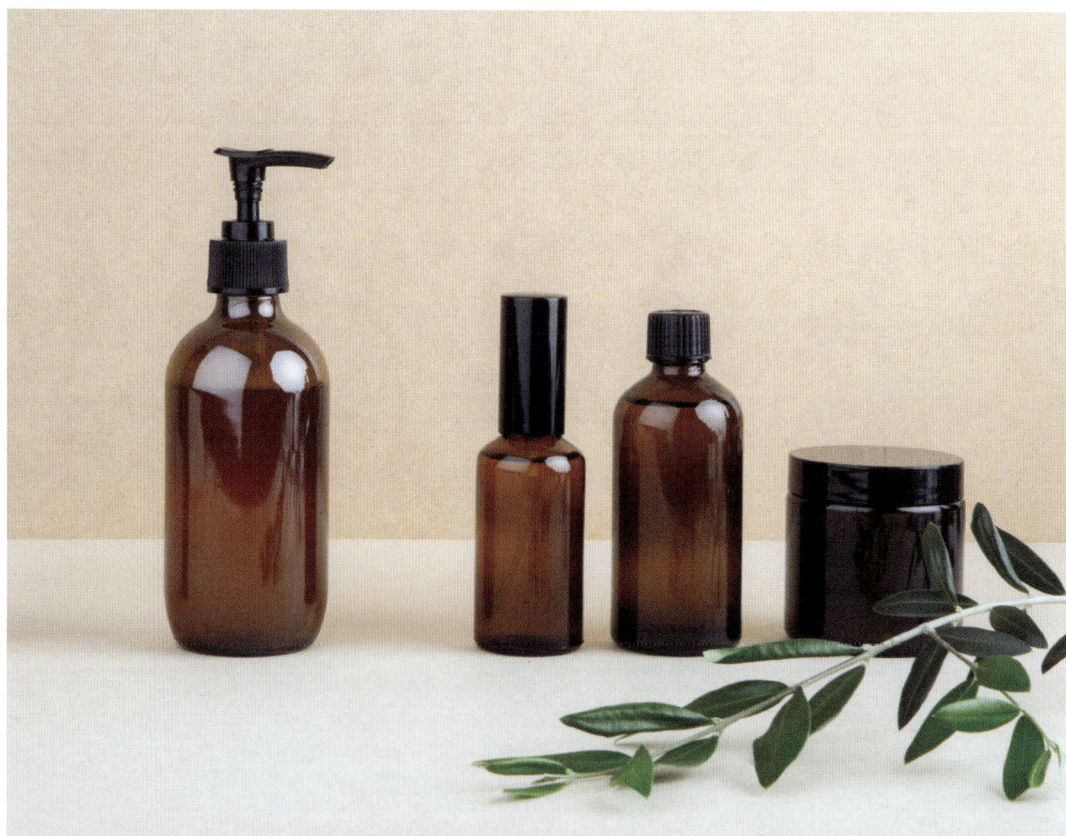

Base Product	Quantity of Active Ingredients
Foaming bases (shampoo, body wash, Castile liquid soap)	To each 100 mL or 100 g of shampoo base, body wash base or Castile liquid soap, the following quantities of ingredients may be added: • essential oils: face — up to 1 g (approx. 20 drops), body — up to 2 g (approx. 40 drops) • vegetable oils: up to 10 g (approx. 2 tsp) • herbal infused oil: up to 10 g (approx. 2 tsp) • herbal extract (glycerol-based): face — up to 5 g (approx. 1 tsp), body — up to 10 g (approx. 2 tsp). To make a shampoo for your hair, see the section on Shampoos (page 255) for recipes. To make a body wash, see the section on Body Washes (page 181) for recipes.
Moisture cream base	To each 100 g of moisture cream base, the following quantities of ingredients may be added: • essential oils: face — up to 1 g (approx. 20 drops), body — up to 2 g (approx. 40 drops) • vegetable oils: up to 10 g (approx. 2 tsp) • herbal infused oil: up to 10 g (approx. 2 tsp) • herbal extract (glycerol-based): face — up to 5 g (approx. 1 tsp), body — up to 10 g (2 tsp). To make a moisture cream base, see the section on Emulsions (page 69) for recipes.
Ointment/balm base	To each 100 g of ointment/balm base, the following quantities of ingredients may be added: • essential oils: face — up to 1 g (approx. 20 drops), body — up to 2 g (approx. 40 drops) • vegetable oils: up to 10 g (approx. 2 tsp) • herbal infused oil: up to 10 g (approx. 2 tsp). To make an ointment/balm base, see the section on Ointments and Balms (page 59) for recipes. If you are intending to add vegetable oil or infused oil to the base after it has been made, make the base with a higher percentage of wax or cocoa butter to ensure that with the addition of the extra oil it won't become too soft. You may prefer to melt the base before adding extra oil so that a firm structure will set up on cooling.

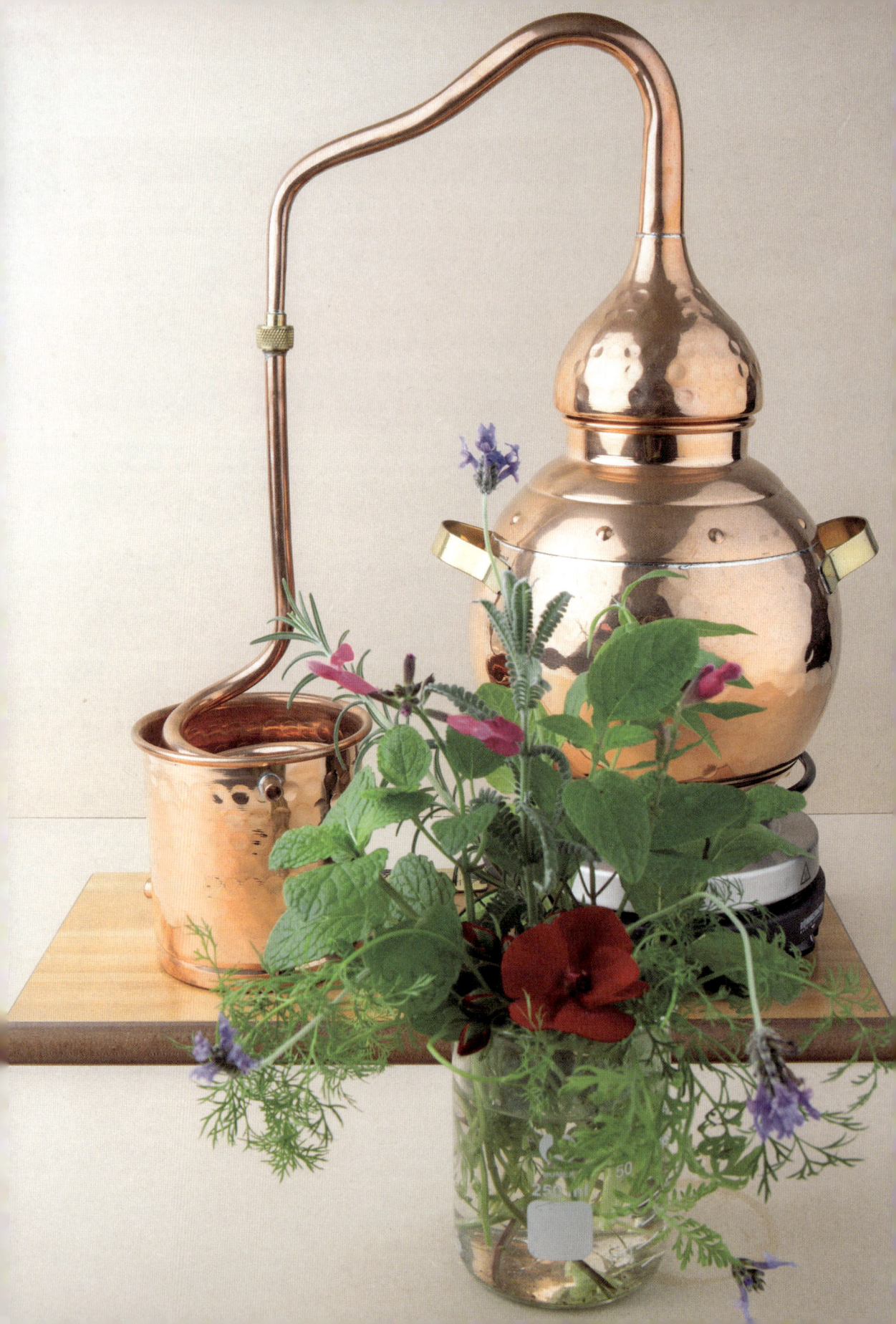

Aromatherapy

Your skin and hair will benefit from carefully selected essential oils blended into your preparations. Applied topically, not only do the essential oils benefit the skin, but they may also penetrate the skin and be absorbed into the body, where they may have further therapeutic benefits. Their odoriferous molecules are inhaled, which means the essential oils can affect us on an emotional and mental level as well.

Aromatherapy Skin Benefits

Essential oils benefit your skin and hair in the following ways, depending on the essential oil. They may:

- support and balance skin functions

- stimulate healthy skin cell production and regeneration. They can aid skin healing when it has been damaged through wounding or from long-term sun exposure, which is evidenced in aging skin

- improve skin hydration

- balance sebum production

- improve circulation in the skin thereby improving the flow of nutrients and oxygen to the skin, as well as the elimination of waste (this property also aids in the dispersion of bruises)

- calm and soothe redness, irritation, itchiness and inflammation

- act as antiseptics or fungicides and be used to treat skin infections

- have astringent properties

- have a relaxing effect and relieve tension

- smell divine.

Essential Oil Dilution

In order to use your essential oils safely and effectively, it is important to use the correct quantity of essential oil in each type of preparation.

Product	Essential Oil Dilution
Facial oils, creams and balms	1% dilution (approx. 20 drops of essential oil per 100 mL or 100 g of base product) when using essential oils therapeutically to treat skin conditions. 0.25–0.5% dilution (approx. 5–10 drops of essential oil per 100 mL or 100 g of base product) for long-term use. This dilution is recommended to prevent the skin from becoming sensitised to a particular essential oil.
Facial moisturising gels	0.25% dilution or less (approx. 5 drops of essential oil per 100 mL or 100 g) is recommended when making a gel.
Direct or neat application	Lavender or tea tree essential oil may be applied directly to a pimple, mosquito bite, wart or cold sore. Do not wipe over the face or over large areas of skin. Direct or neat application is not generally recommended due to the possibility of skin irritation.
Masks	Less than 0.25% dilution (approx. 2–3 drops of essential oil per 100 mL or 100 g) is recommended when making a mask.
Eye products	Avoid using essential oils or use less than 0.25% dilution (approx. 2–3 drops of essential oil per 100 mL or 100 g of oil or cream). Ensure the essential oils you have chosen are non-sensitising or non-stimulating essential oils. The skin around the eyes is particularly thin and sensitive and there is the possibility of essential oils being rubbed into or seeping into the eyes.
Body products (cream, lotion, oil or balm)	1–3% dilution (approx. 20–60 drops of essential oil per 100 mL or 100 g of body product) is generally considered a safe and effective dilution for body oils, creams, lotions, ointments and balms, depending on their purpose. A 1% dilution is more suitable for body lotions being used daily and over large areas of skin, whereas a 3% dilution would be suitable for a balm used every now and then and on small areas of skin.

Product	Essential Oil Dilution
Compresses	Add 3–5 drops of essential oil to 500 mL of water. When wanting to calm an inflamed skin condition, use cool water and re-dip the cloth in the cool water whenever the skin feels as though it is heating up. When using a compress on aching muscles, use warm/hot water and re-dip the cloth in the warm/hot water when the cloth begins to cool down.
Bath products	1–3% dilution (approx. 20–60 drops of essential oil per 100 mL or 100 g of bath product) is generally considered safe. A lower dilution is recommended when treating inflamed skin conditions, and a higher dilution is recommended when making bath preparations for aching muscles.
Foaming products	Foaming products may include unscented Castile liquid soap, bubble baths, shampoos and body washes. A 0.5–1% dilution (approx. 10–20 drops of essential oil per 100 mL or 100 g of foaming product) is recommended. Higher concentrations than this will result in the product's lathering or foaming properties being reduced.
Soaps	Essential oils may constitute 1–4% of the total mixture of a bar soap. The quantity used depends on the essential oil's odour intensity, volatility and skin sensitivity. For example, citrus oils are more volatile and less odour intense than peppermint essential oil. This means more citrus oil needs to be added to fragrance a soap than peppermint oil. Spice essential oils need to be used in lower dilutions and with caution as they may irritate the skin.
Sensitive skin products	Less than 0.25–1% dilution (approx. 5–20 drops of essential oil per 100 mL or 100 g of base product). Essential oil dilution in some particularly sensitive and inflamed conditions may be even less. Your choice of essential oils to be applied to this particular skin type should be made carefully.
Baby and child products	Less than 0.25–1% dilution (approx. 5–20 drops of essential oil per 100 mL or 100 g of base product). It is important to use a very low dilution of essential oil on babies due to their sensitive skins and their body size. Your choice of essential oils for babies is also limited to very safe oils such as German chamomile, Roman chamomile, lavender, mandarin, neroli, sandalwood and tangerine.

Essential Oil Measurement

As very small quantities of essential oil are used in many recipes, their measurements are given in drops, where 20 drops of essential oil approximates 1 g. However, it is worth noting that this can only be an approximation due to variations in dripolator size and viscosity of essential oils. This variability is acceptable for the recipes in this book. However, for accuracy and consistency from batch to batch, it is important to weigh ingredients and convert all measurements to grams.

For the most part, recipes are given as bases into which a range of essential oils may be added. Most recipes are given in increments of 100 g, with the essential oils given as an addition to this. This means if the base is 100 g and a 1% dilution of essential oils is recommended, 1 g of essential oil is added to the 100 g with the entire recipe adding up to 101 g. This has been done for ease of measurement. This means the actual dilution of essential oil will be less than 1%. In this case, it will be 0.9%. For the most part, this lower dilution is acceptable. However, for accuracy and consistency from batch to batch, it is important that the formula adds up to 100%. If the essential oils are 1% of the formula, the base should be converted to 99% of the formula, with the entire formula adding up to 100%.

Precautions

- Ensure that you are using the finest quality essential oils, not perfume, perfume oils, fragrance oils, or essential oils intended for the fragrance industry, food industry or household products. Choosing certified organic essential oils is one way of ensuring your essential oils are free from any synthesised aroma chemicals.

- Essential oils are highly concentrated. Do not apply undiluted essential oils directly onto the skin or take internally unless advised by a qualified practitioner.
- Never exceed the recommended dose or dilutions.
- Do not use the same oil all the time. Use a blend of oils or alternate your essential oils from time to time.

Pregnancy

Many aromatherapists consider it sensible to avoid the use of the following commonly available essential oils during pregnancy, especially during the first three months:

> aniseed, star anise, aniseed myrtle, sweet birch, buchu ct. diosphenol, buchu ct. pulegone, carrot seed, cassia, cinnamon bark, costus, blue cypress, sweet and bitter fennel, ho leaf ct. camphor, hyssop ct. pinocamphone, Spanish lavender, mugwort, myrrh, oregano, parsley leaf and seed, pennyroyal, rue, Dalmatian sage, Spanish sage, savin, tansy, thuja, wintergreen, wormwood

High blood pressure

Many aromatherapists consider it sensible to avoid the use of the following essential oils for anyone with hypertension:

> rosemary, sage and thyme

Photosensitivity

Photosensitising materials cause the skin to burn if exposed to strong UV light from any source, including the sun. Hyperpigmentation of the skin may also result. Cold-pressed citrus essential oils containing furocoumarins are the major group of photosensitising essential oils. Bergamot and cold-pressed lime are two commonly used essential oils that are considered strong photosensitisers, while grapefruit and lemon are mild photosensitisers. To avoid the risk of photosensitising the skin when using these essential oils, do not expose the skin to the sun or UV light for 12 hours after use or ensure the level of these essential oils does not exceed 1% of a formulation. Mandarin, sweet orange and tangerine do not generally pose any issues.

- Strong photosensitisers — bergamot, cold-pressed lime
- Mild photosensitisers — grapefruit, lemon

Skin irritation and sensitivity

Sensitivity to essential oils varies from person to person. Essential oils that are generally considered suitable for use on the skin may not be suitable for a person who has especially sensitive skin or an individual sensitivity to a particular essential oil.

Different parts of the body are more sensitive than others, such as the face and armpits. It is important not to exceed recommended dilutions as higher dilutions are more likely to cause irritation. The following essential oils are considered especially sensitising to the skin and may cause skin irritation. They must be used with caution.

basil, cinnamon bark and leaf, citronella, clove bud, lemongrass, lemon myrtle, lemon-scented eucalyptus, lemon-scented tea tree, may chang, thyme

Babies and children

It is important to use a very low dilution of essential oils on babies due to their sensitive skin and their body size. Your choice of essential oils for babies is also limited to very safe oils such as:

German chamomile, Roman chamomile, lavender, mandarin, neroli, sandalwood and tangerine

Degradation of essential oils

Always use essential oils before their expiry date. Essential oils can degrade over time, especially on exposure to oxygen, heat and light. For this reason, they should be stored in opaque or amber glass bottles in a cool environment. Citrus and pine essential oils should be used within 12–24 months of opening the bottle as they oxidise rapidly. A change in their smell, for example, will indicate that they are no longer fresh and have oxidised. Furthermore, degraded essential oils may lose their therapeutic properties and cause dermal sensitisation.

Essential Oils

Bergamot
Citrus aurantium subsp. *bergamia*

Skin care: Bergamot has antiseptic and wound healing properties. It is used to treat seborrhoea of the skin and scalp including acne, and oily skin and hair. It is also used in formulae for psoriasis and weeping eczema.

Perfume note: top note

Other: uplifting, anti-stress

Black pepper *Piper nigrum*

Skin care: Black pepper has rubefacient properties, which means it stimulates local circulation. This makes it useful, when used in small quantities, for dispersing bruises.

Perfume note: middle note

Other: beneficial for aching muscles, rheumatism and arthritis

Cajeput *Melaleuca cajuputi*

Skin care: Cajeput is antiseptic and is used to relieve the itching from mosquito bites.

Perfume note: middle note

Other: beneficial for aching muscles, rheumatism and arthritis, colds and flu

Cardamom *Elettaria cardamomum*

Skin care: Cardamom is used in perfumery.

Perfume note: middle note

Other: energising and uplifting, aids digestion

Carrot seed *Daucus carota*

Skin care: Carrot seed improves the circulation in the skin and has skin healing properties. It is used to improve skin tone and the health of mature skin, dilated surface capillaries, wounds, eczema and psoriasis.

Perfume note: middle note

Other: hepatic and diuretic

Cedarwood, Atlas *Cedrus atlantica*

Skin care: Atlas cedarwood has antiseptic, astringent and skin healing properties. It is useful in treating acne and oily skin, dandruff and oily hair. It is also used as an insect repellent.

Perfume note: base note

Other: anti-stress, reduces anxiety

Cedarwood, Virginian
Juniperus virginiana

Skin care: Virginian cedarwood has similar properties to Atlas cedarwood. It has antiseptic, astringent and skin healing properties. It is useful in treating acne and oily skin, dandruff and oily hair. It is also used as an insect repellent.

Perfume note: base note

Other: anti-stress, reduces anxiety

Chamomile, German *Matricaria recutita*

Skin care: German chamomile, also known as blue chamomile, has proven anti-inflammatory properties, is antiseptic and has skin healing properties. It calms red, inflamed, irritated skin conditions including acne, dermatitis, eczema and psoriasis. It is suitable for all skin types including sensitive skin. Chamomile is an excellent choice for use on babies and children.

Perfume note: base note

Other: beneficial for muscular aches and pains

Chamomile, Roman *Anthemis nobilis*

Skin care: Roman chamomile is gentle and soothing on sensitive skin and suitable for use all skin types.

Perfume note: middle note

Other: anti-stress, calming

Cinnamon *Cinnamomum verum*

Skin care: Cinnamon bark and leaf are highly antimicrobial. Both are used in perfumery for their warm spice notes. Care must be taken as they can irritate and sensitise the skin.

Perfume note: middle note

Other: emotionally uplifting, warming and energising

Cistus *Cistus ladaniferus*

Skin care: Cistus, also known as rock rose, has antiseptic, astringent and skin healing properties. It is used to heal infected and inflamed skin conditions including acne, eczema, psoriasis, wounds and herpes lesions. It also improves the condition of mature skin. Its intense aroma provides a rich, warm, resinous base note.

Perfume note: base note

Other: emotionally deeply soothing

Citronella *Cymbopogon nardus*

Skin care: Citronella is used as an effective insect repellent.

Perfume note: top note

Other: beneficial for aching muscles, rheumatism and arthritis

Clary sage *Salvia sclarea*

Skin care: Clary sage has antiseptic, astringent and skin healing properties and regulates excess sebum production. It is used to treat acne, oily skin, oily hair and dandruff.

Perfume note: middle note

Other: anti-stress, reduces anxiety and menstrual cramps

Clove bud *Syzygium aromaticum*

Skin care: Clove bud is generally not used in leave-on skin care products as it can be an irritant, but may be used in low dilutions in wash off products. It has traditionally been used in dental care for its analgesic and antibacterial properties. Clove is also used to repel insects.

Perfume note: middle note

Other: beneficial for aching muscles, rheumatism and arthritis

Coriander seed *Coriandrum sativum*

Skin care: Coriander seed is used in perfumery.

Perfume note: middle note

Other: energising and uplifting, aids digestion

Cypress *Cupressus sempervirens*

Skin care: Cypress has antiseptic, astringent, deodorant and vasoconstrictive properties. It can be used to reduce excessive oiliness and perspiration.

Perfume note: middle note

Other: improves circulation

Everlasting *Helichrysum angustifolium*

Skin care: Everlasting, also known as immortelle, has anti-inflammatory, antiseptic, astringent and skin healing properties. It is used to treat sensitive, inflamed skin, eczema and psoriasis. Everlasting is used to heal wounds as well as reduce old scar tissue and stretch marks.

Perfume note: base note

Other: calming and anti-stress

Frankincense *Boswellia carterii*

Skin care: Frankincense has antiseptic, astringent, regenerative and skin healing properties. It is used to improve the tone of mature and damaged skin, heal wounds and improve scars.

Perfume note: middle note

Other: anti-stress, reduces anxiety, calms breathing

Geranium *Pelargonium graveolens*

Skin care: Geranium has antiseptic, astringent and skin healing properties. It helps regulate sebum production, making it especially useful for oily and combination skin, although it is beneficial for all skin types. Geranium encourages wound healing and is also used to improve broken capillaries.

Perfume note: middle note

Other: uplifting and calming

Grapefruit *Citrus paradisi*

Skin care: Grapefruit's antiseptic properties make it useful for treating oily skin, acne and oily scalp.

Perfume note: top note

Other: uplifting and refreshing

Essentials

Hinoki wood *Chamaecyparis obtusa*

Skin care: Hinoki wood may be used in perfumery and has insect repellent properties.

Perfume note: base note

Other: anti-stress, reduces anxiety

Jasmine *Jasminum grandiflorum*

Skin care: Jasmine has antiseptic and skin healing properties and is used to improve the condition of mature skin. Jasmine is usually available as an absolute, which means it has been obtained via solvent extraction. It may be sensitising in some individuals. Jasmine is often used to create rich floral perfumes.

Perfume note: middle note

Other: uplifting, reduces anxiety

Juniper *Juniperus communis*

Skin care: Juniper has antiseptic and astringent properties, making it suitable for use on oily skin and acne. Assists in healing weepy eczema and psoriasis.

Perfume note: middle note

Other: diuretic, lymphatic decongestant

Lavender *Lavandula angustifolia*

Skin care: Lavender has anti-inflammatory, antiseptic and skin healing properties. It is especially successful in the treatment of burns, whether from hot objects, liquids or the sun. Lavender is particularly soothing for inflamed skin conditions such as eczema, dermatitis and psoriasis and is used to encourage wound healing. Acne conditions benefit from lavender's anti-inflammatory, antiseptic and skin healing properties. It is also used to relieve itching and can be used as an effective insect repellent.

Perfume note: middle note

Other: relaxing, reduces anxiety

Lavender, spike *Lavandula spica*

Skin care: Spike lavender has antiseptic, wound healing and insect repellent properties.

Perfume note: middle note

Other: beneficial for headaches and sore muscles

Lemon *Citrus limon*

Skin care: Lemon has antiseptic, astringent, wound healing and mild circulatory stimulating properties. It also helps to dissolve sebum. Lemon is used to treat oily, congested skin and devitalised skin. Its astringent and mild circulatory stimulating properties improve the condition of varicose veins.

Perfume note: top note

Other: uplifting and refreshing

Lemongrass *Cymbopogon citratus*

Skin care: Lemongrass is added to soaps to create an intense, refreshing lemony aroma. In other skin care products, it may be sensitising to some people and may be best used in wash off products only or in very low dilutions.

Perfume note: top note

Other: uplifting and energising, antiseptic

Lime *Citrus aurantifolia*

Skin care: Cold-pressed lime has antiseptic and astringent properties making it suitable for use on oily skin and acne. Lime is used in perfumes for its refreshing fragrance.

Perfume note: top note

Other: refreshing and uplifting, improves lymph flow

Mandarin/tangerine *Citrus reticulata*

Skin care: Mandarin assists in treating acne and oily skin.

Perfume note: top note

Other: uplifting, reduces anxiety

Manuka *Leptospermum scoparium*

Skin care: Manuka's gentle antimicrobial properties make it beneficial for treating acne and wound healing.

Perfume note: middle note

Other: colds and flu

Marjoram, sweet *Origanum marjorana*

Skin care: While sweet marjoram is not used in skin care, it is often used in massage and bath preparations to relax the body, mind and spirit.

Perfume note: middle note

Other: anti-stress, reduces anxiety

May chang *Litsea cubeba*

Skin care: May chang has antibacterial properties which make it useful for acne. Care must be taken as it may irritate sensitive skin. It is an effective deodorant and gives fresh, lemony notes to perfume blends.

Perfume note: top note

Other: refreshing, uplifting

Melissa *Melissa officinalis*

Skin care: Melissa possesses antiviral properties against the *Herpes simplex* virus (cold sores). It should be applied undiluted directly to the lesion. Also known as lemon balm.

Perfume note: top note

Other: uplifting and calming

Myrrh *Commiphora myrrha*

Skin care: Myrrh has anti-inflammatory, antiseptic, astringent, regenerative, skin and wound healing properties. It is used to heal wounds and ulcers, weeping eczema, tinea, and deep cracks on the heels and hands. Myrrh's regenerative properties also make it useful in improving the condition of mature skin.

Perfume note: base note

Other: deeply calming

Neroli *Citrus aurantium* var. *amara*

Skin care: Neroli is used for its antiseptic and skin healing properties. It is suitable for use on all skin types, especially dry, sensitive skin and broken capillaries.

Perfume note: top note

Other: uplifting and reduces anxiety, anti-stress

Niaouli *Melaleuca quinquenervia*

Skin care: Niaouli has antiseptic and skin healing properties. It is useful in treating acne and wounds. It is also used as an insect repellent.

Perfume note: middle note

Other: beneficial for muscular aches and pains, arthritis and respiratory conditions

Orange, sweet *Citrus sinensis*

Skin care: Sweet orange may be used on most skin types. It has antiseptic properties.

Perfume note: top note

Other: uplifting and calming

Palmarosa *Cymbopogon martini*

Skin care: Palmarosa has antiseptic and skin healing properties that make it useful in treating acne, eczema, herpes, infected skin conditions and wounds. It is suitable for use on all skin types.

Perfume note: middle note

Other: calming and uplifting

Patchouli *Pogostemon cablin*

Skin care: Patchouli has anti-inflammatory, antiseptic, astringent, regenerative and skin healing properties. It stimulates the growth of skin cells and assists in the formation of scar tissue. It assists in the healing of sores and wounds, and rough cracked skin,. It is used in the treatment of acne, eczema, mature skin, fungal infections and scalp disorders. Patchouli also makes a wonderful deodorant.

Perfume note: base note

Other: calming and grounding

Peppermint *Mentha piperita*

Skin care: Peppermint has analgesic, antiseptic, astringent and vasoconstrictive properties. It can be used to relieve skin inflammation, irritation or itching. For this purpose, it is used in a 1% dilution or less; otherwise the irritation may be worsened. It may be used to relieve the pain of sunburn and shingles and the itching of dermatitis and eczema. It cools the skin by constricting the capillaries and makes a very refreshing body spray.

Perfume note: middle note

Other: relieves digestive disorders

Petitgrain *Citrus aurantium* var. *amara*

Skin care: Petitgrain has antiseptic, astringent and deodorant properties. This makes it useful in treating acne, oily skin and hair, and excessive perspiration.

Perfume note: middle note

Other: uplifting and calming

Pine *Pinus sylvestris*

Skin care: Pine is not used for face care. However, it is used in a range of body care preparations where a clean, fresh pine note is appealing. It has insect repellent properties and its antiseptic and deodorising properties make it useful in room fresheners and cleaning preparations.

Perfume note: middle note

Other: beneficial for respiratory disorders, colds and flu, muscular aches and pains

Rose *Rosa damascena* and *Rosa centifolia*

Skin care: Rose has antiseptic, astringent, regenerative and skin healing properties. It may be used on all skin types, especially mature skin. Its astringent properties make it useful for strengthening surface capillaries. Its healing properties encourage wound healing. Rose is available as rose otto, which is obtained via distillation of the rose petals, or absolute, which is obtained via solvent extraction. Rose otto is recommended for use in skin care, while both rose otto and rose absolute may be used in perfumery.

Perfume note: middle note (absolute), top note (otto)

Other: brings joy to the heart, uplifting, reduces anxiety

Rosemary *Rosmarinus officinalis*

Skin care: Rosemary is astringent and stimulates the circulation. It has traditionally been used in the treatment of hair and scalp conditions, such as dandruff and hair loss.

Perfume note: middle note

Other: promotes clear thinking and concentration, relieves aching muscles

Sage *Salvia officinalis*

Skin care: Sage is antiseptic and regenerates the skin. It is useful in the treatment of wounds, acne, eczema, dermatitis and dandruff.

Perfume note: middle note

Other: beneficial for rheumatism and arthritis

Sandalwood *Santalum album*

Skin care: Sandalwood has anti-inflammatory, antiseptic and hydrating properties. It encourages the retention of moisture within the skin layers, and this makes it useful in the treatment of dehydrated skin and dry, inflamed conditions such as eczema, dermatitis and psoriasis. Its antiseptic and anti-inflammatory properties also make it beneficial in the treatment of acne and for the treatment of wounds. Australian sandalwood essential oil (*Santalum spicatum*) can be used for similar purposes and substituted into recipes where sandalwood essential oil is called for. Please note that its odour is a little more intense, drier and more resinous.

Perfume note: base note

Other: calming and relaxing

Tansy, blue *Tanacetum annum*

Skin care: Blue tansy has anti-inflammatory properties and is soothing to the skin. It assists in healing and rejuvenating damaged skin. It is beneficial for sensitive, inflamed and mature skin and assists in wound healing.

Perfume note: middle note

Other: calming, reduces nervous tension and anxiety

Tea tree *Melaleuca alternifolia*

See Australian essential oils on page 47.

Thyme *Thymus vulgaris* ct. *linalool*

Skin care: Thyme has antiseptic, astringent and wound healing properties. It is used to treat acne, boils, wounds and other skin infections. Thyme oil is available in several chemotypes. The chemotype most useful in skin care is *Thymus vulgaris* ct. linalool. It is particularly good for healing and treating infections on sensitive and inflamed skin, whereas other thyme chemotypes including *Thymus vulgaris* ct. thymol, which is most commonly available, can be a strong skin irritant.

Perfume note: middle note

Other: beneficial for colds and flu, energising

Vetiver *Vetiveria zizanoides*

Skin care: Vetiver stimulates the circulation and improves the strength of connective tissue. It is useful in improving skin tone and devitalised skin.

Perfume note: base note

Other: calming and grounding

Yarrow *Achillea millefolium*

Skin care: Yarrow has anti-inflammatory, antiseptic, astringent and wound healing properties. It is used to treat wounds, sores, acne, eczema, inflamed and irritated skin, and sensitive skin.

Perfume note: middle note

Other: calming and balancing

Ylang ylang *Cananga odorata*

Skin care: Ylang ylang has antiseptic properties and is reputed to have a balancing effect on sebum production. This makes it suitable for both oily and dry skin. It has been used in hairdressing preparations to help promote healthy hair growth and improve scalp conditions.

Perfume note: middle note

Other: anti-stress, reduces anxiety

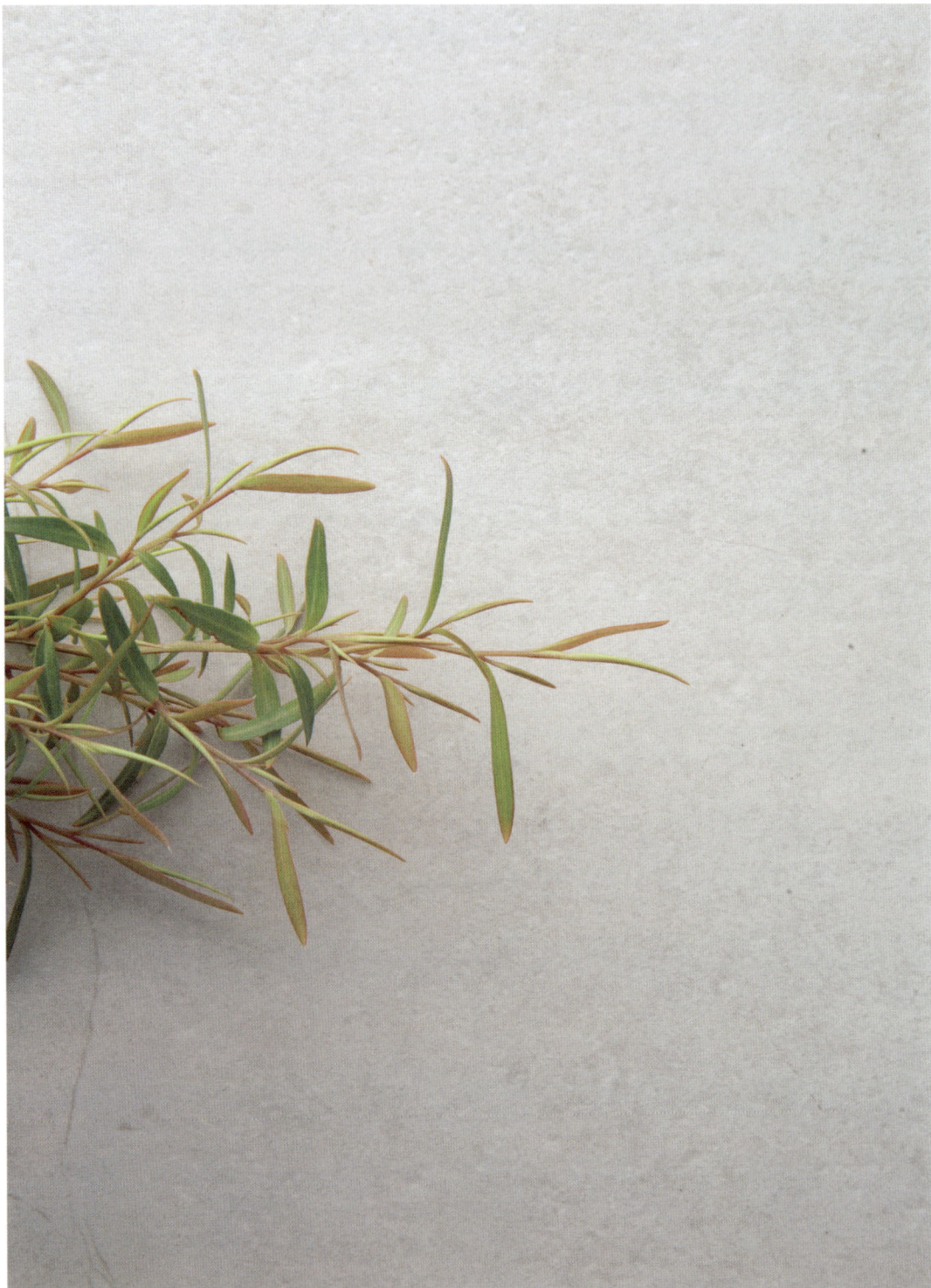

AUSTRALIAN ESSENTIAL OILS

Buddha wood *Eremophilia mitchellii*

Skin care: Buddha wood is used in perfumery and has insect repellent properties.

Perfume note: base note

Other: beneficial for muscular aches and pains

Eucalyptus, blue Mallee
Eucalyptus polybractea

Skin care: Blue Mallee eucalyptus is not used for face care as it can be sensitising to the skin. It is used in body care products such as soaps, body washes and scrubs that are refreshing to the senses and stimulate circulation. It is used in insect repellent preparations.

Perfume note: middle note

Other: beneficial for respiratory disorders, colds and flu, muscular aches and pains

Eucalyptus, lemon-scented
Corymbia citriodora

Skin care: Lemon-scented eucalyptus is not used for face care as it can be sensitising to the skin. It is used in body care products such as soaps, body washes and scrubs that are refreshing to the senses.

Perfume note: top note

Other: antimicrobial, antifungal, insect repellent

Eucalyptus, peppermint
Eucalyptus dives

Skin care: Peppermint eucalyptus is not used for face care as it can be sensitising to the skin. It is used in body care products such as soaps, body washes and scrubs that are refreshing to the senses.

Perfume note: middle note

Other: antimicrobial

Fragonia *Agonis fragrans*

Skin care: Fragonia is useful in the treatment of acne.

Perfume note: middle note

Other: beneficial for respiratory conditions, antifungal, calming

Ironbark, lemon-scented
Eucalyptus staigeriana

Skin care: Lemon-scented ironbark has antimicrobial and antiseptic properties.

Perfume note: top note

Other: uplifting and relaxing

Kunzea *Kunzea ambigua*

Skin care: Kunzea can be helpful for the relief of eczema and dermatitis. It has a fresh Australian bush scent.

Perfume note: middle note

Other: beneficial for mild anxiety, muscular and arthritic pain

Lemon myrtle *Backhousia citriodora*

Skin care: Lemon myrtle is not used for face care as it can be sensitising to the skin. It is often used in body care preparations such as soaps, body washes and scrubs that are antimicrobial and refreshing to the senses.

Perfume note: top note

Other: antimicrobial, uplifting

Rosalina *Melaleuca ericifolia*

Skin care: Rosalina is gentle on the skin and has antibacterial properties that make it useful for acne and helping to calm rashes. Its antifungal properties may assist with dandruff.

Perfume note: middle note

Other: relaxing, beneficial for colds, flu and sinusitis

Tea tree *Melaleuca alternifolia*

Skin care: Tea tree has antifungal, antibacterial, antiseptic and wound healing properties. It is also an effective insect repellent. Tea tree is used in the treatment of acne, cold sores (herpes), dandruff, infected wounds, insect bites, rashes and tinea.

Perfume note: middle note

Other: beneficial for respiratory conditions

The following essential oil compositions are ideal for use on the indicated skin types. The quantities specified here are to be added to each 100 g or 100 mL of base. Once you become familiar with the essential oils, you may like to make up your own personalised composition.

Essential oil compositions for skin care

Normal skin
9 drops geranium
6 drops jasmine absolute
5 drops ylang ylang

Sensitive skin
6 drops sandalwood
3 drops everlasting
2 drops German chamomile

Dry skin
10 drops sandalwood
6 drops rose otto
4 drops neroli

Broken capillaries
15 drops cypress
5 drops German chamomile

Oily skin
12 drops lemon
4 drops geranium
4 drops juniper

Combination skin
8 drops grapefruit
4 drops geranium
4 drops patchouli
4 drops petitgrain

Dehydrated skin
10 drops sandalwood
6 drops lavender
4 drops ylang ylang

Mature skin
12 drops rose otto
5 drops frankincense
3 drops patchouli

Acne skin
7 drops lavender
5 drops palmarosa
5 drops tea tree
3 drops German chamomile

Devitalised skin
16 drops lemon
4 drops vetiver

Herbal Extracts and Preparations

Herbal preparations extract the active constituents of the herbs and can be incorporated into skin care and hair care preparations and, as a result, benefit the skin, scalp and hair. Simple extraction methods include infusions, decoctions, tinctures, infused oils and herbal vinegars.

When making your herbal preparations, keep in mind that herbs vary in their density. For example, the same weight in rose petals as that of ginger root will fill a much larger volume. The quantities given in each of these preparations are standard. However, if the herb is particularly lightweight, you may find that you will have to reduce the quantity used as the quantity of liquid indicated will not cover the herb.

Less dried herb is required than fresh herb as water makes up a large component of a fresh herb.

Herbal Infusions

Infusions are very simple preparations to make and will keep in the refrigerator for around 2 days. They are used to make skin toners, hair rinses and compresses.

If you have ever made a cup of tea, you have made an infusion. The softer and more delicate parts of the plant are used to make an infusion. This includes the flowers and leaves. Water-soluble active constituents are readily extracted from these parts of the plant

by infusion. Cut or crush the herb into small pieces before making the infusion.

Equipment

- digital scales
- kettle
- teapot
- strainer and muslin
- glass bottle

Method for making herbal infusions

1. In a teapot, pour 250 mL of boiling water over 15 g of dried herb or 45 g of fresh herb (reduce the amount of fresh herb if too bulky to be covered with the boiling water).
2. Place a lid on the teapot to ensure minimal loss of volatile substances such as essential oils.
3. Allow the herb to steep for 10–15 minutes.
4. Strain the herb material out of the infusion and filter through a double layer of muslin if necessary.
5. The infusion may be used on the skin either warm or cool depending on its purpose.

Herbal Decoctions

The preparation of a decoction is similar to an infusion except that the herb material is boiled. This is necessary when extracting active constituents from the harder parts of the plant such as the roots, wood, bark, seeds and berries. However, an infusion

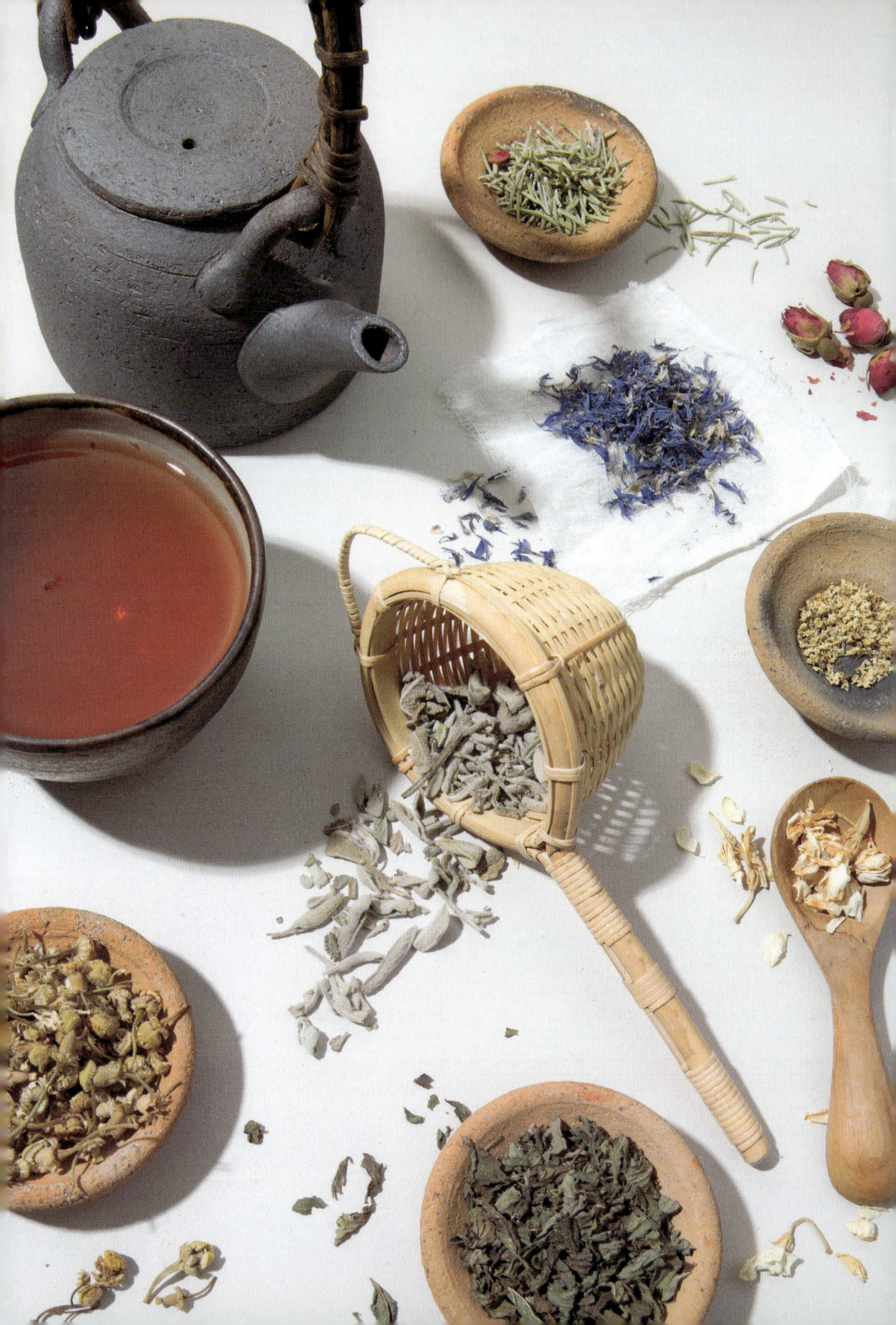

can be made from these parts of the plant if they are finely powdered. When making a decoction, ensure that the roots, wood or bark are chopped up well and that any seeds or berries are crushed.

Equipment

- digital scales
- saucepan
- stovetop or hot plate
- heat-resistant jug
- strainer and muslin
- glass bottle

Method for making herbal decoctions

1. Put 15 g of dried herb or 45 g of fresh herb and 300 mL of water into a saucepan (reduce the amount of fresh herb if too bulky to be covered with the water).

2. Bring to the boil and simmer for 20 minutes. Do this with a loose lid on the saucepan.

3. Remove from the heat and let the mixture stand for 10 minutes.

4. Strain the herb material out of the decoction and filter through a double layer of muslin if necessary.

5. The herbal decoction may be used on the skin either warm or cool depending on its purpose.

Your infusion or decoction is now ready for immediate use or can be used over the next day or two if kept in the refrigerator. Do not keep any longer than this as microbial growth will occur.

Herbal Tinctures

Tinctures can be added to creams and shampoos and to water to make toners.

Tinctures are herbal extracts made using alcohol and water. The herbs are steeped in water and alcohol over a period of time in order to extract their active constituents. The mixture of water and alcohol will extract a broader range of active constituents from the herbs than just the water in an infusion or decoction. A tincture is more concentrated than an infusion or decoction. There is no heat involved and tinctures will keep for at least 2 years.

Vodka can be used to make tinctures for skin care preparations and is readily available. The minimum concentration of alcohol needed in a herbal tincture to keep it preserved is around 20–30% and vodka has at least this alcohol concentration. It is also relatively odourless and does not contain unsuitable additives.

A second method for making tinctures for perfumery purposes is covered on page 246.

Equipment

- digital scales
- large glass jar with lid
- jug
- strainer, muslin, coffee filter paper
- glass bottle

Method for making herbal tinctures

1. Place approximately 50 g of finely cut or ground dried herb or 150 g of chopped fresh herb into a glass container and cover with approximately 250 mL of vodka (reduce the amount of fresh herb if too bulky to be covered with the vodka).

2. Secure the lid.

3. Gently swirl the jar to ensure the vodka is in contact with all the plant material.

4. Place in a cool, dark place and leave for 2 weeks, gently swirling it daily.

5. After 2 weeks, strain and filter the tincture firstly through a strainer lined with a double layer of muslin and then through dampened coffee filter paper.

6. Store in a glass bottle in a cool, dark place.

Herbal Infused Oils

Infused oils are made by placing herbs into a vegetable carrier oil and allowing the active constituents, such as essential oils and resins, to be extracted by the oil (maceration). There are hot and cold methods of making infused oils. The hot method may be used for the leafier parts of the herb and the cold method should be used for delicate flowers.

Infused oils may be used directly on the skin or blended with other vegetable oils and essential oils. They can be added to balm and moisture cream recipes.

Cold-infused oil

Equipment

- large glass jar with lid
- jug
- strainer and muslin
- glass bottle

Method for making a cold-infused oil

1. Fill a glass jar loosely with fresh chopped herbs or undamaged flowers or half fill with dried herbs or flowers. If using fresh herbs or flowers, do not use them when they are wet with moisture such as rain or dew. Spread them over a tea towel and allow any small amounts of moisture to evaporate for approximately one hour. The addition of moisture to an infused oil can provide a medium on which microbes can grow.

2. Cover the plant material with a cold-pressed vegetable oil of your choice, preferably one with as little odour as possible, until the jar is full. The oil should sit a couple of centimetres above the herbs or flowers. Jojoba oil is particularly suitable as it does not turn rancid. However, other vegetable oils such as sweet almond or apricot kernel oil may also be used.

3. Secure the lid.

4. Gently swirl the jar to ensure the oil is in contact with all the plant material.

5. Leave in a warm place for 1—6 weeks. If the jar is placed in direct sunlight, especially in summer, the vegetable oil is likely to turn rancid. Leave the following parts of the plant to infuse for approximately these times.

   - Flowers — 1 week. Watch for any change in the flowers such as turning brown or transparent and remove immediately.

   - Soft leaves and citrus rinds — 2 weeks.

   - Hard leaves, spices and seeds — 6 weeks or more. Crush the plant material before infusing in the vegetable oil.

6. Gently swirl the jar twice daily.

7. Check to see if any moisture has been released from any of the fresh plant material. If it has, you will see a layer of water on the bottom of the jar. You will need to carefully remove the plant material and pour off the oil leaving the water

behind with some of the oil to ensure your infused oil is not contaminated. You can put your plant material and infused oil into a fresh jar to continue infusing.

8. Once the infusion has been completed, strain the mixture through a strainer lined with a double layer of muslin. If you feel the infused oil is not strong enough, repeat the process with a fresh lot of herbs or flowers using the same oil. This can be done several times.

9. Pour the strained oil into a jar and keep it in the refrigerator. After a few days, you will see sediment at the bottom of the jar. Carefully decant the oil into a glass bottle, leaving the small amount of sediment behind.

10. Refrigerate the infused oil until you are ready to use it.

Hot-infused oil

Equipment

- saucepan
- heat-resistant jug
- metal trivet
- stovetop or hot plate
- thermometer
- strainer and muslin
- glass bottle

Method for making a hot-infused oil

The following method is more suitable for the leafier and harder parts of the herb such as roots and seeds, and not suitable for delicate flowers.

1. Place a handful of dried or fresh plant material into a heat-resistant jug and pour in enough cold-pressed vegetable oil to cover it. If using fresh plant material, do not use the plant when it is wet with moisture such as rain or dew. Spread it over a tea towel and allow any small amounts of moisture to evaporate for approximately one hour. The addition of moisture to an infused oil can provide a medium on which microbes can grow.

2. Place the jug on a metal trivet in a saucepan that has been filled to approximately halfway with water and place on a hot plate or stove (this is called a *bain-marie*).

3. Allow the plant material to gently infuse for up to 3 hours. Maintain the temperature of the oil at around 40°C. From time to time you will need to add more water to the saucepan.

4. Remove the jug from the heat.

5. Once the oil has cooled, continue as for the cold-infused method from step 8.

Bain-Marie

Bain-marie is a French term for a double boiler or a water bath. It is used to heat ingredients gently and reduce the risk of over-heating or burning the ingredients. A simple *bain-marie* used to make the recipes in this book consists of a saucepan and heat-resistant glass jug. The saucepan is first filled to about halfway with water then a metal trivet is placed on the bottom of the saucepan. The glass jug is then sat on the trivet in the saucepan. The saucepan is then heated on a hot plate.

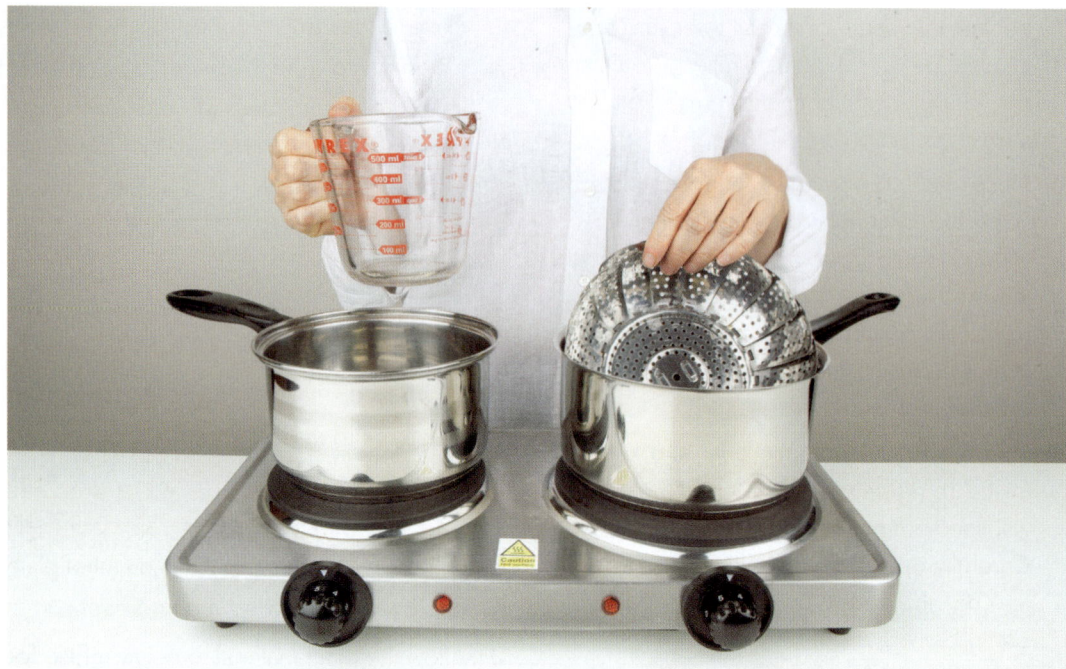

Bain-marie — double boiler or water bath

Herbal Vinegars

Herbal vinegars can be diluted to create hair rinses and a range of skin care preparations such as bath vinegars and skin toners. Apple cider vinegar is most often used, especially the kind that still contains the 'mother', as it combines beneficial yeast and bacteria, along with acetic acid, citric acid, vitamins, minerals and other micronutrients.

Equipment

- large glass jar with a glass lid such as a preserving jar
- jug
- strainer, muslin, coffee filter paper
- glass bottle

Method for making herbal vinegars

1. Fill a glass jar loosely with fresh chopped herbs or undamaged flowers or half fill with dried herbs or flowers. If using fresh herbs or flowers, do not use them when they are wet with moisture such as rain or dew. Spread them over a tea towel and allow any small amounts of moisture to evaporate for approximately one hour. The addition of moisture to a vinegar can provide a medium on which microbes can grow.

2. Pour in enough vinegar to cover the plant material and fill the jar.

3. Secure the lid.

4. Gently swirl the jar to ensure the vinegar is in contact with all the plant material.

5. Leave in a dark place for 1–6 weeks. Leave the following parts of the plant to infuse for approximately these times.

- Flowers — 1 week. Watch for any change in the flowers such as turning brown or transparent and remove immediately.
- Soft leaves and citrus rinds — 2 weeks.
- Hard leaves, spices and seeds — 6 weeks or more. Crush the plant material before infusing in the vinegar.

6. Gently swirl the jar twice daily.

7. Once completed, strain the mixture through a strainer lined with a double layer of muslin. If you feel the vinegar is not strong enough, repeat the process with a fresh lot of plant material using the same vinegar. This can be done several times.

8. Filter the final vinegar through dampened coffee filter paper and store in a glass bottle.

9. Refrigerate the vinegar until you are ready to use it.

Using Herbal Extracts

Many skin care preparations can be made using herbal extracts. Infusions, decoctions, tinctures, herbal infused oils and vinegars contain active constituents that can treat and improve the condition of your skin. Please note that the addition of herbal infusions and decoctions will reduce the life of your preparations due to their high water content and plant matter that bacteria, yeast and mould thrive on. Preparations made using infusions and decoctions should be stored in the refrigerator and used within a couple of days.

This chart describes many of the skin care preparations that can be made using herbal extracts.

Product	Herbal Extract
Skin toners/fresheners	Infusions and decoctions can be used directly on your skin as skin toners or fresheners. They can be wiped over your face with cotton pads or misted over your face from a spray bottle. Herbal vinegars make excellent skin toners. Add 5 mL (1 tsp) to 250 mL water (1 cup) and wipe or spray over your face.
Face masks	Infusions and decoctions can be mixed with clays and gums to thicken them and then be applied as face masks.
Creams	Infusions, decoctions, tinctures and infused oils can be incorporated into creams and moisturising preparations.
Deodorants	Herbal vinegars and tinctures that are made using antiseptic, astringent and fragrant herbs can be used in deodorant preparations.
Colognes and aftershaves	Fragrant infusions and decoctions, herbal vinegars and tinctures can be used in formulae for colognes, and those that are also astringent, healing and soothing can be used in or as aftershave preparations.
Hair rinses	Herbal infusions, decoctions and vinegars can be used as hair rinses to treat scalp problems or to add highlights to and condition the hair.
Bath preparations	Infusions, decoctions, tinctures, herbal vinegars and infused oils can be added to the bathwater and foot baths for their therapeutic benefits and their fragrance.
Compresses and fomentations	Soothing, healing compresses and fomentations can be made using infusions and decoctions.
Ointments and balms	Infused oils can be incorporated into ointments and balms.

Fomentations

Fomentation is the traditional word used for a hot compress. To make a fomentation, soak a cloth or towel in a hot infusion or decoction, wring out the excess liquid and apply while still hot to the affected area of skin. Reapply the fomentation several times as it begins to cool down.

Fomentations that are not excessively hot can be placed over the face to soften the skin, soften sebum build-up and encourage perspiration. This can be performed once or twice a week during a facial and after cleansing.

Ginger is commonly used in fomentations to create warmth and stimulate the circulation, especially over sore joints and muscles, which benefit from heat.

Compresses

Soak a cloth or towel in an infusion or decoction that has cooled, wring out the excess liquid, and apply to the affected area of skin. Reapply the compress several times as it begins to warm up.

Compresses are used to reduce inflammation and irritation. A soothing cream may be applied afterwards.

These days the term compress seems to refer to a fomentation as well and is defined as either a hot or cold compress.

Chamomile is commonly used in compresses for inflamed skin.

Poultices

A poultice is a moist, hot herb pack applied to the skin.

If using a fresh herb, crush it into a pulpy mass and warm it up. If using a dried herb, mix it with hot water into a paste. The addition of a small amount of slippery elm powder may be useful to bind the herb material together.

A poultice may be applied directly to the skin or between two pieces of gauze or similar material. This may then be covered with a hot damp cloth.

- Comfrey leaves are commonly used in poultices to encourage skin healing and bone healing.
- Slippery elm and linseeds are often used to draw out boils.
- Bruised cabbage leaves are also used in drawing poultices.

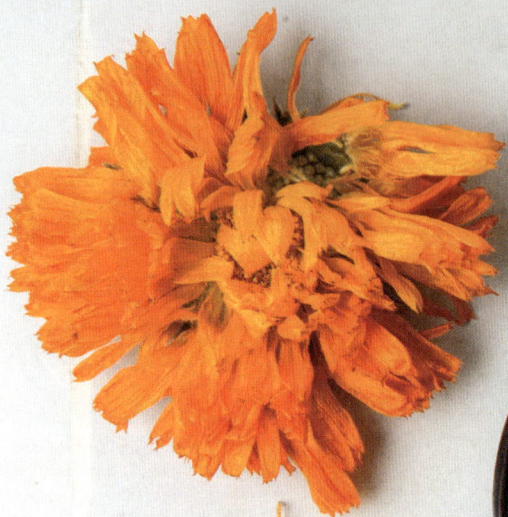

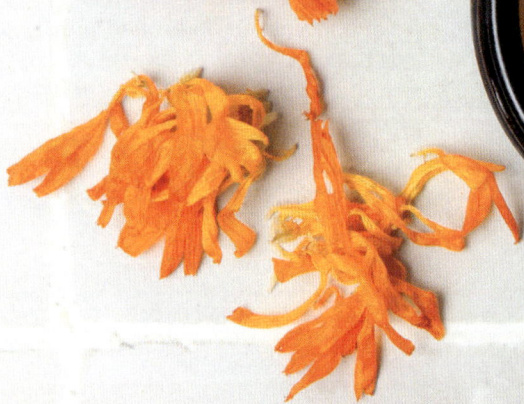

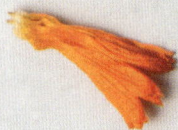

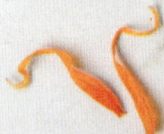

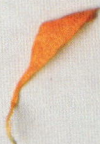

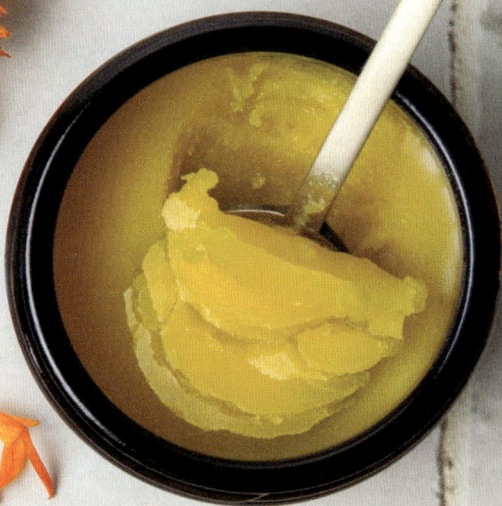

Ointments and Balms

Ointments and balms are made from oils, waxes and butters, and contain no water. They tend to remain on the surface of the skin longer than a cream and can afford protection to the skin and reduce moisture loss from the skin. Examples include lip balms, body balms and nappy rash balms. Other names for ointments and balms include salves and unguents.

The ratio of oil to wax or oil to butter will determine the hardness or softness of the balm. The higher the wax and butter content, the firmer the balm will be. You would consider making a balm with a higher wax content if, for example, you live in a warm climate where the heat will make the balm much softer or if you are making a balm in stick form. On the other hand, you would reduce the amount of wax in a cold climate where temperature will make the balm much harder or if you are making a soft balm in a jar.

The wax you choose will alter the texture and skin-feel of a balm. For example, beeswax will produce a more pliable balm and can feel thicker on the skin, whereas candelilla wax is a brittle wax and produces a balm that feels thinner on the skin and absorbs more rapidly. The texture of a balm will also be affected by the choice and amount of butters added to a balm. Shea butter adds softness and creaminess to a balm, whereas cocoa butter will make a balm stiffer. This means you can make unique textured balms with thicker, richer textures that are more protective or thinner, more rapidly absorbed balms. The ointment and balm bases given in this book may be modified through altering ratios and combinations of oils, butters and waxes to provide a variety textures. All of the ointments and balms are vegan, except for those containing beeswax.

It is important to wait for your balm to set up properly before deciding on whether or not it is soft or hard enough for your purposes. Generally, wait at least 4 days if you are allowing your balm to set up at room temperature. Alternatively, put the balm in the freezer for 2 hours and then allow to return to room temperature.

Ointment and Balm Bases

Choose from a combination of these simple ingredients to make herbal and aromatherapy ointments and balms: vegetable oil, beeswax, candelilla wax, carnauba wax, shea butter and cocoa butter. Four combinations of these ingredients are given on page 60. The first base uses beeswax, whereas the other three are all vegan. They all vary slightly in their texture and feel on the skin.

The first three recipes give you a range of ingredient ratios, where the least amount of wax or butter will yield a softer balm suitable for packaging in a jar, and the highest amount of wax or butter will yield a very firm balm suitable for making a stick. Always ensure the two ingredients add up to 100%. For example, if you intend making a softer balm using *Beeswax balm base* recipe with

15 g of beeswax, ensure you use 85 g of vegetable oil to add up to 100 g. The fourth recipe, based on shea butter, is suitable for packaging in a jar.

Sweet almond oil, apricot kernel oil and jojoba oil are the oils of choice as they remain relatively stable when heated. Olive oil and coconut oil may also be used. However, they feel heavier and thicker and are not as readily absorbed by the skin. They are best used where skin protection is a priority.

Beeswax balm base

15–20 g beeswax
80–85 g vegetable oil

Candelilla or carnauba wax balm base

15–20 g candelilla wax or carnauba wax
80–85 g vegetable oil

Cocoa butter balm base

50–60 g cocoa butter
40–50 g vegetable oil

Shea butter balm base

100 g shea butter

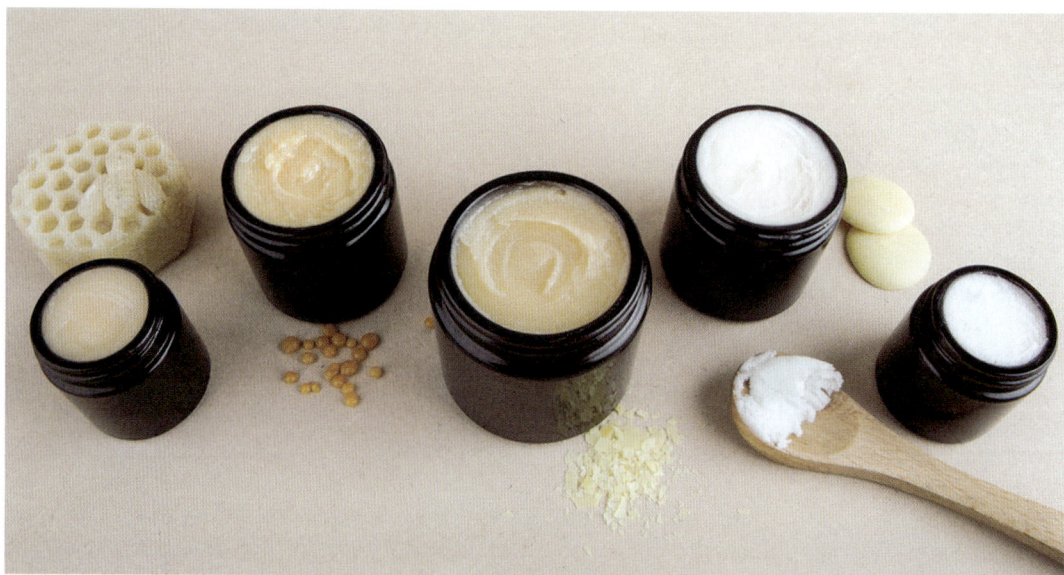

Beeswax, candelilla, carnauba, cocoa butter and shea butter balm bases

Herbal Ointments and Balms

The simplest of herbal ointments and balms have been made with local herbs and ingredients for millennia for soothing, protecting and healing the skin. The techniques and ingredients are still used today.

Useful herbs

The following herbs are commonly used to make ointments and balms:

- arnica — bruising and swelling
- calendula — soothing and healing for eczema, dermatitis, nappy rash and wounds
- chickweed — soothing and healing for rashes and inflammations including eczema, dermatitis and wounds
- comfrey leaves — soothing and healing for cuts, wounds and skin damage
- yarrow — healing for cuts and wounds.

Care needs to be taken that no moisture from fresh herbs remains in the balm to cause the growth of mould, yeasts and bacteria. If using fresh plant material, do not use the plant when it is wet with moisture such as rain or dew. Spread it over a tea towel and allow any small amounts of moisture to evaporate for approximately 1 hour.

Equipment

- digital scales
- measuring glass or beaker
- saucepan
- heat-resistant jug
- metal trivet
- stovetop or hot plate
- strainer and muslin
- metal stirring spoon
- jars

Methods for making herbal ointments and balms

Choose from the following methods for making a herbal ointment or balm. The different methods allow for different kinds of herbal extracts to be added.

Herbal ointment and balm method 1

This method extracts the active constituents of the herb into the ointment or balm while you are making it. *Beeswax, Candelilla, Carnauba* or *Cocoa butter balm bases* can be used with this method.

1. Place a handful of dried or fresh plant material into a heat-resistant jug and pour in enough cold-pressed vegetable oil to cover it.
2. Place the jug on a metal trivet in a saucepan that has been filled to approximately halfway with water and place on a hot plate or stove (this is called a *bain-marie*).
3. Gently heat until the herb loses its normal colour. This indicates that most of the active constituents have been absorbed by the oil. Maintain the temperature of the oil at around 40°C during this process. From time to time you may need to add more water to the saucepan.
4. Remove the jug from the heat and strain the herbs from the mixture using muslin or a double layer of cheesecloth lining a strainer.
5. Add the beeswax, candelilla wax, carnauba wax or cocoa butter to the jug with the herbal infused oil and heat until melted.
6. Pour the mixture into glass jars.
7. Allow to cool to room temperature before adding lids. The jars of ointment can be

put in the freezer for 2 hours to speed up solidification time, but allow to come back to room temperature before adding lids.

Herbal ointment and balm method 2
Using herbal infused oils

A pre-made infused oil is used to make this herbal ointment or balm. It is by far the easiest method of making a herbal ointment or balm. *Beeswax, Candelilla, Carnauba* or *Cocoa butter balm bases* can be used with this method.

1. In a *bain-marie,* melt the beeswax, candelilla wax, carnauba wax or cocoa butter and add a pre-made herbal infused oil either totally or partially in place of vegetable oil.
2. Mix thoroughly to ensure all ingredients are melted.
3. Pour the mixture into glass jars.
4. Allow to cool to room temperature before adding lids. The jars of ointment can be put in the freezer for 2 hours to speed up solidification time, but allow to come back to room temperature before adding lids.

Herbal ointment and balm method 3
Using shea butter

This method is similar to *Method 1* but has been modified to make it suitable for *a* base that is made entirely of shea butter. If shea butter is heated to over 40°C, when it cools, granular crystals may form throughout the ointment or balm rather than it feeling smooth and buttery. This is due to its various fatty acids solidifying at different rates as it slowly cools down. To avoid grainy shea butter, heat it up until it has completely liquefied; then once you have finished making the balm, place it in the freezer immediately. This will ensure it sets up quickly and homogenously, avoiding grainy crystals.

1. In a *bain-marie*, melt the shea butter.
2. Once the shea butter has melted, add in enough herb so that the melted shea butter covers it.
3. Maintain the temperature of the shea butter at around 40°C until the herb loses its normal colour. This indicates that most of the active constituents have been absorbed by the melted shea butter. From time to time you may need to add more water to the saucepan.
4. Remove the jug from the heat and strain the herbs from the liquid shea butter using muslin or a double layer of cheesecloth lining a strainer.
5. Pour into glass jars and place in the freezer immediately. Leave for 2 hours allowing the ointment to solidify quickly.
6. Allow to come back to room temperature before adding lids.

Instead of infusing the herb into the heated shea butter, a pre-made infused oil can be added to the melted shea butter at 10% of the entire recipe. This is similar to *Method 2.* Alternatively, in warmer climates, small quantities of shea butter can often be stirred and softened without additional heat before stirring in an infused oil or herbal tincture (similar to *Method 4* below) at 10% of the entire recipe without making it too soft.

Herbal ointment and balm method 4
Using herbal tinctures

This method incorporates herbal tinctures into a herbal ointment or balm and is suitable for *Beeswax, Candelilla, Carnauba* or *Cocoa butter balm bases.*

1. Melt the ointment or balm base in a *bain-marie.*
2. Add 10 mL of herbal tincture, stirring it in thoroughly as the mixture cools down.

3. Pour or spoon into glass jars.

4. Allow to cool to room temperature before adding lids. The jars of ointment can be put in the freezer for 2 hours to speed up solidification time, but allow to come back to room temperature before adding lids.

Please note: If the ointment or balm heats up due to exposure to heat or warm weather, the tincture may separate out.

Herbal ointment and balm method 5
Using powdered herbs

Trituration is a method of making a herbal ointment by mixing a finely powdered herb into an ointment base. Either melt the base ingredients first and stir in the powder as it begins to solidify or, if the ointment base is soft enough, stir the powder into it directly. All balm bases are suitable for this method.

Aromatherapy Balms

Aromatherapy balms include massage balms, healing ointments, beauty balms, cleansing balms, lip balms, body balms, deodorant balms, hair balms or perfume balms. The ingredients used to make aromatherapy balm bases are the same as those used to make herbal ointment and balm bases.

Depending on the purpose of the balm, 0.25–5% essential oils can be added to the balm base, i.e. approximately 5–100 drops of essential oil can be added to 100 g of base.

Equipment

- digital scales
- measuring glass or beaker
- saucepan
- heat-resistant jug
- metal trivet
- stovetop or hot plate
- metal stirring spoon
- jars

Methods for making aromatherapy balms

Choose from the following methods for making an aromatherapy balm.

Aromatherapy balm method 1
Using beeswax, candelilla, carnauba wax or cocoa butter balm bases

1. Add beeswax, candelilla wax, carnauba wax or cocoa butter and vegetable oil to a heat-resistant jug.

2. Place the jug on a metal trivet in a saucepan which has been filled to approximately halfway with water and place on a hot plate or stove (this is called a *bain-marie*).

3. Gently heat the saucepan until the hard ingredients melt.

4. Once the hard ingredients have melted into the vegetable oil, remove the jug from the heat, add the essential oils and stir thoroughly.

5. Pour into glass jars.

6. Allow to cool to room temperature before adding lids. The jars of balm can be put in the freezer for 2 hours to speed up solidification time, but allow to come back to room temperature before adding lids.

Aromatherapy balm method 2
Using shea butter balm base

If shea butter is heated to over 40°C, when it cools, granular crystals may form throughout the balm rather than it feeling smooth and buttery. This is due to its various fatty acids solidifying at different rates as it slowly cools down. To avoid grainy shea butter, heat it up until it has completely liquefied; then once you have finished adding the essential oils, place it in the freezer immediately. This will ensure it sets up quickly and homogenously, avoiding grainy crystals.

1. In a *bain-marie*, melt the shea butter.
2. Once the shea butter has melted, add the essential oils and stir thoroughly.
3. Pour into glass jars and place in the freezer immediately. Leave for 2 hours allowing the balm to solidify quickly.
4. Allow to come back to room temperature before adding lids.

Alternatively, small quantities of shea butter can often be stirred and softened without additional heat before stirring in essential oils. Additional vegetable or infused oils can be also be added using this method at 10% of the entire recipe without making the balm too soft.

Gels

Gels are used to hydrate, soothe and cool the skin. They are a great way to introduce essential oils to the skin where an aqueous base is desired rather than an oily base.

Gels can be made from a range of plants, such as linseeds, pectin, guar gum and xanthan gum.

Gels make excellent moisturisers for oily skin as they are oil-free. Gels can also be used under a moisturiser as a hydrating skin treatment for dehydrated skin. The addition of glycerin provides a humectant which holds moisture to the skin.

Eye gels are cooling and soothing to the eyes. However, essential oils are not added to eye gels as they may irritate the eyes and the delicate skin around them.

Essential oils that are anti-inflammatory, healing and antiseptic can be added to a gel base to help clear the skin of pimples and reduce break-outs.

Gel masks help hydrate, cool and calm the skin as the moisture is held against the skin for some time.

Natural hair gels work well for keeping hair styles in place even though they do not give the same strong hold as some commercial hair gels.

Gel Bases

Gel bases can be made by hydrating powdered gums such as guar or xanthan. They swell and thicken in the water to form a gel.

The higher the proportion of powdered gum used, the thicker the gel will be and the more film forming the gel will be on the skin or hair. The lower the proportion of powdered gum used, the thinner and more liquid the gel will be and the more readily it will be absorbed by the skin.

Pre-dispersing the powdered gums in glycerin before adding water to hydrate the gum makes it easier to create a smooth gel, as oftentimes the powder can form lumps that are difficult to dissolve in the water.

Due to the water content and nutrient content provided by the gums, a preservative is necessary to reduce the risk of microbial growth. Otherwise, the gel must be used within a day or two.

The following gum gel bases, depending on the proportion of gum to water, can be used for face moisturising gels, eye gels, blemish gels, hydrating masks and hair gels.

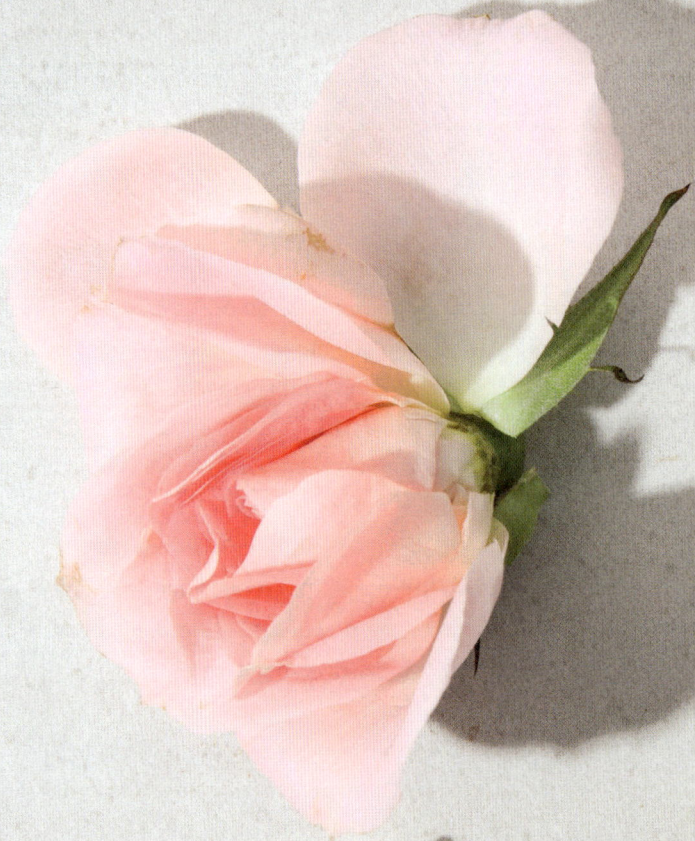

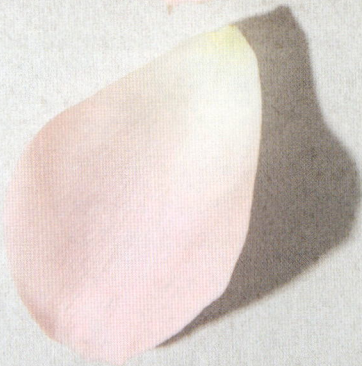

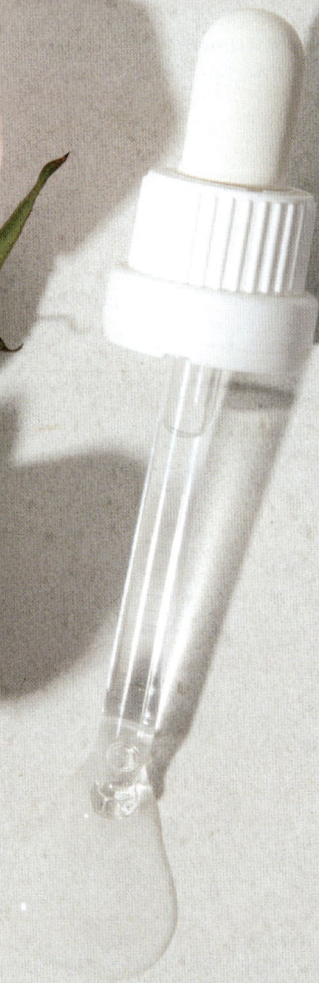

Gel base 1
*for face moisturising gels, eye gels,
blemish gels*

**0.5 g powdered gum: xanthan or guar
3 g vegetable glycerin
95.5 g purified water
1 g preservative**

pH adjustment
qs citric acid + purified water solution

Gel base 2
for gel masks

**3 g powdered gum: xanthan or guar
9 g vegetable glycerin
87 g purified water
1 g preservative**

pH adjustment
qs citric acid + purified water solution

Gel base 3
for hair gels

**4 g powdered gum: xanthan or guar
12 g vegetable glycerin
83 g purified water
1 g preservative**

pH adjustment
qs citric acid + purified water solution

Equipment

- digital scales
- 2 glass jugs or beakers
- electric stick mixer
- metal stirring spoon
- pH strips or meter
- glass beaker
- jars or bottles

Method for making gel bases

1. In one jug, stir the powdered gum into the vegetable glycerin.

2. In another jug, add the preservative to the water. (Find more information on preservatives on page 72.)

3. Slowly add small amounts of the water to the gum and glycerin mixture, stirring as you go, until you have added all the water.

4. Continue stirring, then very briefly use an electric stick mixer to create a smooth gel. Be careful not to over-aerate the mixture.

5. Allow the mixture to fully hydrate and thicken over several hours — up to 24 hours.

6. Add up to 1% essential oil to the gel and disperse with a whisk or electric stick mixer for a few seconds.

7. Check the pH and adjust with a citric acid and purified water solution if required. While the gels are compatible with the skin's pH range, it may be necessary to lower the pH a little, depending on the additional ingredients added, to ensure the preservative is effective. Follow the instructions for adjusting pH on page 74.

Powdered dehydrated aloe vera gel can also be added to these gel bases. Mix the aloe vera powder with your chosen powdered gum first, then follow the instructions for adding water (add 1 g powdered dehydrated aloe vera gel to each 200 g water as an approximate guide, or follow the suppliers' recommendations).

Floral waters make a beautiful substitute for the purified water in these recipes.

Linseed Gel Base

Linseed gel is made by simmering the linseeds in water to release a gel, which is then strained to remove the seeds.

Linseed gel base

20 g crushed linseeds
200 g boiling water
2 g preservative

pH adjustment

qs citric acid + purified water solution

Equipment

- digital scales
- saucepan
- heat-resistant bowl or jug
- muslin
- stovetop or hot plate
- metal stirring spoon
- pH strips or meter
- glass beaker
- jars or bottles

Method for making linseed gel base

1. In a small saucepan, bring the linseeds and water to boiling point. Then simmer for 3 or so minutes until you see the gel starting to be released from the seeds.

2. Take off the heat and allow the gel to continue to be released and thicken.

3. Strain the seeds from the gel using muslin over a bowl or jug. Pour the mixture into the muslin and squeeze the gel through the muslin into the bowl or jug.

4. Add more water and work through if a thinner consistency is desired.

5. Stir in the preservative. (Find more information on preservatives on page 72.)

6. Check the pH and adjust with a citric acid and purified water solution if required. While the gel is compatible with the skin's pH range, it may be necessary to lower the pH a little, depending on the additional ingredients added, to ensure the preservative is effective. Follow the instructions for adjusting pH on page 74.

Emulsions

Many skin care preparations are emulsions — especially creams and lotions. Cleansing milks, cleansing creams, face creams, eye creams, hand creams and body lotions are examples of skin care preparations that are emulsions.

What is an Emulsion?

Three key ingredients are required to make an emulsion — oil, water and an emulsifier. An emulsion is a mixture of oil and water blended together with an emulsifier to form a stable homogenous mixture. For example, an emulsion can be tiny droplets of oil surrounded by emulsifier molecules, which remain dispersed throughout water.

To make an emulsion, two phases — oil phase and water phase — are heated. Once the desired temperature is reached, the two phases are mixed together and the emulsion is formed.

Oil phase

The oil phase may include any of the following oil/fat/wax ingredients:

- cold-pressed vegetable oils
- infused oils
- vegetable butters
- waxes
- emulsifying wax.

Water phase

The water phase may include any of the following aqueous or water-soluble ingredients:

- purified, distilled or deionised water
- floral waters
- infusions and decoctions
- glycerin
- some water-soluble preservatives.

Water that is free of microbes such as purified water that has been boiled, distilled water or deionised water will reduce the amount of bacteria, yeast and mould introduced to an emulsion. This will help prolong the life of an emulsion and reduce any potential risk to the user.

Types of Emulsions

There are two basic types of emulsions, 'oil-in-water' emulsions and 'water-in-oil' emulsions.

Oil-in-water emulsions

- Contain mostly water and a small amount of oil.
- Feel moist on the skin but not greasy.
- Include cleansing milks, face and body lotions, face and body creams, lightweight moisturisers.

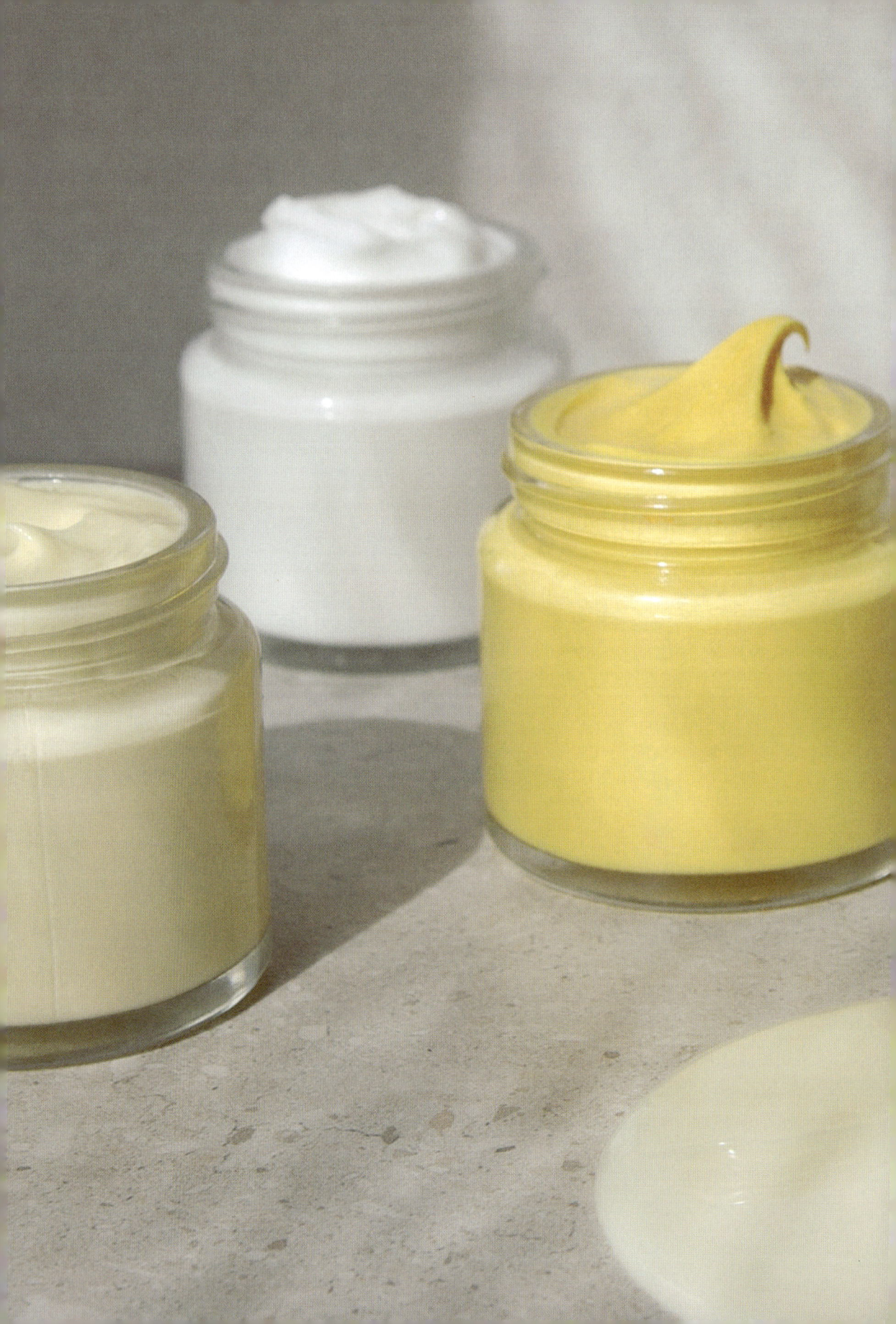

Water-in-oil emulsions

- Contain mostly oil and a small amount of water.
- Have an oilier, thicker feeling on the skin.
- Include cold creams, ointments, barrier creams, heavy moisturisers.

Basic Ingredients

Emulsifiers

The emulsifier is the ingredient that holds the oil and water together in a stable homogenous emulsion. It is both hydrophilic (attracted to water) and lipophilic (attracted to oil). The ratio of oil to water in an emulsion may determine your choice of emulsifier, as certain emulsifiers work better if there is more oil in a formula and others work better if there is more water. However, there are emulsifiers or emulsifier blends available that work across a range of water to oil ratios.

Lecithin

Lecithin is available in granule or liquid form and is a natural emulsifier. Making emulsions using lecithin is much like making a mayonnaise, where small additions of the water phase are added into the oil phase while being continually blended. It is best used in conjunction with a gum, such as xanthan, to assist in stabilising the emulsion. Otherwise, beeswax will aid in giving structure to the emulsion. Lecithin has skin conditioning properties that make it desirable in skin care preparations. An emulsion made using lecithin can be made entirely without heating unless you include a fat or wax, which requires heating to liquefy it.

Emulsifying wax

There are many emulsifying waxes from which to choose. However, those listed here are certified natural, plant-derived, mostly readily available and easy to work with, and serve most general emulsification purposes.

These emulsifiers include:

> cetearyl glucoside & cetearyl alcohol, cetearyl olivate & sorbitan olivate, glyceryl stearate, glyceryl stearate SE and glyceryl stearate citrate

At this point in time, it is difficult to find plant-derived emulsifiers that are palm oil-free. Of the emulsifiers mentioned above, glyceryl stearate citrate is the only one where a palm oil-free version is available. Check with cosmetic ingredient suppliers regarding the palm-free status of the emulsifiers they supply if you would like to avoid using palm oil.

Cetearyl glucoside and glyceryl stearate citrate are often combined with wax alcohols such as cetearyl alcohol or brassica alcohol to provide extra structure to an emulsion and to reduce its chances of separating. Xanthan gum is also often included in emulsion formulas to increase viscosity and improve stability.

Your ingredient supplier may assist you in choosing the best emulsifier for the purpose for which you wish to use it.

EMULSIFIER: CETEARYL OLIVATE & SORBITAN OLIVATE

Where emulsifying wax has been included in any of the recipes in this book, a readily available emulsifier, which is a combination of cetearyl olivate and sorbitan olivate, has been used. It is relatively easy to work with and is effective in creating a range of oil-in-water emulsions. It may emulsify up to 25% lipids (vegetable oils and butters). It is used at levels of 2–8% and is added to the oil phase and heated to 70–75°C. It is effective across a wide pH range of 3–12. Xanthan gum at 0.3% may be added to a formula if further emulsion stability is required. It is a certified natural emulsifier. Alternative emulsifiers can be used but must be used according to the manufacturer's instructions as the quantity used and method of use may differ.

Preservatives

Preservatives are used in personal care preparations to reduce their deterioration resulting from contamination by and growth of microorganisms such as bacteria, yeasts and moulds. Their use also helps ensure products won't cause harm or pose health risks to the user.

During the research and development phase of commercially produced emulsions, and other products, a Preservative Efficacy Test (PET) is carried out to test the efficacy of product preservation. Bacteria (gram-negative and gram-positive), yeasts and moulds are used to test the broad-spectrum efficacy of preservatives.

For a detailed discussion on preservatives, the Australian Society of Cosmetic Chemists provides a paper on its website: https://ascc.com.au/preservatives-used-in-personal-care-products-2/.

There are a number of factors that need to be considered when seeking to prolong the shelf life of your skin and hair care preparations besides the addition of preservatives:

- Fresh fruits, vegetables and herbs used in preparations will contribute to rapid deterioration. Preparations using fresh fruits, vegetables and herbs should be used immediately or stored in the refrigerator and used within a couple of days.

- Preparations made with dry plant ingredients such as flours, starches and granules will keep well if stored in sealed airtight containers, away from moisture, heat and light. They may be prone to weevil and insect infestation, and granules made from seeds and kernels may become rancid after some time if not kept cool.

- Any preparations containing vegetable oils will oxidise and become rancid after some time. Rancidity will happen more rapidly if the preparation is not stored in a sealed airtight container, away from heat and light. Antioxidants, such as tocopherol (vitamin E), are often added to preparations containing vegetable oils to reduce oxidation and rancidity.

- Clean equipment and storage containers will reduce contamination of your preparations and thus deterioration.

- A product is easily contaminated with microorganisms from your fingers. A pump-action bottle or a bottle that can be poured or squeezed from will reduce contamination and deterioration. If storage of a preparation in a jar is necessary due to the viscosity of a product, use a clean spatula or spoon to remove your preparation.

- Any water or moisture in a product will provide a suitable medium in which bacteria, yeast and mould can grow.

- In addition to water, common ingredients such as lecithin, aloe vera, starches, gums and herbal extracts provide further nutrients for the growth of bacteria, yeast and mould.

- Warm temperatures combined with moisture will further enhance the growth of bacteria, yeast and mould. Storing preparations in the refrigerator may slow their growth.

Antimicrobials

Antimicrobial preservatives reduce or prevent the growth of bacteria, yeast and mould in your preparations. It is desirable to use a combination of preservatives and preventative measures to reduce the possibility of contamination and spoilage of your preparations.

Alcohol/ethanol

Ethanol may be used in cosmetic preparations as a preservative at concentrations of 20% or above.

Preparations in which alcohol is the sole preservative include perfumes, deodorants, hand sanitisers and room sprays, where the alcohol also has other functions such as acting as the solvent.

Herbal tinctures made on alcohol are also preserved by their alcohol content.

To reduce the drying effect of alcohol, glycerin (glycerol) can be included in a formulation, where appropriate, if it is applied to the skin.

Essential oils

Essential oils that are incorporated into cosmetic preparations will have an antimicrobial effect and thus assist in preserving a preparation. This effect will vary from essential oil to essential oil. However, as the amount of essential oil usually incorporated into preparations is relatively low, they will not be effective preservatives by themselves.

It has been suggested that essential oils such as lemongrass, tea tree, oregano and clove bud can be used as preservatives in cosmetics as they provide sufficient antimicrobial activity. However, these essential oils present a high risk of skin irritancy, especially at the levels required to be effective.

COSMOS-approved preservatives

COSMOS is an independent and international certifying body that has developed accepted standards for certified natural and certified organic cosmetics.

COSMOS-approved preservatives include a range of safe, naturally derived or nature-identical preservatives including:

- acids and salts, such as benzoic acid, sodium benzoate, salicylic acid, sorbic acid, potassium sorbate, glyceryl caprylate, sodium levulinate, ethyl lactate, anisic acid, sodium anisate and dehydroacetic acid

- alcohols, such as benzyl alcohol and phenethyl alcohol.

The addition of a preservative to a product is no guarantee that it won't grow microbes. Each preservative will be suitable for particular types of preparations and may be affected by the final pH of a product. Keep in mind natural fragrance compound preservatives, such as phenethyl alcohol that smells like roses, will have an aroma that will affect the final aroma of your product. It is also important to consider any potential skin irritancy a preservative may have. Commercial product manufacturers carefully test their products for preservative efficacy, product stability and skin irritancy before releasing to the market.

PRESERVATIVE: SODIUM BENZOATE & POTASSIUM SORBATE

Where a dedicated preservative has been recommended for recipes in this book, a readily available preservative which is a combination of sodium benzoate and potassium sorbate in an aqueous base, has been recommended. It is relatively easy to work with and is effective against bacteria, yeast and mould. It is used at levels of up to 1% and is added into the water phase where the temperature does not rise above 80°C. It also requires a pH of 4.5–5.5 in order to be effective. It is a COSMOS-approved preservative. Alternative and additional preservatives can be used but must be used according to the manufacturer's instructions.

Glyceryl caprylate

Glyceryl caprylate is a naturally-derived preservative that can be used to enhance the preservative action of the combination of sodium benzoate, potassium sorbate, aqua and other preservatives. It is added to the water phase where the temperature does not rise above 80°C and requires a pH between 4.5–7 to be effective. It is important to use this preservative at levels below 0.5% as it may irritate the skin and make emulsions thinner.

ADJUSTING PH

It is important to test the pH of an emulsion for a couple of reasons — firstly, to ensure it is compatible with that of the skin, and secondly, for the preservative used in recipes to function effectively.

pH strips (or a pH meter) can be used to measure pH. Once an emulsion has been completed, dip a pH strip into it, wait for 10 seconds or so, then remove any excess so that you can see the strip change colour. Match it with the pH chart provided with the strips to determine the pH.

With the ingredients used in the emulsion recipes in this book, you may need to lower the pH for the preservative to be effective while still being compatible with the pH of the skin. To lower the pH, make up a solution of citric acid in water — 5 g citric acid in 25 g of purified water. Then using a dropper, add a drop or so to your emulsion and stir in well. Test the emulsion again with a fresh pH strip. Continue to repeat this process of adding a drop or so of the solution and stirring in well and retesting with a fresh strip each time until you have a pH of around 5. It is important not to add too much citric acid solution at once as you may suddenly lower the pH too much.

This same method of adjusting pH can be used for other preparations, such as gels and mists, where a preservative has been added.

Antioxidants

Antioxidants are used in preparations to prevent vegetable oils and fats from oxidative rancidity.

Tocopherol

A commonly available antioxidant is tocopherol, also referred to as vitamin E. Mixed tocopherols (D-alpha, D-beta, D-delta and D-gamma) are especially suitable for this application. They are available from sources of plant origin and from both GMO and non-GMO sources.

Rosemary oleoresin

Rosemary oleoresin is another commonly used antioxidant used to prevent vegetable oil rancidity.

Jojoba oil is a particularly stable oil, as it is actually a liquid wax, and does not require antioxidants to prevent oxidation.

ANTIOXIDANT: MIXED TOCOPHEROLS

Where a dedicated antioxidant has been recommended for recipes in this book, mixed tocopherols of non-GMO plant origin has been recommended. This mixture is used at levels of up to 0.2–0.5% and is mixed thoroughly with the vegetable oil content. If the vegetable oils are being added to a balm or an emulsion, this antioxidant must be added before they are heated. Alternative tocopherols and other antioxidants such as rosemary oleoresin can be used but must be used according to the manufacturer's instructions.

Making an Emulsion with Emulsifying Wax

Use these instructions to make the emulsion preparations throughout this book that contain the **plant-derived emulsifying wax — cetearyl olivate & sorbitan olivate**. The ingredients in each recipe will be listed as either 'oil phase' ingredients or 'water phase' ingredients to ensure your ingredients are combined correctly.

It is important when heating the ingredients that the correct temperature is reached to ensure emulsification occurs and therefore reduce the chances of separation.

Equipment

- digital scales
- measuring glass or beaker
- 2 saucepans
- 2 heat-resistant jugs
- 2 metal trivets
- stovetop or hot plate with 2 plates
- 2 cooking thermometers
- electric stick mixer
- metal stirring spoon
- pH strips or meter
- jars or bottles

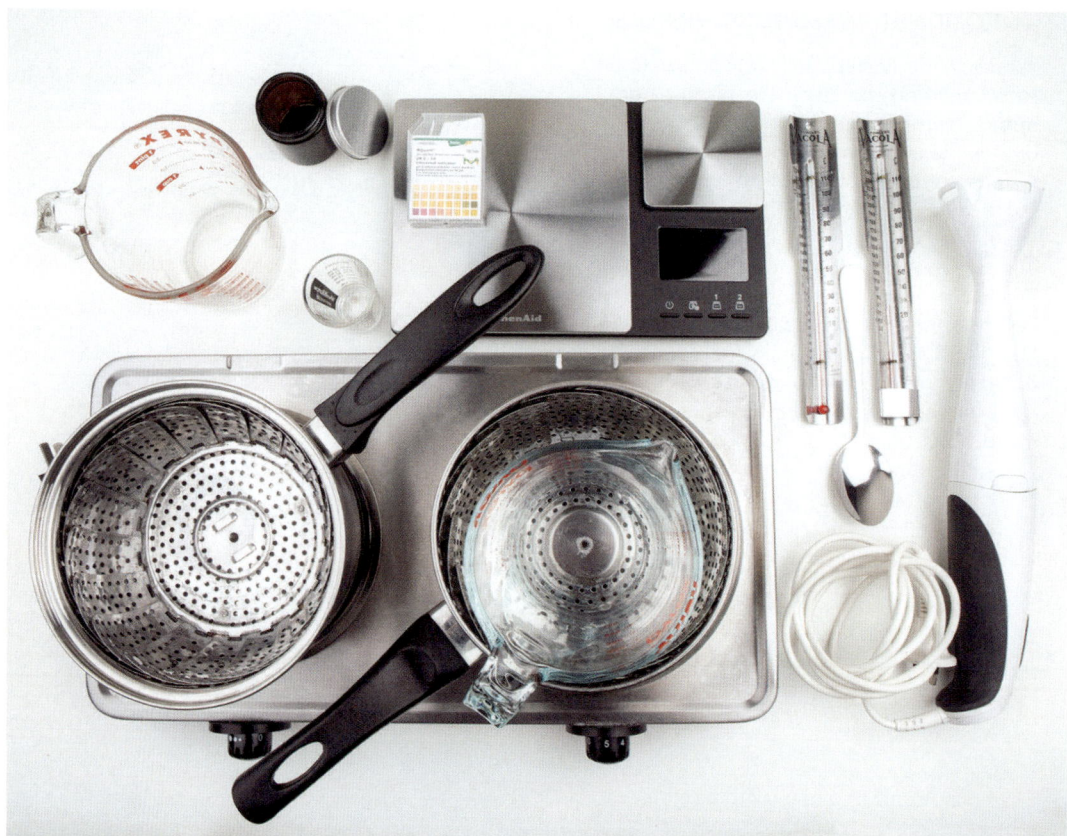

Base cream

This is an all-purpose base cream. It can be kept on hand and customised with essential oils, infused oils, cold-pressed oils, floral waters, herbal infusions, herbal tinctures or herbal extracts. Small amounts can be used at any one time and customised with your choice of these ingredients.

To work out how much of each additional ingredient to add, see page 33.

It can also be used as it is as a simple moisturising cream.

Ingredients

Oil phase

> 10 g plant-derived emulsifying wax
> 30 g sweet almond oil
> 1 g antioxidant

Water phase

> 6 g vegetable glycerin
> 151 g purified water
> 2 g preservative

Add at 40°C

> essential oils
> active ingredients

pH adjustment

> qs citric acid + purified water

To make this cream, follow the *Method for making an emulsion with emulsifying wax* on page 79.

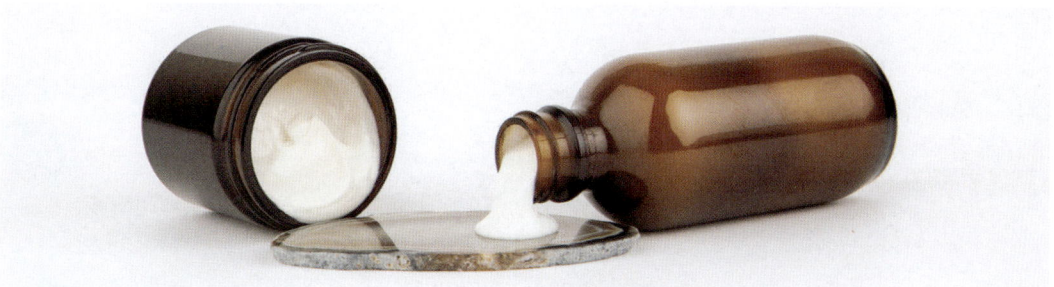

Base lotion

This is a lightweight base lotion into which essential oils can be added. It can be kept on hand and customised with essential oils according to your requirements. It has less emulsifying wax, which means the addition of ingredients other than essential oils may cause it to separate. It is an alternative to a base cream where a lighter weight, more water-based lotion is required.

It can be poured out in small amounts at a time and customised with your choice of essential oils. Alternatively, it can be used as a simple moisturising lotion.

Ingredients

Oil phase

> 6 g plant-derived emulsifying wax
> 12 g jojoba oil
> 1 g antioxidant

Water phase

> 6 g vegetable glycerin
> 0.5 g xanthan gum
> 172.5 g purified water
> 2 g preservative

Add at 40°C

> essential oils
> active ingredients

pH adjustment

> qs citric acid + purified water

To make this lotion, follow the *Method for making an emulsion with emulsifying wax* on page 79.

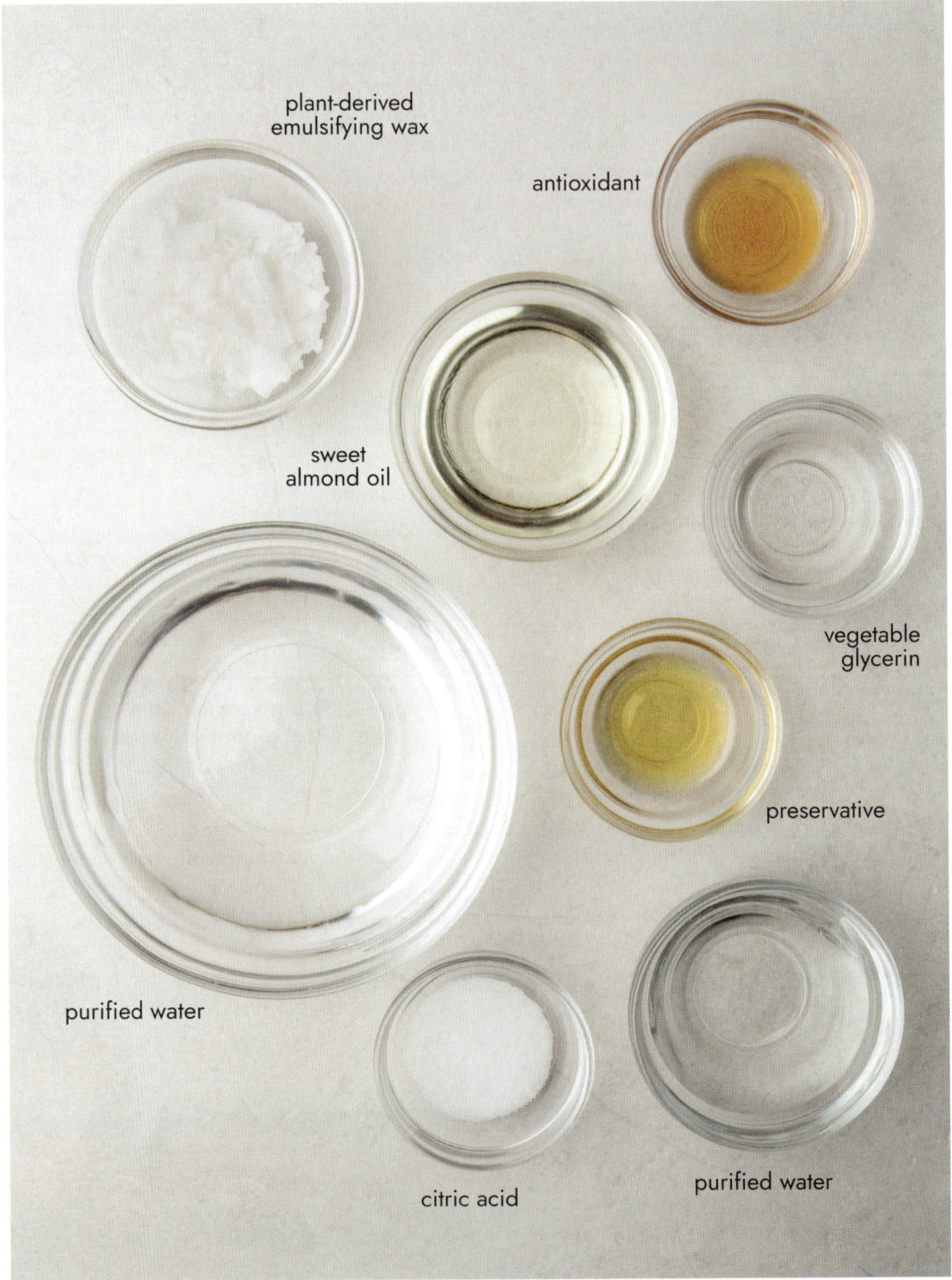

plant-derived
emulsifying wax

antioxidant

sweet
almond oil

vegetable
glycerin

preservative

purified water

citric acid

purified water

Base cream ingredients

Method for making an emulsion with emulsifying wax

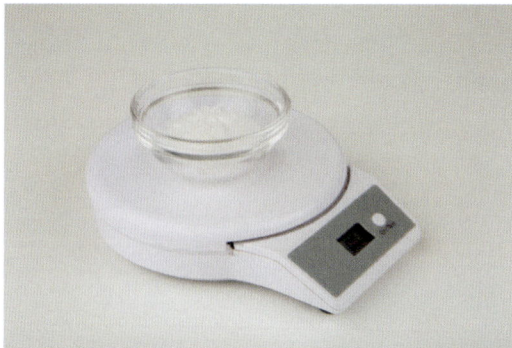

1. Weigh out your ingredients.

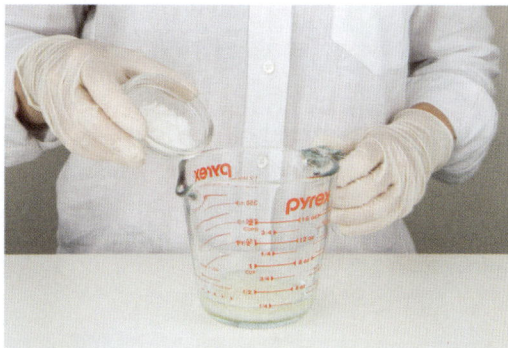

2. Place the emulsifying wax and other solid fats from your 'oil phase' into a heat-resistant jug.

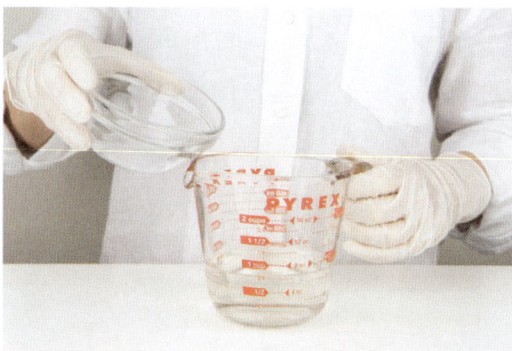

3. Place your 'water phase' ingredients into another heat-resistant jug.

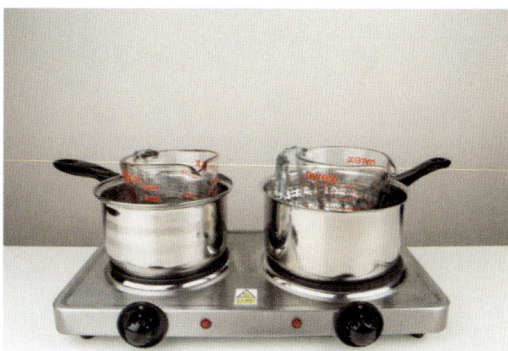

4. Place both jugs into large saucepans filled to approximately half with water. This is called a *bain-marie*. Then place the saucepans onto a stove or hot plate and heat gently.

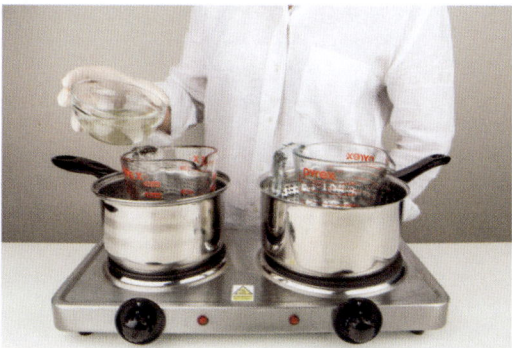

5. Once your waxes and solid fats have melted in your 'oil phase' jug, add the vegetable oils and antioxidant to this jug.

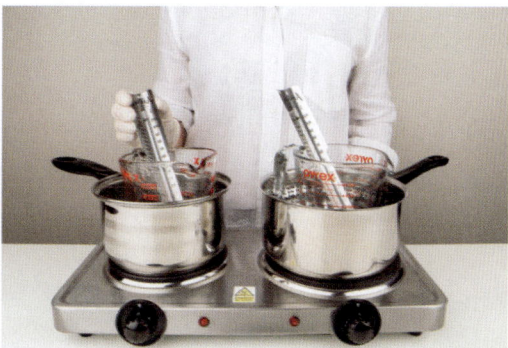

6. Heat both your 'oil phase' and 'water phase' ingredients to 70–75°C.

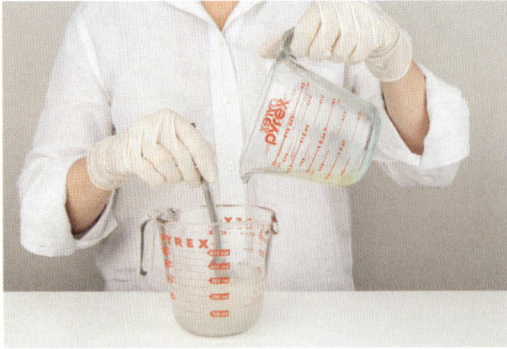

7. Now that both 'oil phase' and 'water phase' ingredients have reached 70–75°C, turn off the heat and remove the jugs from the *bain-marie*.

8. Slowly pour the 'oil phase' into the 'water phase'. Stir continuously while doing this.

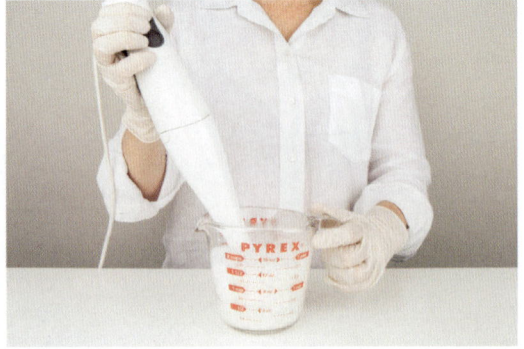

9. Use an electric stick mixer for a short time, approximately 20–30 seconds, to ensure emulsification takes place. This is important for emulsion stability as the oil is dispersed in fine droplets throughout the water phase, reducing its ability to come back together and separate out from the water phase.

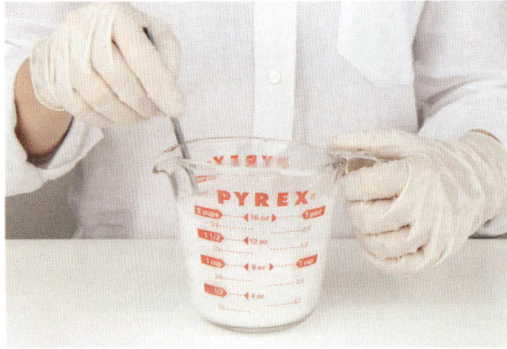

10. Stir regularly with a spoon as the emulsion cools.

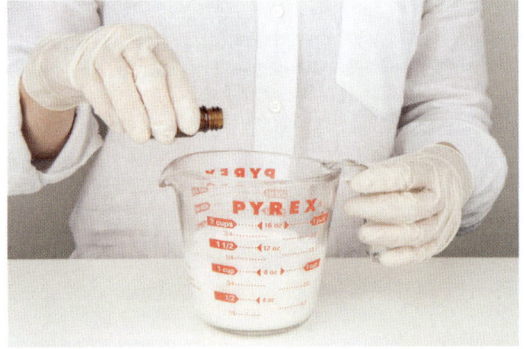

11. When the emulsion cools down to 40°C, add your essential oils and other heat-sensitive active ingredients and stir in thoroughly.

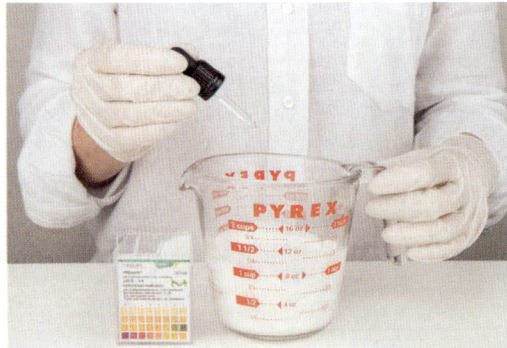

12. Check the pH and adjust if necessary by following the instructions on page 74.

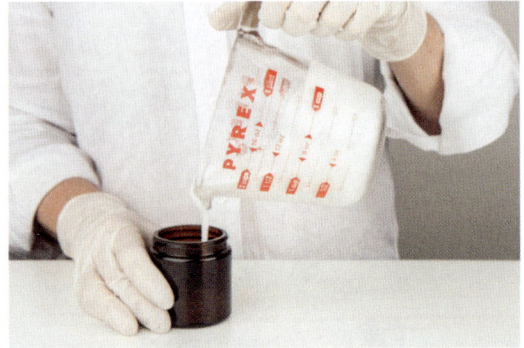

13. Once you see the emulsion begin to thicken but still remaining pourable, pour into jars or bottles. It will take around 24 hours for an emulsion to reach full viscosity.

14. Cap and label your containers when the emulsion has cooled to room temperature. Include on your label the name, purpose of the emulsion, ingredients and date.

EMULSION TIPS

Stabilising with xanthan gum
Step 3: Your emulsion may require further stabilisation with xanthan gum if it has a high water content to reduce the chances of separation. If this is the case, you would stir the xanthan gum into the glycerin ensuring it is evenly dispersed, then slowly add and stir in the water to form a liquid gel. Any other water phase ingredients would then be added and mixed in. You would then heat this mixture as you normally would your water phase and continue on with the other steps of making an emulsion.

Using heat sensitive oils
Step 6: If your recipe requires any vegetable oils that are high in essential fatty acids such as evening primrose oil or rosehip oil, add them once the other ingredients in your 'oil phase' have reached 70–75°C. They are added at this point as prolonged heating will cause their deterioration.

Avoid spilling
Step 9: If the stick blender causes the emulsion to spill, either transfer the emulsion to a larger vessel or pulse the stick blender rather than running it at a constant speed.

Avoid whipping air into the mixture
Step 9: Do not use an electric stick mixer for too long as air will be whipped into the emulsion, reducing its stability.

Avoid condensation
Step 14: If you cap your emulsion while it is still warm, condensation will form on the inside of the lid and the droplets will provide an environment for mould, yeast and bacteria to grow in.

Making an Emulsion with Lecithin

Lecithin is considered a truly natural emulsifier. It is more difficult to work with than an emulsifying wax and emulsions have more potential to separate. However, it is especially skin-compatible and an effective skin conditioner. Creams can be made with liquid lecithin or lecithin granules. Emulsions made with lecithin can be made without heating the ingredients using a cold-process method similar to making mayonnaise. Ingredients are stirred and slowly incorporated into an emulsion. It can be quite a time-consuming process. Emulsions with lecithin can also be created using a hot-process method, which is faster. The two processes are described below.

Lecithin Emulsion Cold-Process Method

This method requires patience and is much slower than the hot-process method.

Equipment

- digital scales
- 3 glass beakers or jugs
- metal stirring spoons
- small hand egg whisk
- electric stick mixer
- pH strips or meter
- jars or bottles

Liquid lecithin emulsion

This recipe will create a lightweight emulsion.

Ingredients

10 g liquid lecithin
150 g purified water
8 g vegetable glycerin
1 g xanthan gum
28 g vegetable oil
1 g antioxidant
2 g preservative
essential oils
active ingredients

pH adjustment

qs citric acid + purified water

To make this lightweight emulsion lotion, follow the *Cold-process method for making an emulsion with lecithin* on page 83.

Lecithin granules emulsion

This recipe will create a rich, emollient emulsion.

Ingredients

5 g lecithin granules
105 g purified water
8 g vegetable glycerin
1 g xanthan gum
78 g vegetable oil
1 g antioxidant
2 g preservative essential oils
active ingredients

pH adjustment

qs citric acid + purified water

To make this rich, emollient emulsion, follow the *Cold-process method for making an emulsion with lecithin* on page 83.

Cold-process method for making an emulsion with lecithin

1. **Using liquid lecithin:** In this first step, you will create a hydrated lecithin emulsifier into which the oil and water phase are then incorporated. This first step takes time and requires patience in order to form a high-quality emulsifier. In one glass beaker or jug, add 20 g of the purified water and pour the liquid lecithin into it. Using a spoon, give the liquid a slow, brief stir every 10 minutes or so over the first hour. The first time you stir the water and lecithin, the lecithin will look syrupy. Then, over time, it will start to swell a little and the syrupy lecithin will start to look lumpy and sticky. Don't be tempted to over-stir. Just give it a gentle, brief stir each time. If the lecithin sticks to the spoon, scrape the lecithin back into the water with another spoon. Eventually, the lecithin will start to break up into smaller lumps. After about an hour of this intermittent stirring, the water will start to look milky. Using a small hand egg whisk, increase the speed of stirring, then whisk to fully dissolve the lecithin. Continue to wait about 10 minutes in between stirring. It will take around 3 hours for your hydrated lecithin emulsifier to be ready to use. It will be smooth and creamy and a light caramel colour when it is ready.

Using lecithin granules: Using lecithin granules to make an emulsion is similar to making an emulsion with liquid lecithin. However, in step 1, the lecithin granules are added to 25 g of water and allowed to hydrate and swell for about half an hour or so. The mixture is stirred every 10 minutes or so during this time to fully dissolve the granules, and will eventually form a smooth, creamy paste. Do not over-stir or whip to the point where the hydrated lecithin becomes a thick rubbery mass. Creating your emulsifier with lecithin granules is faster than using liquid lecithin.

2. In another glass beaker or jug, mix the vegetable glycerin and xanthan gum together, ensuring the xanthan gum is well-dispersed throughout the glycerin.

3. Slowly add and stir the rest of the purified water into the glycerin and xanthan gum mixture, allowing it to fully hydrate into a gel.

4. Add the preservative to this gel mixture and stir in thoroughly.

5. In the third glass beaker, mix the vegetable oil with the antioxidant.

6. Add a small amount, about a teaspoon or so, of the vegetable oil and tocopherol mixture into the hydrated lecithin emulsifier and mix well using the small hand egg whisk. Continue to do this gradually until all of the oil mixture is incorporated into the hydrated lecithin. Each time you add a teaspoon of oil, you need to make sure it is fully incorporated before adding the next teaspoon of oil. It should look creamy and smooth once completed.

7. Add a small amount, about a teaspoon or so, of the gel mixture into the lecithin/oil mixture and stir well using the small hand egg whisk. Continue to do this gradually until all the gel mixture is incorporated into the lecithin/oil mixture. Each time you add a teaspoon of gel, you need to make sure it is fully incorporated before adding the next teaspoon of gel. It will be a smooth, creamy liquid once completed.

8. Using an electric stick mixer, emulsify the mixture for a minute or so. Do not use an electric stick mixer for too long as air will be whipped into the emulsion and its stability will be reduced.

9. Stir in any essential oils and other active ingredients and mix briefly, approximately 5–10 seconds, with the electric stick mixer.

10. Check the pH and adjust if necessary by following the instructions on page 74.

11. Pour into jars or bottles.

12. Cap and label your containers. Include on your label the name, purpose of the emulsion, ingredients and date.

Lecithin Emulsion Hot-Process Method

This method is faster than the cold-process method and is similar to making an emulsion using an emulsifying wax.

Equipment

- digital scales
- measuring glass or beaker
- 2 saucepans
- 3 heat-resistant jugs
- 2 metal trivets
- 2 cooking thermometers
- stovetop or hot plate with 2 plates
- electric stick mixer
- metal stirring spoons
- pH strips or meter
- jars or bottles

Lightweight lecithin emulsion

This recipe will create a lightweight emulsion. The xanthan gum supports the lecithin emulsifier in maintaining emulsion stability.

Ingredients

Water phase

8 g lecithin granules
149 g purified water
2 g xanthan gum
8 g vegetable glycerin
2 g preservative

Oil phase

30 g vegetable oil
1 g antioxidant

Add at 40°C

essential oils
active ingredients

pH adjustment

qs citric acid + purified water

To make this lightweight emulsion lotion, follow the *Hot-process method for making an emulsion with lecithin* below.

Hot-process method for making an emulsion with lecithin

1. In the first jug, add the water, lecithin granules and preservative. Allow the lecithin granules to fully hydrate and mix homogenously with the water. This will take half an hour or so with regular stirring every 10 minutes. It should look like slightly gelled milky water with no granules visible.

2. In a second jug, mix the xanthan gum and glycerin.

3. In a third jug, add the vegetable oil and tocopherols.

4. Add the mixture of lecithin and water in the first jug to the mixture of xanthan gum and

glycerin in the second jug. Do this slowly while stirring.

5. Heat the jug with the 'water phase' mixture to 70°C in a *bain-marie*.

6. Heat the jug with the 'oil phase' to 70°C in a separate *bain-marie*.

7. Once both 'water phase' and 'oil phase' ingredients have reached 70°C, turn off the heat.

8. Slowly pour the 'oil phase' into the 'water phase' while keeping the water phase sitting in the saucepan in the hot water. Stir continuously while doing this.

9. Once all the 'oil phase' ingredients have been incorporated into the 'water phase', remove the jug containing the emulsion from the saucepan.

10. Use an electric stick mixer for a short time, approximately 20–30 seconds, to ensure emulsification takes place. Do not use an electric stick mixer for too long as air will be whipped into the emulsion and its stability will be reduced.

11. When the emulsion cools down to 40°C, add your essential oils and other heat-sensitive active ingredients and stir in thoroughly.

12. Check the pH and adjust if necessary by following the instructions on page 74.

13. Pour into jars or bottles.

14. Cap and label your containers when the emulsion has cooled to room temperature. Include on your label the name, purpose of the emulsion, ingredients and date.

Making an Emulsion with Beeswax

Beeswax is not an emulsifier, but provides a structure throughout which a small amount of water can be dispersed and held in suspension. Consequently, this kind of cream will have a rich, thick, oily skin-feel. Its stability is relatively low, which means that over time or if exposed to heat, it will separate. For this reason, it is recommended that small batches are made, stored in the refrigerator and used within a month or so.

Equipment

- digital scales
- measuring glass or beaker
- 2 saucepans
- 2 heat-resistant jugs
- 2 metal trivets
- 2 cooking thermometers
- stovetop or hot plate with 2 plates
- electric stick mixer
- metal stirring spoons
- jars

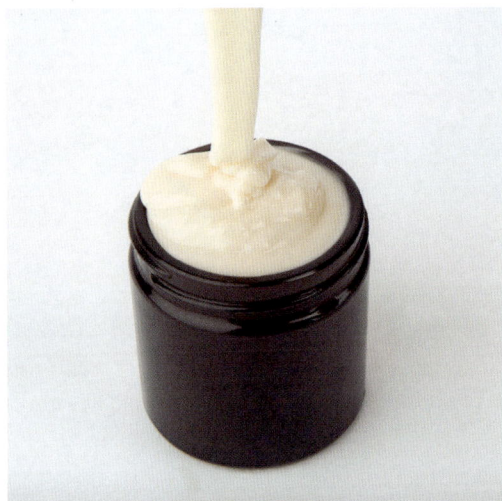

Ultra-rich beeswax cream

This is a rich emollient cream for dry skin exposed to the elements. It is recommended that this cream is made in small batches and stored in the refrigerator. As no preservative has been added, it should be used within a month or so.

Ingredients

Oil phase

20 g beeswax
124 g vegetable oil
1 g antioxidant

Water phase

55 g purified water

Add at 40°C

essential oils

Method for making an emulsion with beeswax

1. Melt the beeswax in a heat-resistant jug in a *bain-marie*.

2. Once the beeswax has melted, add the vegetable oil and tocopherols and heat to 70°C.

3. Add the water and preservative to the other heat-resistant jug and heat in a *bain-marie* to 70°C.

4. Once both phases have reached 70°C, slowly add the water to the oil phase while stirring.

5. Once all of the water has been added, remove from the heat and blend well with an electric stick mixer for a minute or so.

6. Continue stirring by hand until the mixture cools down to 40°C and add in any essential oils.

7. Continue stirring until the mixture reaches room temperature.

8. It will take up to 24 hours for the beeswax structure to fully set up. During this time, give the cream a gentle stir. If you

see any water separation, rapidly stir to reincorporate the water.

9. At the end of 24 hours, scoop the cream into jars, cap and label your containers. Include on your label the name, purpose of the emulsion, ingredients and date.

Butter rich skin cream

This rich moisturiser has a texture similar to creamy butter. It is relatively stable due to the addition of lecithin.

Ingredients

Oil phase

20 g beeswax
79 g vegetable oil
1 g antioxidant (mixed tocopherols)

Water phase

94 g purified water
4 g lecithin granules
2 g preservative

Add at 40°C

essential oils
active ingredients

pH adjustment

qs citric acid + purified water

Method for making an emulsion with beeswax and lecithin

1. Add the water, lecithin granules and preservative to a heat-resistant jug and allow the lecithin granules to fully dissolve into the water. It will take half an hour or so, during which time the mixture should be stirred every 10 minutes or so. The granules will eventually dissolve and the water will look milky and a little thickened.

2. Heat the water phase in a *bain-marie* to 70°C.

3. Melt the beeswax in another *bain-marie*.

4. Once the beeswax has melted, add the vegetable oil and tocopherol and heat to 70°C.

5. Once both phases have reached 70°C, slowly add the oil to the water phase while stirring.

6. Once all of the oil phase has been added, blend well with an electric stick mixer for 30 or so seconds.

7. Continue stirring by hand until the mixture cools down to 40°C and add in any essential oils and other heat-sensitive active ingredients and stir in thoroughly.

8. Check pH and adjust if necessary by following the instructions on page 74.

9. Continue stirring until the mixture reaches room temperature.

10. It will take up to 24 hours for the beeswax structure to fully set up. During this time, give the cream a gentle stir. If you see any water separation, rapidly stir to reincorporate the water.

11. At the end of 24 hours, scoop the cream into jars, cap and label your containers. Include on your label the name, purpose of the emulsion, ingredients and date.

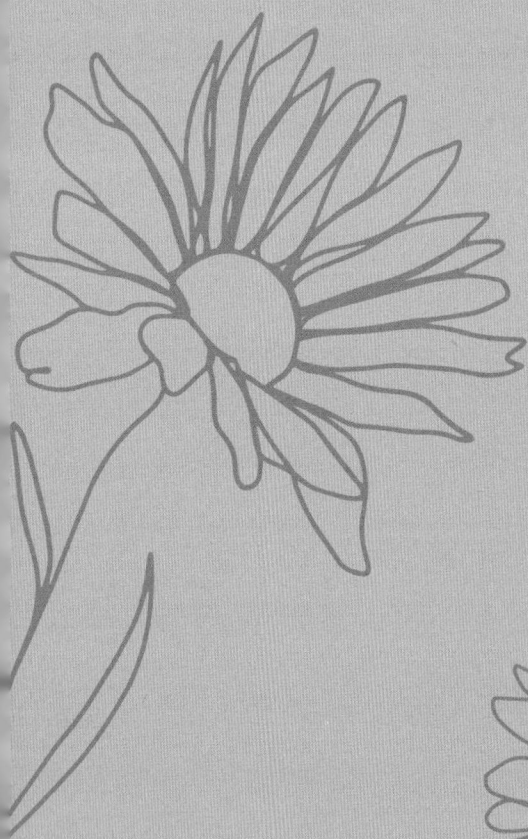

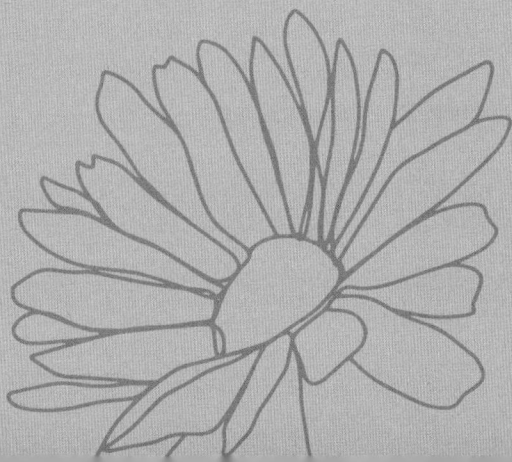

Clean & Minimal

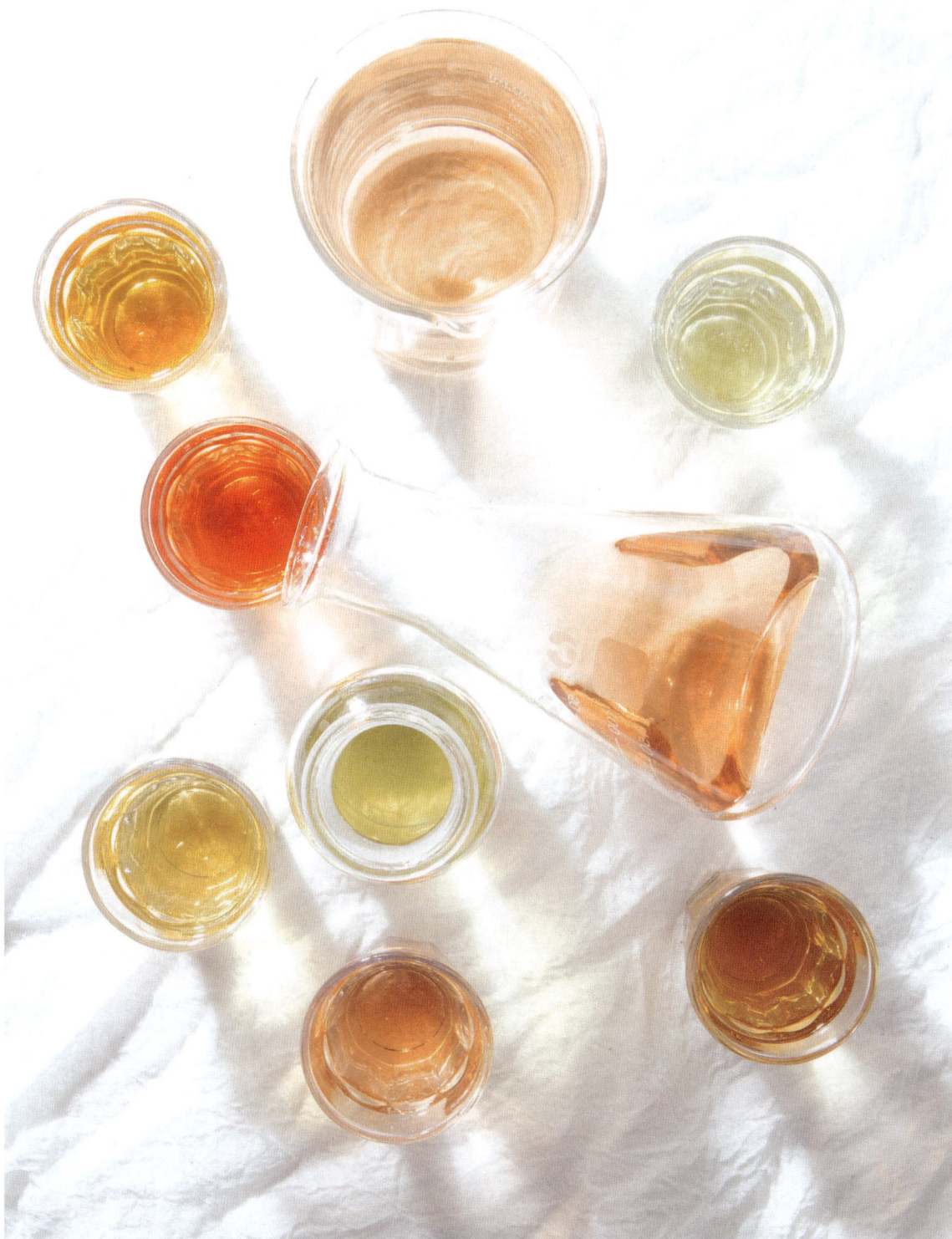

Clean and minimal skin care preparations are made with minimal, pure, unprocessed or minimally processed ingredients, and are preservative-free. They are simple mixtures and are made effortlessly in a minimum amount of time. They are clean, effective inclusions to your daily skin care ritual.

Beauty Infusions

Make use of the healing benefits of your dried herbs by combining them and storing them in a jar where they are ready for use at any time. Simply make up a fresh infusion whenever you need it.

Facial Toners and Skin Fresheners

Use half a teaspoon of one of the dried herb mixes on this page and half a cup of boiling water to make a facial toner or skin freshener. They can also be used to make facial compresses.

1. Place the herb mix into a tea infuser and place into a cup, pour the boiling water over the herbs and infuse for approximately 5 minutes.
2. Allow to cool and decant into a bottle or spray bottle. Or simply dip a cotton pad into the cup.
3. Mist over your face or apply to cotton pads and wipe over your face.
4. Keep your infusion in the refrigerator and use within 2 days before it deteriorates and becomes unhealthy.

Find more information and recipes for toners on page 129.

Antiseptic infusion
for blemished skin

1 tbsp calendula flowers
1 tbsp sage
1 tbsp thyme
1 tbsp yarrow

Soothing infusion
for sensitive skin

1 tbsp calendula flowers
1 tbsp chamomile flowers
1 tbsp elderflowers
1 tbsp rolled oats

Hydrating infusion
for dehydrated skin

1 tbsp aloe vera powder
1 tbsp calendula flowers
1 tbsp lavender flowers
1 tbsp rose petals

Healing and repair infusion
for damaged, scarred skin

1 tbsp calendula flowers
1 tbsp gotu kola
1 tbsp green tea
1 tbsp comfrey leaves

Hair Rinses

Use 1 teaspoon of one of the dried herb mixes below and 1 cup of boiling water. (This is enough for one application.) These infusions improve hair shine and scalp health.

1. Place the herb mix into a tea infuser and place into a cup, pour the boiling water over the herbs and infuse for approximately 5 minutes.
2. Allow to cool and decant into a bottle or spray bottle.
3. Pour or spray over your scalp and through your hair after shampooing and conditioning.
4. Leave on for 2 minutes, then rinse.

Blonde hair shine infusion

4 tbsp chamomile

Dark hair shine infusion

4 tbsp sage

Healthy scalp infusion

1 tbsp nettle
1 tbsp peppermint
1 tbsp rosemary

Bath Infusions

Add 4 tablespoons or so of the dried herb mix (this is enough for one bath) to a large tea infuser or muslin square and tie. Infuse in your bathwater while you soak.

Relaxing bath infusion

1 tbsp calendula flowers
1 tbsp lavender flowers
1 tbsp lemon verbena
1 tbsp rose petals

Skin soothing bath infusion

1 tbsp calendula flowers
1 tbsp chamomile flowers
1 tbsp lavender flowers
1 tbsp rolled oats

Energising bath infusion

1 tbsp lemon myrtle
1 tbsp peppermint
1 tbsp rosemary
1 tbsp sage

Beauty Powders and Pastes

Combine a range of nature's finest powdered ingredients and simply add water to create face and body masks, and face and body scrubs. Create dry deodorant powders and dry shampoo powders too.

Dried herbs and botanicals can be powdered in an electric coffee grinder. To make your beauty powders, mix the dry ingredients together in a bowl. If necessary, sieve to break down any lumps in the powder. Then add any drops of essential oils that may be in a recipe, ensuring you sprinkle them uniformly over the mixture then stir them in. Sieve again a couple of times to ensure any lumps are broken down and the essential oils are evenly distributed throughout the mixture.

Store the perfect combination of active powdered ingredients for your skin type in an airtight jar, then add a teaspoon or so of the powder to your hand or bowl and simply add water to activate and use as a mask or scrub. A deodorant powder or dry shampoo powder is applied directly to your body or hair as is.

No preservative is necessary to preserve these products and you only need to add water to the quantity you require to activate and make a fresh product whenever you need it.

Powdered ingredients you may like to combine include clays; dried, powdered herbs and flowers; flours; ground seeds; powdered milks and yoghurts; dehydrated, powdered fruits and vegetables; powdered seaweeds; activated charcoal; brewer's yeast — just for starters!

Mask Powders and Pastes

Add a heaped teaspoon of one of the mask powders on page 95 to a small bowl and stir in 1–2 teaspoons of water to activate and use. Smooth over clean skin and leave on for 5 minutes for dry, dehydrated skin, and up to 10 minutes for combination and oily skin. Remove with a damp cloth and follow with a facial mist and moisturiser.

To make a scalp mask, add a heaped teaspoon of the mask powder to a small bowl and stir in 1–2 teaspoons of water to activate and use. Massage into the scalp and leave on for 3–5 minutes before rinsing well.

Find more information and recipes for face masks on page 149 and body masks on page 187.

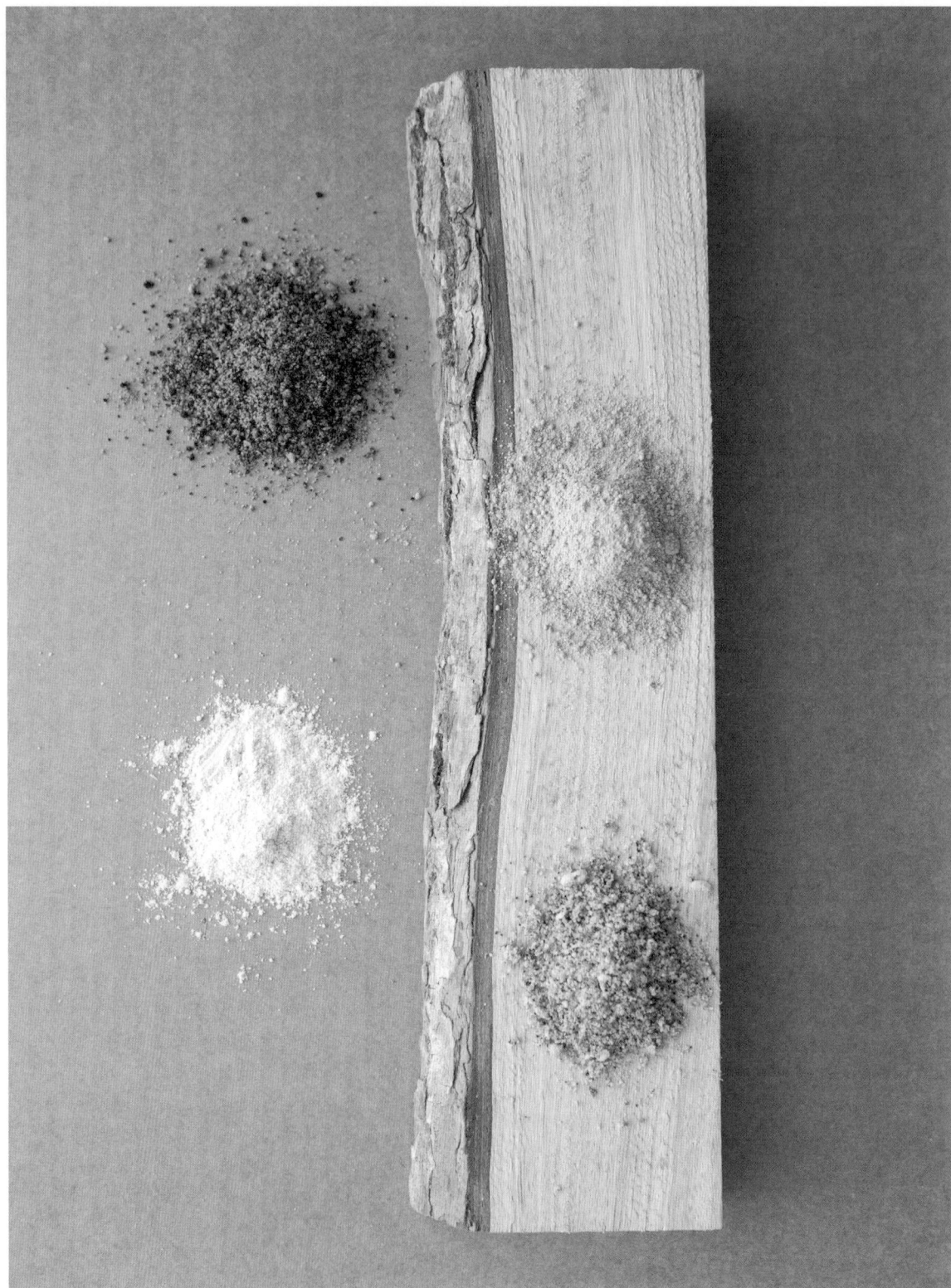

Detox and cleanse mask
for oily and blemished skin

3 tsp green Argiletz clay
1 tsp bentonite clay
1 tsp kaolin clay
1 tsp activated charcoal powder
1 tsp neem leaf powder
1 drop lavender essential oil
1 drop tea tree essential oil

Skin therapy mask
for pimples and blemished skin

3 tsp Australian olive green clay
¼ tsp calendula flower powder
¼ tsp comfrey leaf powder
¼ tsp gotu kola powder
¼ tsp myrrh gum powder

Hydration mask
for dry, dehydrated skin

3 tsp kelp powder
1 tsp oat flour
½ tsp aloe vera powder

Radiance mask
for mature skin

2 tsp coconut milk powder
1 tsp red Argiletz clay
1 tsp rose petal powder
¼ tsp Kakadu plum powder

Lift and revitalise mask
for dull and devitalised skin

3 tsp yellow Argiletz clay
1 tsp yoghurt powder
¼ tsp brewer's yeast
¼ tsp matcha powder

Calm and smooth mask
for sensitive skin

2 tsp kaolin clay
2 tsp oat flour
½ tsp aloe vera powder
¼ tsp calendula flower powder
¼ tsp comfrey leaf powder

Soft and velvety mask
for dull, dry skin

2 tsp Australian yellow clay
2 tsp full cream milk powder
1 tsp strawberry powder

Face and body cleanse and tone mask

3 tsp green Argiletz clay
2 tsp kelp powder
1 tsp bentonite clay
1 tsp rhassoul clay
1 tsp matcha powder

Healthy scalp mask

2 tsp rhassoul clay
1 tsp neem leaf powder

Exfoliant Powders and Pastes

Add a heaped teaspoon of one of the exfoliant powders below to your hand or bowl and stir in 2 teaspoons of water to activate and use. Massage over clean skin and rinse to remove. Some exfoliants may be left on as masks for up to 10 minutes or so before removing with a damp cloth.

Find more information and recipes for facial exfoliants on page 155 and body exfoliants on page 183.

Fresh skin facial scrub
for oily and blemished skin

3 tsp kaolin clay
1 tsp tomato powder
1 tsp white rice flour

Creamy coconut facial exfoliant
for normal to dry skin

2 tsp coconut flour
2 tsp dried coconut milk
1 tsp white rice flour

Refined skin facial polish
for dry and mature skin

3 tsp almond meal
2 tsp coconut flour
½ tsp ground wattle seeds
½ tsp pomegranate juice powder

Gentle touch facial exfoliant
for all skin types

3½ tsp kaolin clay
1 tsp besan flour
1 tsp sandalwood powder
½ tsp white rice flour

Hazelnut and coffee body scrub

2 tsp ground coffee
2 tsp hazelnut meal
2 tsp white rice flour
3 drops sweet orange essential oil

Pink poppy hand scrub

3 tsp pink Argiletz clay
2 tsp walnut shell granules
1 tsp poppy seeds
3 drops geranium essential oil

Pumice refreshing foot scrub

3 tsp ground pumice
2½ tsp kaolin clay
1 tsp spirulina
2 drops lemon essential oil
1 drop peppermint essential oil

Deodorant Powders

Dust a little on your armpits to help absorb perspiration, deodorise and keep you smelling fresh.

Find more information and recipes for deodorants on page 197.

Active underarm deodorant powder

3 tsp bentonite clay
3 tsp kaolin clay
2½ tsp arrowroot flour
1½ tsp sodium bicarbonate
3 drops petitgrain essential oil
2 drops cypress essential oil

Sensitive underarm deodorant powder

4 tsp kaolin clay
2 tsp arrowroot flour
1 tsp bentonite clay
2 drops patchouli essential oil
2 drops ylang ylang essential oil

Foot deodorant powder

3 tsp bentonite clay
3 tsp kaolin clay
2½ tsp arrowroot flour
1½ tsp sodium bicarbonate
5 drops peppermint essential oil

Dry Shampoo Powders

Massage a small quantity into the roots of your hair and brush throughout the length of your hair to absorb oil in between shampooing. A couple of drops of your favourite essential oil can be added. If you add essential oil, break down any lumps that form and run the powder through a sieve a couple of times to ensure even distribution of the essential oil.

Dry shampoo powder — dark

3 tsp cacao powder
1 tsp activated charcoal
½ tsp arrowroot flour
½ tsp kaolin clay

Dry shampoo powder — light

3 tsp kaolin clay
1 tsp arrowroot flour
1 tsp corn starch

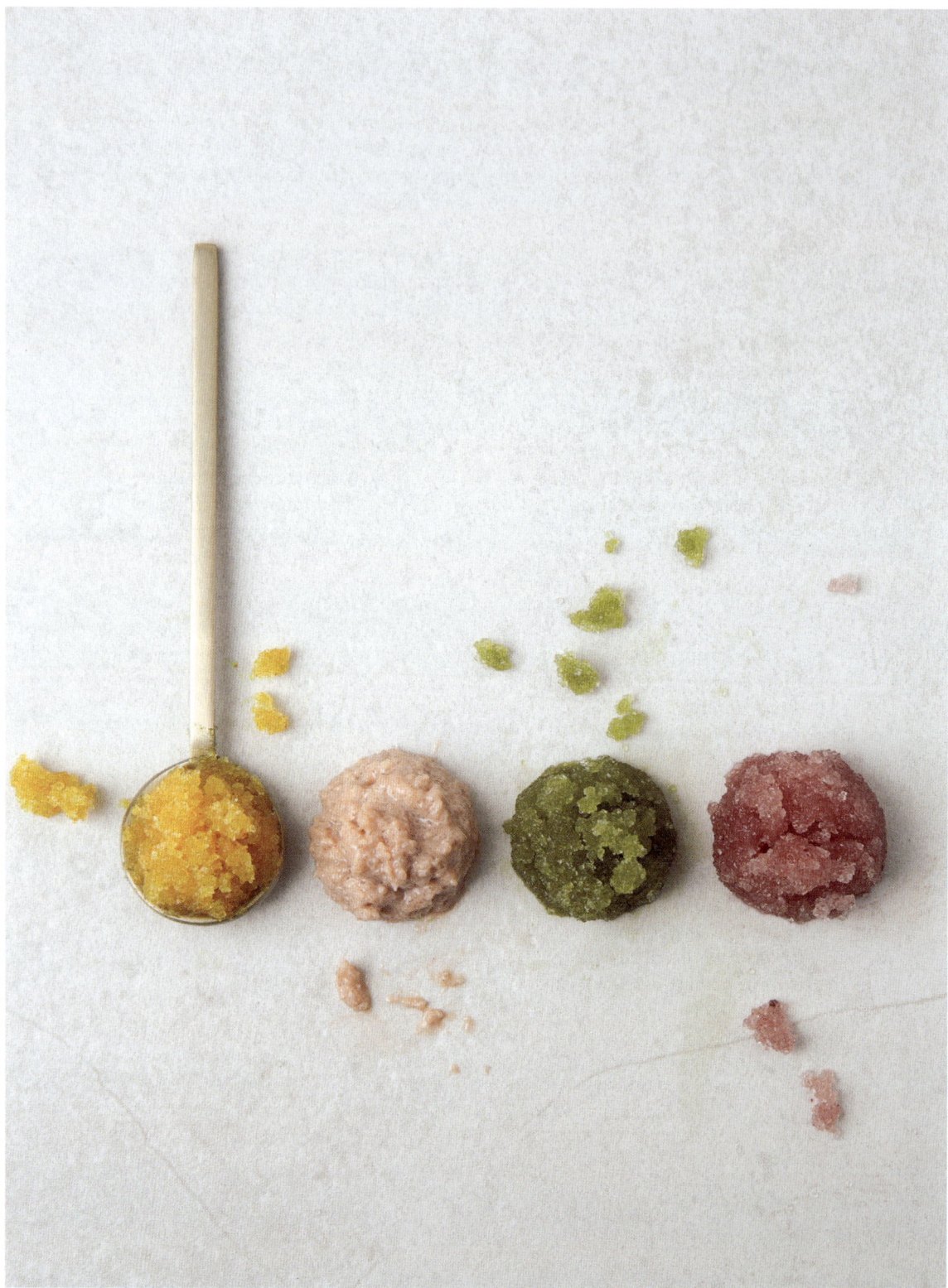

Beauty Sugar and Salt Scrubs

Buff away dry, rough skin and reveal fresh smooth skin with a sugar or salt scrub.

Make these recipes by simply mixing these ingredients together and storing them in a jar ready for use. After cleansing, massage over damp skin and rinse. The sugar or salt will dissolve and be rinsed away in the water while the oil remains on the skin to soften and moisturise.

Find more information and recipes for facial exfoliants on page 155 and body exfoliants on page 183.

Sugar Scrubs

Rose facial scrub

4 tsp caster sugar
¼ tsp rose petal powder
2 tsp jojoba oil
1 drop rose otto

Cinnamon lip scrub

4 tsp caster sugar
¼ tsp cinnamon powder
1 tsp jojoba oil
½ tsp coconut oil

Matcha green tea body scrub

4 tsp caster sugar
¼ tsp matcha powder
2 tsp sweet almond oil
3 drops bergamot essential oil

Coffee body scrub

3 tsp coconut sugar
2 tsp dried coffee grounds
2 tsp apricot kernel oil

Coconut ice body scrub

3 tsp caster sugar
1 tsp kaolin clay
¼ tsp pink Argiletz clay
1 tsp desiccated coconut
1 tsp coconut oil
1 tsp sweet almond oil

Chocolate orange body scrub

4 tsp coconut sugar
1 tsp cacao powder
1½ tsp sweet almond oil
20 drops sweet orange essential oil

Salt Scrubs

Fresh mint lime body scrub

4 tsp salt
1 tsp dried peppermint
¼ tsp spirulina
2 tsp jojoba oil
4 drops cold-pressed lime essential oil
1 drop peppermint essential oil

Charcoal patchouli body scrub

4 tsp salt
½ tsp activated charcoal powder
2 tsp apricot kernel oil
3 drops patchouli essential oil

Seaweed detox body scrub

4 tsp salt
1 tsp green Argiletz clay
¼ tsp kelp powder
2 tsp sweet almond oil
4 drops grapefruit essential oil
1 drop cypress essential oil

Soft pink body scrub

4 tsp ground Murray River salt
1 tsp kaolin clay
⅛ tsp pink Argiletz clay
2 tsp sweet almond oil
3 drops geranium essential oil

Ginger turmeric body scrub

4 tsp salt
⅛ tsp turmeric
2 tsp sesame oil
3 drops lemongrass essential oil
1 drop ginger essential oil

Earth energy body scrub

4 tsp ground Murray River salt
¼ tsp Australian yellow clay
2 tsp macadamia oil
2 drops lemon myrtle essential oil
2 drops peppermint eucalyptus
essential oil

Golden goddess hand scrub

4 tsp salt
1 tsp calendula petals
1½ tsp apricot kernel oil
½ tsp calendula infused oil
2 drops grapefruit essential oil
2 drops lemon essential oil
2 drops mandarin essential oil

Mint rush foot scrub

4 tsp salt
1 tsp green Argiletz clay
2 tsp macadamia oil
2 drops cypress essential oil
2 drops peppermint essential oil

Beauty Washes

Castile soap is available in hard bar soap form and in liquid soap form. It is named after a region called Castile in Spain where olive oil is produced. It is used to cleanse the face and body. Castile liquid soap is the base of these clean and minimal beauty washes.

Castile liquid soap can be used just as it is to wash the skin. However, if your skin is dry, a vegetable oil can be added to reduce any drying effects. You will need to shake before use if adding vegetable oils. Essential oils to suit your skin type or for other aromatherapy benefits can simply be stirred into it.

Find more information and recipes for face cleansers on page 121 and body washes on page 181.

Facial Washes

Oily skin wash

100 mL Castile liquid soap
10 drops lime essential oil
6 drops mandarin essential oil
4 drops cypress essential oil

Normal to dry skin wash

80 mL Castile liquid soap
20 mL apricot kernel oil
12 drops sweet orange essential oil
6 drops petitgrain essential oil
2 drops ylang ylang essential oil

Hand and Body Washes

Serenity hand and body wash

90 mL Castile liquid soap
10 mL apricot kernel oil
8 drops lavender essential oil
6 drops Atlas cedarwood essential oil
6 drops clary sage essential oil

Forest retreat hand and body wash

100 mL Castile liquid soap
8 drops spruce essential oil
5 drops eucalyptus essential oil
5 drops pine essential oil

Botanical antiseptic hand and body wash

100 mL Castile liquid soap
13 drops grapefruit essential oil
3 drops manuka essential oil
3 drops tea tree essential oil
1 drop clove bud essential oil

Gentle hand and body wash

90 mL Castile liquid soap
10 mL macadamia oil
10 drops lavender essential oil
3 drops German chamomile essential oil

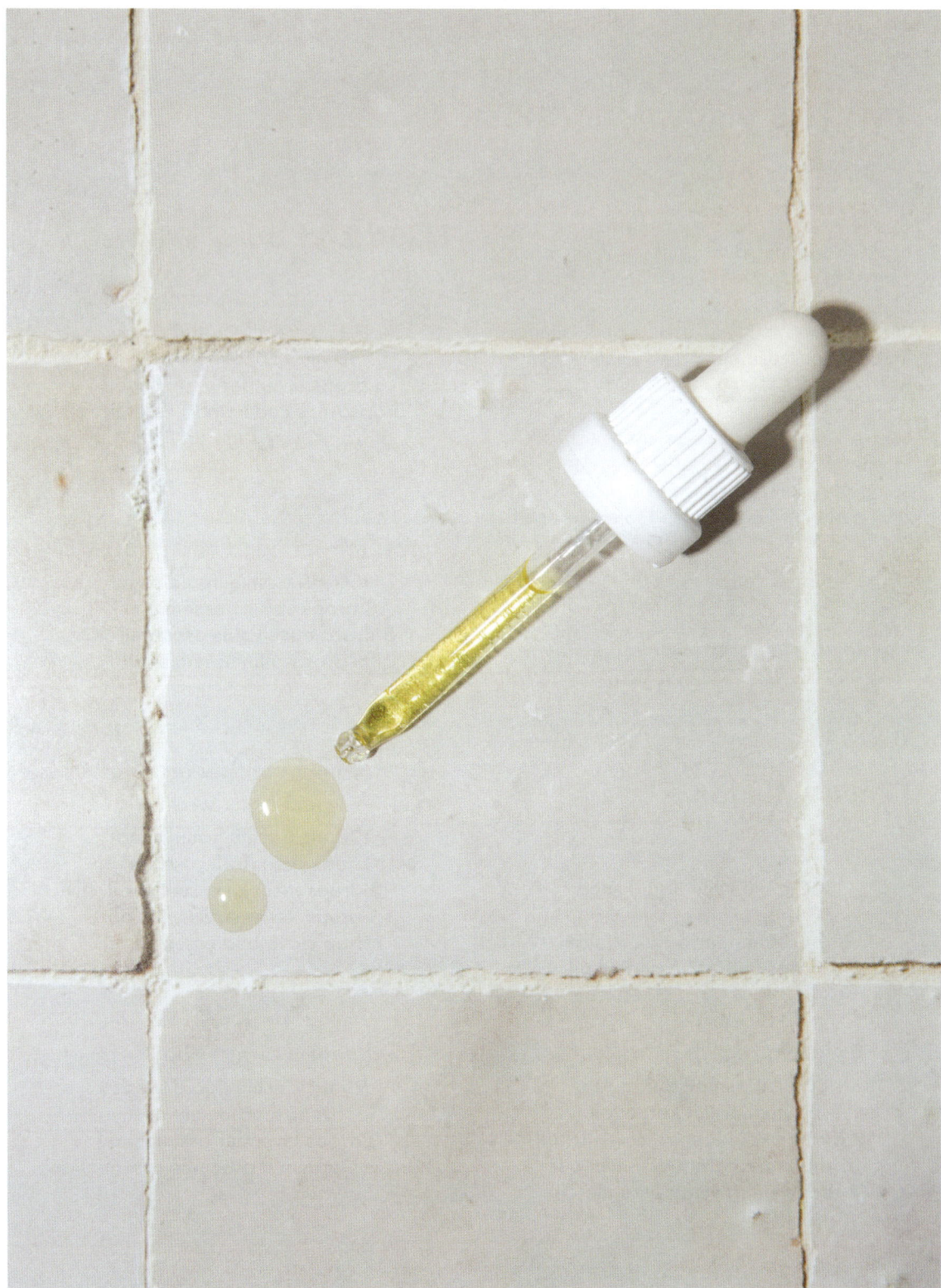

Beauty Oils and Elixirs

Beauty oils are simple recipes of vegetable oils blended with infused oils and essential oils to cleanse, heal, nourish, rejuvenate and improve the moisture levels of your skin. Simply add all ingredients to a glass bottle and shake well to ensure the ingredients are thoroughly blended.

Facial Cleansing Oils

A single vegetable oil that suits your skin type can be used as a simple cleansing oil. Alternatively, you can choose one of the luxurious recipes below. A facial cleansing oil removes make-up, grime and pollution without drying the skin. Cleansing oils are especially recommended for dry and sensitive skin types. They leave the skin feeling clean, fresh and smooth. To make, simply add all ingredients to a glass bottle and shake well to ensure the ingredients are thoroughly blended.

How to Use

Eye make-up removal

1. If you are wearing eye make-up, remove it first before cleansing the rest of your face. Add a few drops of jojoba oil to a cotton pad dampened with warm water and gently wipe the make-up from your eyelids and lashes. Be careful not to wipe into your eyes. Use jojoba oil without any added essential oils to avoid eye irritation.

Face cleansing

2. Then, massage your facial cleansing oil over your face using circular movements. Ensure you use enough oil to cover your skin well.

3. Wet the palms of your hands with warm water and massage over your face.

4. Soak a clean face cloth in warm water, wring out the excess water, place it over your face and press it into your skin. Then, using the cloth, wipe away the cleansing oil.

5. Follow by thoroughly wiping over your face with a cotton pad dampened with a toner or floral water suited to your skin type.

Find more information and recipes for cleansers on page 121.

Rose cleansing oil
for dry skin

95 mL apricot kernel oil
5 mL avocado oil
5 drops rose otto

Sandalwood cleansing oil
for sensitive skin

50 mL apricot kernel oil
50 mL jojoba oil
10 drops sandalwood essential oil

Lavender cleansing oil
for all skin types

50 mL apricot kernel oil
50 mL macadamia oil
10 drops lavender essential oil

Eye make-up remover oil
jojoba oil

Facial Treatment Oils, Serums and Elixirs

Use these facial oils to heal, replenish, rejuvenate, protect your skin, and diminish skin dryness. They are often referred to as oil serums and elixirs. To make, simply add all ingredients to a glass bottle and shake well to ensure the ingredients are thoroughly blended.

After cleansing and toning, massage and press 5–7 drops into your face and neck. Follow with a moisturiser if required.

Find more information and recipes for facial oils on page 139.

Rejuvenation oil serum
for dry, mature skin

10 mL apricot kernel oil
10 mL rosehip oil
5 mL avocado oil
3 drops rose otto
1 drop frankincense essential oil
1 drop sandalwood essential oil

Skin repair oil
for damaged skin

20 mL rosehip oil
5 mL calendula infused oil
2 drops everlasting essential oil
2 drops lavender essential oil
1 drop frankincense essential oil

Calming facial oil
for sensitive skin

15 mL jojoba oil
5 mL apricot kernel oil
5 mL calendula infused oil
3 drops neroli essential oil
1 drop everlasting essential oil

Light silk facial elixir
for most skin types

25 mL jojoba oil
2 drops geranium essential oil
2 drops jasmine absolute
1 drop ylang ylang essential oil

Body Oils

Soften, protect and reduce skin dryness with these body oils.

Simply add all ingredients to a glass bottle and shake well to ensure the ingredients are thoroughly blended.

After showering and while your skin is still a little damp, massage over your skin. They are especially effective when used after exfoliation.

Find more information and recipes for body and massage preparations on page 191.

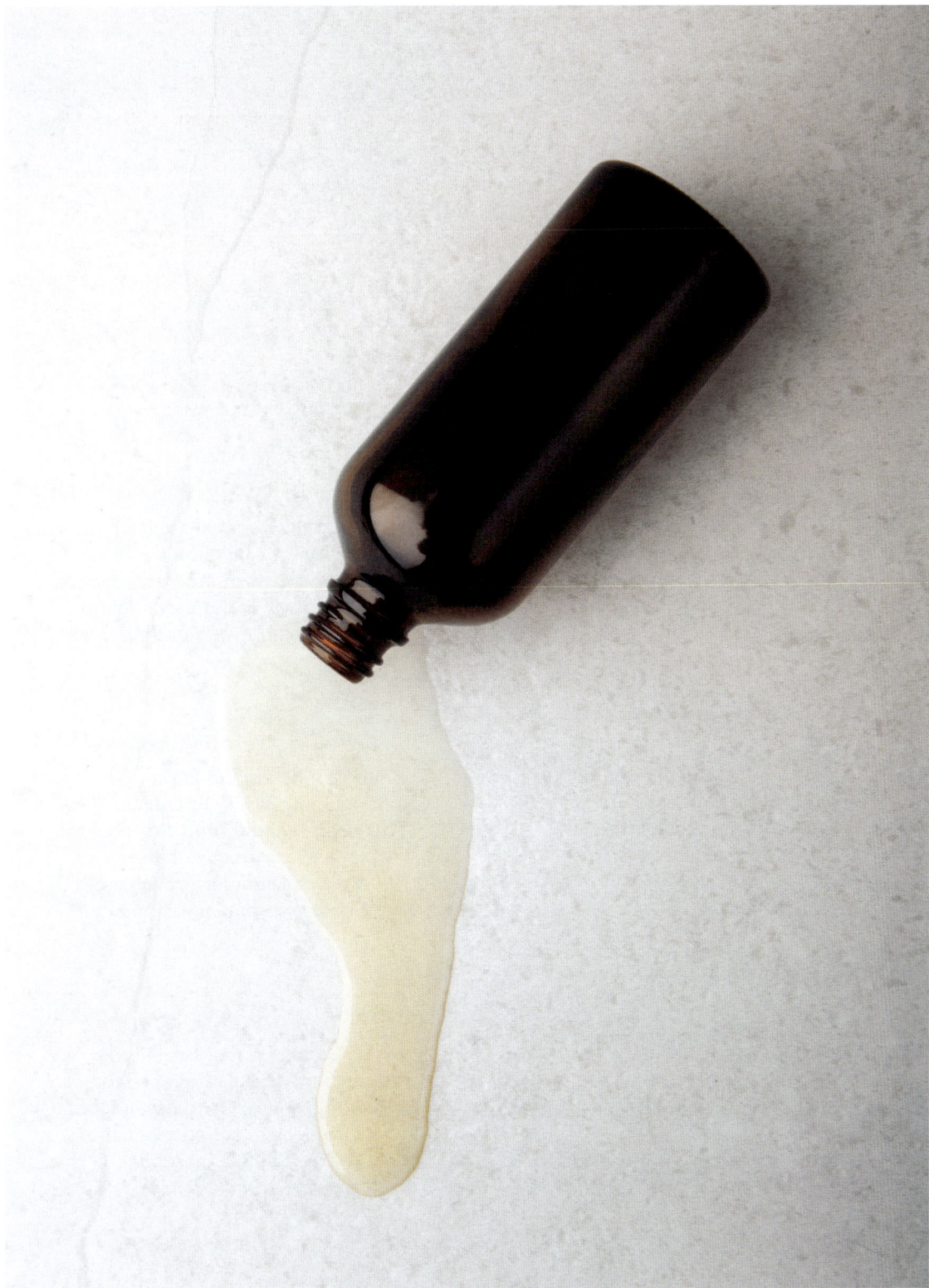

Ultra-nourishing body oil
for dry skin

50 mL apricot kernel oil
25 mL coconut oil
15 mL avocado oil
5 mL calendula infused oil
5 mL rosehip oil
10 drops sandalwood essential oil
8 drops lavender essential oil
7 drops geranium essential oil
3 drops patchouli essential oil

Silken body elixir
for normal to dry skin

50 mL apricot kernel oil
50 mL sweet almond oil
19 drops sweet orange essential oil
15 drops sandalwood essential oil
4 drops jasmine absolute

Gorgeous body oil
for most skin types

100 mL sweet almond oil
5 drops neroli essential oil
4 drops rose otto
3 drops jasmine absolute

Bath Oils

Baths are a wonderful way to relax and unwind. These bath oil recipes are designed to disperse essential oils throughout the water so that you can enjoy their therapeutic benefits.

Method

Simply blend the essential oils and vegetable oils with the Castile liquid soap to form a homogenous creamy liquid. The addition of the Castile liquid soap ensures the essential oils disperse throughout the water rather than float on top.

Shake the mixture prior to use. Then add 1 tablespoon to a warm bath and swish throughout the water to fully disperse.

Find more bath recipes on page 221.

Floating on clouds bath oil

25 mL sweet almond oil
25 mL Castile liquid soap
15 drops sweet orange essential oil
6 drops lavender essential oil
4 drops clary sage essential oil

Feel the serenity bath oil

25 mL apricot kernel oil
25 mL Castile liquid soap
10 drops sandalwood essential oil
5 drops rose otto
3 drops lavender essential oil
2 drops geranium essential oil

Calm goddess bath oil

25 mL apricot kernel oil
25 mL Castile liquid soap
12 drops ylang ylang essential oil
4 drops clary sage essential oil
4 drops vetiver essential oil

Hair and Scalp Oils

Hair and scalp oils can be used to treat scalp conditions such as dryness and dandruff, and will add a conditioning shine and lustre to the hair.

Simply add all ingredients to a glass bottle and shake well to ensure the ingredients are thoroughly blended.

Massage the oil into your scalp and smooth along the length of your hair. Use enough oil to ensure you have covered your scalp and hair without being excessive. Leave in for at least half an hour before double shampooing.

Find more hair care recipes on page 265.

Dandruff scalp oil
50 mL jojoba oil
5 drops Atlas cedarwood essential oil
5 drops rosemary essential oil
5 drops sage essential oil

Conditioning hair oil
50 mL coconut oil
7 drops ylang ylang essential oil

Leave-in hair smoothing oil
50 mL jojoba
10 drops lime essential oil

To use the *Leave-in hair smoothing oil,* massage a drop or two over your fingers and lightly run throughout your hair. Start at the ends before smoothing over the rest of your hair. It may be used on damp hair to help seal in moisture or on dry hair simply to smooth the hair.

Beauty Vinegars

Prepare a herbal vinegar according to the *Method for making herbal vinegars* on page 54, then make up a range of preparations for your skin and hair following the directions below.

Facial Toner Herbal Vinegars

Dilute 1 teaspoon of herbal vinegar in 100 mL of purified water and store in a glass bottle. It may be stored in the refrigerator for up to a week. Simply make up a fresh bottle of toner each week.

Use by wiping over your face after cleansing.

The following combinations can be used to make facial toner vinegars.

Oily and blemished skin herbal vinegar toner
geranium + thyme

Normal to dry skin herbal vinegar toner
chamomile + lavender

Hair and Scalp Herbal Vinegars

If you wash your hair with a shampoo soap bar or liquid soap, the relatively high pH of these products may cause your scalp to become dry and itchy. A diluted herbal vinegar can be poured throughout your hair and over your scalp to readjust the pH and reduce the effects of the soap.

Dilute 1 tablespoon (20 mL) of herbal vinegar in 500 mL of purified water. Pour into a bottle, then pour throughout your hair and over your scalp. Massage into the scalp and rinse with clean water.

Hair conditioning herbal vinegar rinse
chamomile + lavender + rosemary + sage

Dandruff scalp herbal vinegar
rosemary + sage + thyme

Follow the directions above and leave on for 10 minutes before rinsing.

Bath Herbal Vinegars

Add up to half a cup of your fragrant bath herbal vinegar to your bathwater and disperse well before enjoying your bath.

Botanical boost bath vinegar
geranium + lavender + peppermint

Deodorant Herbal Vinegar

Add 1 tablespoon (20 mL) of herbal vinegar to 100 mL purified water and store in a glass spray bottle. This may be stored in the refrigerator for up to a week. As your undiluted herbal vinegar can be stored for quite some time, simply make up a fresh bottle of herbal deodorant vinegar each week.

Garden fresh deodorant vinegar
lavender + sage

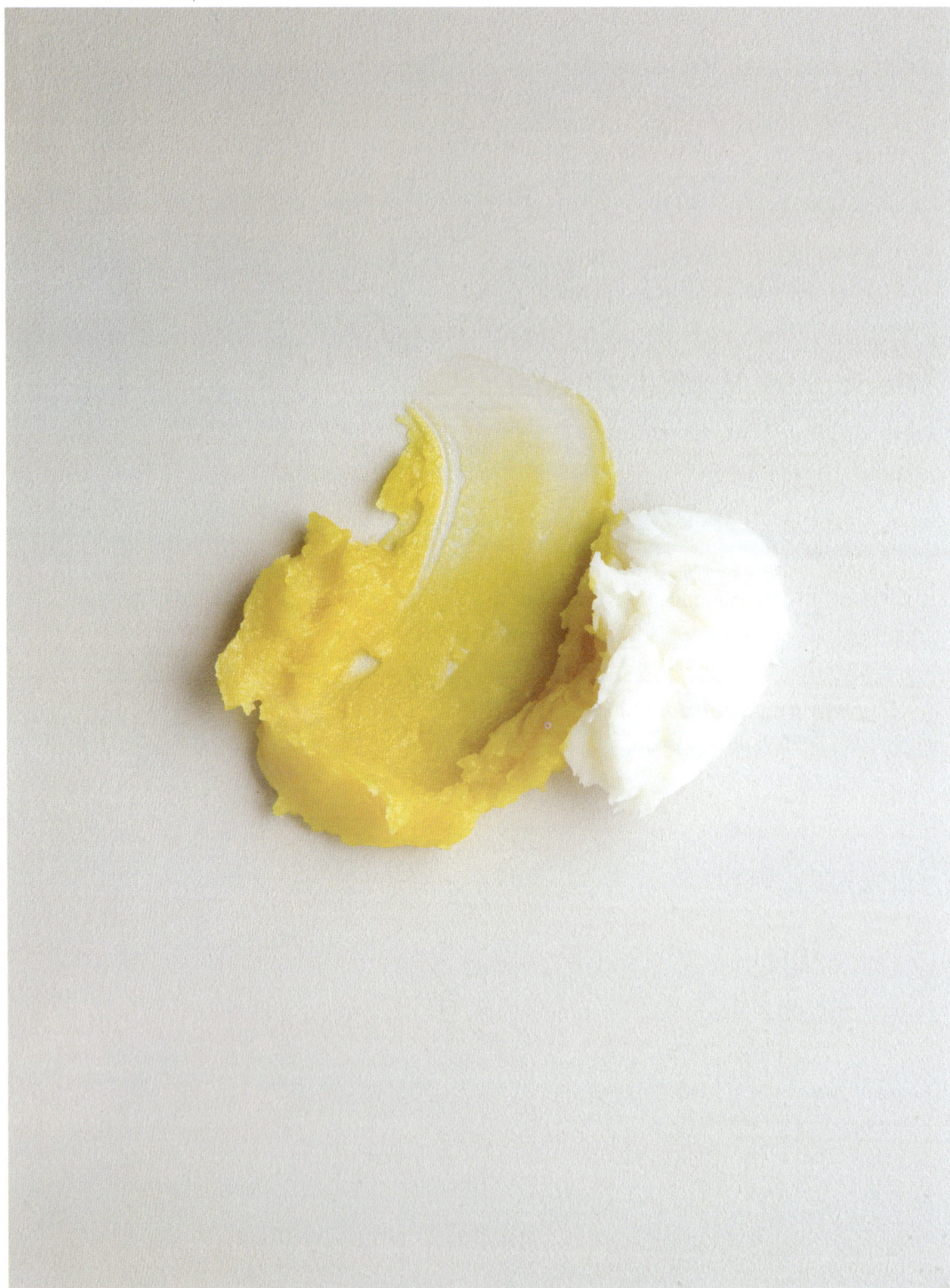

Beauty Balms

Simple aromatherapy balms are easy-to-make recipes of essential oils blended with vegetable oils, infused oils, plant butters and natural waxes to heal, nourish and protect your skin and impart aromatherapy benefits.

Lip Balms

Create protective, moisturising lip balms from skin nourishing ingredients.

Follow the *Methods for making aromatherapy balms* on page 63, combining the ingredients in the following recipes.

Find more lip balm recipes on page 141.

Lip conditioning balm

40 g shea butter
5 g candelilla wax
3 g liquid lecithin
2 g castor oil

Fresh mint lip balm

50 g shea butter
10 drops peppermint essential oil

Citrus zest lip balm

50 g shea butter
5 drops sweet orange essential oil
4 drops lemon essential oil
3 drops lime essential oil

Body Balms

Create a body balm to moisturise, repair and protect your skin.

Follow the *Methods for making aromatherapy balms* on page 63, combining the ingredients in the following recipes.

Nourishing body balm

A rich nourishing balm to protect and soften your skin.

50 g cocoa butter
10 g shea butter
25 g avocado oil
5 g carrot infused oil
8 drops patchouli essential oil
3 drops Roman chamomile essential oil
2 drops ylang ylang essential oil

Hand and cuticle repair balm

Repairs and protects hands exposed to harsh conditions.

90 g shea butter
10 g calendula infused oil
12 drops lavender essential oil
5 drops tea tree essential oil
3 drops everlasting essential oil

All-purpose healing balm

Repairs, soothes, protects the skin on any part of the body.

90 g shea butter
5 g calendula infused oil
5 g rosehip oil
6 drops everlasting essential oil
6 drops patchouli essential oil
5 drops geranium essential oil
3 drops German chamomile essential oil

Beauty Balms

Create these beautiful facial balms by following the *Methods for making aromatherapy balms* on page 63, and combining the ingredients in the following recipes.

Rose cleansing balm
for dry and mature skin

Massage over your face using circular movements to cleanse and remove make-up. Wet the palms of your hands with warm water and massage over your face. Soak a clean face cloth in warm water, wring out the excess water, place it over your face and press it into your skin. Then, using the cloth, wipe away the cleansing balm. Follow by thoroughly wiping over your face with a cotton pad dampened with a toner or floral water suited to your skin type.

30 g cocoa butter
20 g jojoba oil
5 drops rose otto

Ultra-rich skin restoration balm
for dry and mature skin

An ultra-rich balm to protect and rejuvenate dry, depleted skin.

40 g shea butter
5 g calendula infused oil
5 g rosehip oil
5 drops lavender essential oil
3 drops everlasting essential oil
2 drops frankincense essential oil

Perfume Balms

Create a gorgeous little take anywhere aromatherapy perfume balm to lift your spirits and bring pleasure to your day.

Follow the methods for *Making aromatherapy balms* on page 63, combining the ingredients in the following recipes.

Find more information and recipes for perfumes on page 241.

Fresh energy perfume balm

A fresh, herbaceous, uplifting scent.

10 g beeswax
40 g jojoba oil
27 drops lemon essential oil
10 drops lavender essential oil
9 drops Atlas cedarwood essential oil
4 drops sage essential oil

Warm earth perfume balm

A warm, earthy, grounding perfume.

30 g cocoa butter
20 g jojoba oil
30 drops sweet orange essential oil
10 drops patchouli essential oil
5 drops geranium essential oil
5 drops ginger essential oil
5 drops vetiver essential oil

Flourish perfume balm

A soft, sweet, floral fragrance.

10 g beeswax
40 g jojoba oil
15 drops sandalwood essential oil
10 drops geranium essential oil
10 drops rose otto
5 drops ylang ylang essential oil

Lime and coconut curl shaping balm

60 g cocoa butter
40 g coconut oil
40 drops lime essential oil

Sage and cedar hair texturising balm

45 g kaolin clay
55 g shea butter
15 drops Atlas cedarwood essential oil
5 drops sage essential oil

Hair Balms

Use a tiny amount of one of these balms to add shine to your hair, shape your curls or texturise your hair.

Follow the *Methods for making aromatherapy balms* on page 63, combining the ingredients in the following recipes.

Find more hair balm recipes on page 269.

Sandalwood hair shine balm

15 g beeswax
85 g jojoba oil
30 drops sandalwood essential oil

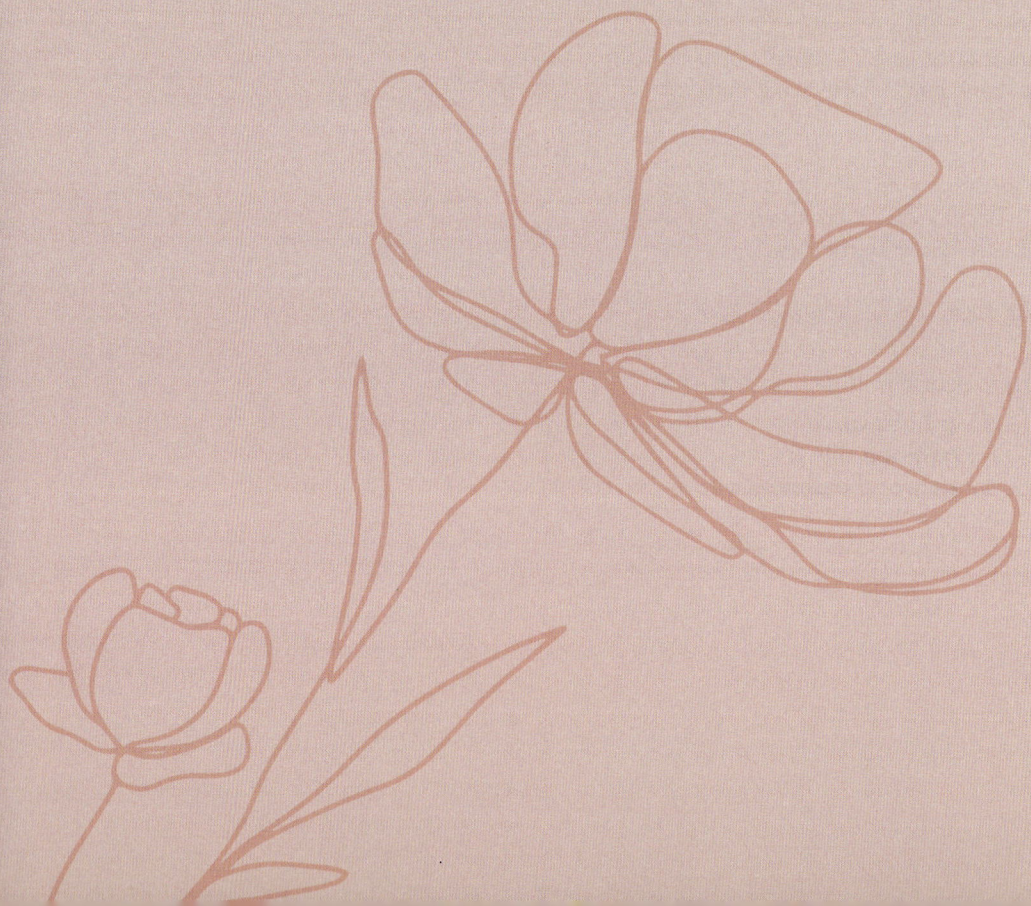

Face

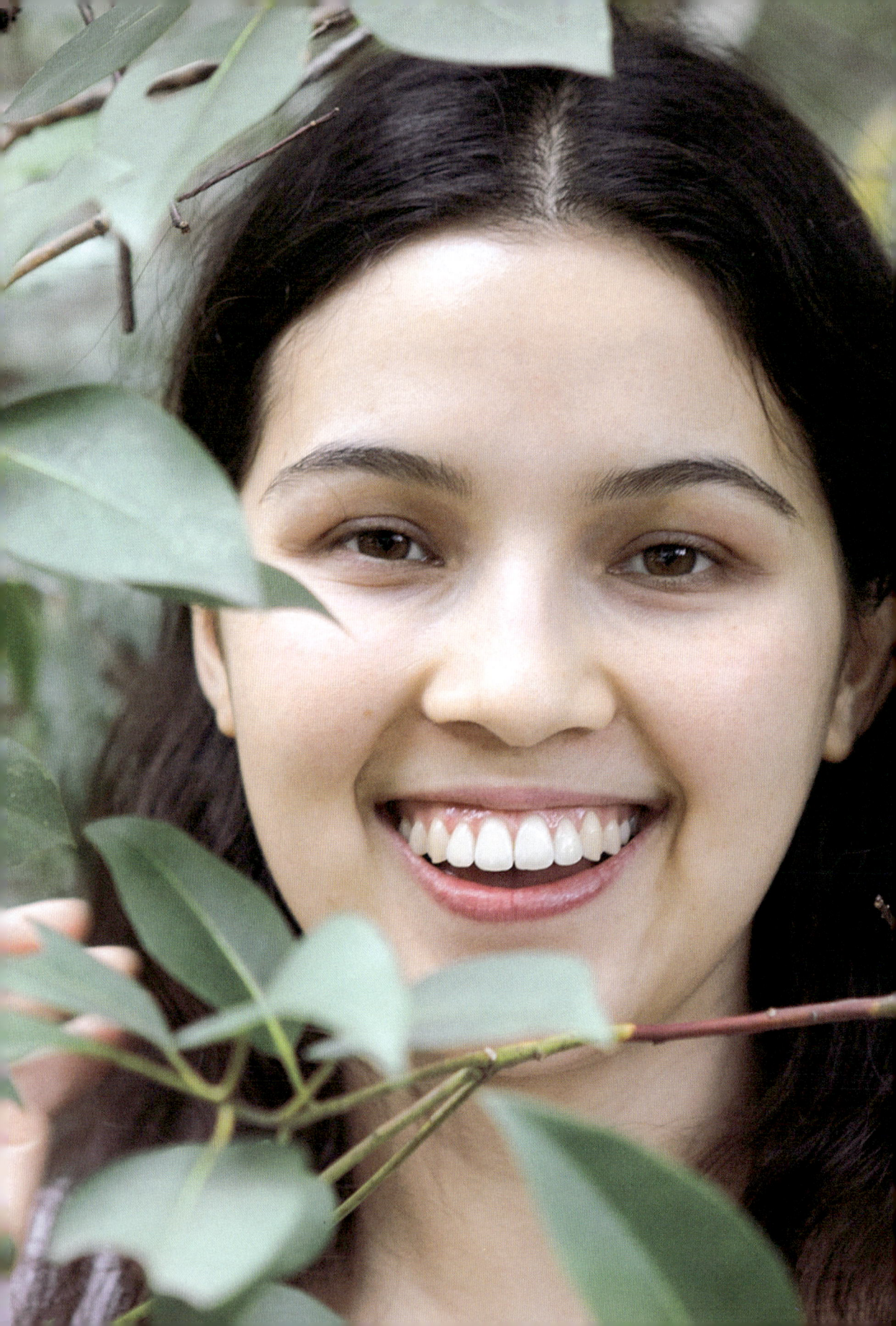

Skin Types and Conditions

Understanding your skin type along with any conditions it may have is key to identifying the skin care preparations most suitable for your skin. While your skin type and any skin conditions that may develop are dependent on your genetics, various health, lifestyle and environmental factors play an important part in determining the wellbeing of your skin. These factors include:

- climate — including exposure to heat, sun, humidity, cold, wind, dry conditions
- UV radiation
- indoor heating and air conditioning
- long, hot baths and showers
- cosmetic ingredients and formulations
- medications
- emotional wellbeing, including stress
- sleep
- diet
- illness
- hormones
- smoking
- pollution.

Skin Types

Skin type is dependent on the skin's sebaceous activity and it is common to have more than one skin type at any one time. Skin type changes as we age and is also affected by climate. For example, your skin may be oily in summer and may be relatively normal in winter.

Normal skin

So-called normal skin looks soft, moist, plump, dewy and firm, and has a healthy glow and even colour. It is neither excessively oily nor dry and is hydrated. The surface of the skin shows a fine texture, and there are no visible wrinkles, fine lines or open pores.

Dry skin

Dry skin is the result of sebaceous gland underactivity. It is hereditary but can also result from the aging process. Dry skin also tends to be dehydrated. Its lack of oil diminishes its ability to retain moisture. It tends to be very fine, with almost invisible pores, and tends to wrinkle easily. It may become rough and scaly.

Oily skin

Oily skin develops due to overactive sebaceous glands. This activity is controlled by the androgen hormones. Oily skin can be recognised by its shiny, oily appearance with enlarged pores. It can be exacerbated by climatic influences such as heat and humidity. It also tends to be affected by blocked pores and acne.

Combination skin

Combination skin is characterised by the existence of two or more different skin types or conditions. A classic combination skin has oily skin around the nose, forehead and chin, but normal or dry on the rest of the face. This is one of the most common skin types.

When treating combination skin, each area is treated for its particular needs. For example, when applying a mask, a mask formulated for oily skin is applied to the oily areas of the face and a mask formulated for dry skin is applied to dry areas. A combination skin may only need a touch of moisturiser in the oily zone with a heavier application to the rest of the face.

Skin Conditions

Skin conditions may occur with all skin types. Skin conditions develop over time or may be due to other factors such as those listed on page 117.

Dehydrated skin

This is one of the most common skin conditions. It indicates a lack of sufficient moisture in the cells and intercellular channels and looks dull with fine lines. It can become scaly or flaky and may feel itchy or become inflamed if dehydration worsens.

Dehydration may be caused and aggravated by excessive perspiration, lack of sufficient sebum to prevent evaporation of natural moisture, insufficient water intake, taking diuretics, illness and medications, atmospheric conditions, including exposure to sun and wind and a lack of moisture in the air, air conditioning, not using moisturisers, and cleansing with harsh soaps and water. Both dry and oily skins can be dehydrated.

Mature skin

Skin ages intrinsically (over time and due to genetic factors) and extrinsically (due to external factors such as exposure to UV radiation, diet and lifestyle).

It loses its elasticity and tone and sags with deepening lines and wrinkles. The skin becomes thinner, drier, dehydrated and dull, although some people with mature skin may still experience some oiliness. Growths and pigmentation appear along with small capillaries. This all happens in varying degrees as we age. Sun exposure is a major contributor to the premature aging of the skin. Changes occur in the epidermal, dermal and subdermal layers of the skin.

The junction of the epidermis and dermis is altered, with a reduction in blood supply to the epidermis resulting in reduced nutrients, metabolites and oxygen to this outermost layer of skin. The epidermis atrophies as cell production decreases. Skin cells are not replaced as regularly, causing drier and rougher skin and slower healing. The skin becomes dull and lacks a healthy glow. The number of melanocytes is reduced, resulting in skin that looks paler and has a reduced tolerance to sun exposure. The melanocytes that remain increase in size causing patches of pigmentation and age spots. Furthermore, the cumulative effects of chronic sun exposure mean the risk of skin cancer increases.

The dermis contains capillaries, which supply nutrients and oxygen vital to the skin cells. It comprises an extracellular matrix containing collagen and elastin fibres, which gives skin its strength, elasticity and resilience. Fibroblast cells produce collagen, elastin and other structural molecules in the extracellular matrix. It also contains mast cells that are responsible for the production of histamine.

As we age, the thickness of the dermis reduces with a decrease in the number of mast cells and a reduction in blood flow. Fibroblast cells shrivel and their activity decreases over time. This means collagen production decreases, and subsequently the number of fibres. The organised bundles of fibres atrophy, rupture and become fragmented, degraded and disorganised, with losses in their interwoven connections with elastin fibres. They cross-link and become stiff. Their capacity to bind water is diminished along with a decrease in the mucopolysaccharides in the extracellular matrix. This contributes to skin sagging, wrinkle formation and impairment in wound healing. Sebaceous and sweat gland activity is also reduced. The protection against infection provided by the acidity of sebum is reduced.

The subdermis experiences a loss of and redistribution of subcutaneous fat, with reduction around the cheeks and deposition around the nasolabial folds and below the chin. This means the skin looks thinner in some areas and sags more in others. It also becomes less resistant to trauma and has reduced thermoregulation. Mature skin tends to benefit from richer, thicker, more protective and nourishing creams.

Sensitive skin

Sensitive skin is hyperreactive and easily irritated. It can express itself with the following range of reactions — redness, itching, stinging and burning, all the way through to rashes, papules and scaling.

It is aggravated by environmental stressors such as wind, sun and heat, and certain products that it may come into contact with including industrial, household, skin care and cosmetic products.

Skin care and cosmetic product ingredients such as perfume, preservatives and even some essential oils may be irritating to sensitive skin. Overwashing with soap and hot water, facial scrubbing, and the use of astringents with a high level of alcohol will aggravate this skin condition, especially through the removal of the skin's lipid barrier.

Some people are born with skin that is generally more sensitive, while others have various genetic inflammatory skin conditions, including acne, rosacea, eczema and psoriasis, that make the skin more sensitive. A person who has contact dermatitis has become sensitised to specific allergens due to repeated exposure and will continue to be triggered by them. Someone who is normally unreactive to skin care products may temporarily become sensitive if their skin has recently been treated harshly or become compromised. It will return to normal once given proper care. As skin ages, it becomes more sensitive.

Certain parts of the body such as eyelids and armpits are often more sensitive than other parts of the body.

Acne

Acne is a chronic inflammatory disease of the sebaceous glands and hair follicles. It is characterised by comedones (closed — whiteheads, and open — blackheads), papules, pustules and cysts.

A combination of related factors produces acne, including increased sebum production, a proliferation of *Propionibacterium acnes* in the follicles and sebaceous glands, and an increase in skin cell production and inflammation.

Acne vulgaris is the most common form of acne, especially during the teenage years. Most adolescents have some manifestation of acne, with peak incidence occurring in the mid to late teens. Other more severe forms of acne such as cystic acne, acne conglobata and rosacea require medical attention.

For many people, acne is a mild and short-lived condition. Most of those with acne are free of the condition by their early 20s. However, it can persist into the 30s and 40s with premenstrual flare-ups. Some people find that it persists beyond menopause.

Hormones, stress, cosmetic and skin care products, medications and diet can exacerbate acne. Some people find that dairy products and refined sugar exacerbate acne. It may be worse in hot humid climates.

Acne-prone skin should avoid thick moisturisers and heavy oils and balms. While cleansing and exfoliation is important, overdoing it will cause other skin problems such as irritation, inflammation and dehydration.

Rosacea

Rosacea appears as red skin generally in the middle part of the face, with the appearance of dilated blood vessels on the nose and cheeks, and can affect the eyelids. Pimples and bumps containing pus may also develop and the skin may feel hot, tender and sensitive. Over time, the skin on the nose may thicken and appear bulbous.

Rosacea may be triggered or aggravated by a variety of stressors such as sun exposure and other climatic conditions including heat, cold and wind; emotional stress; exercise; dietary triggers such as spices, alcohol, food additives and hot beverages; and cosmetic ingredients such as perfumes and fragrance additives. It may subside and reappear, becoming worse over time. The causes of rosacea are unknown but may involve genetics, damaged blood vessels, and a sensitivity to a skin mite called *Demodex folliculorum* or a proliferation of it. Other studies suggest gut bacteria may raise gastrin levels, which may cause the skin to look flushed. Avoiding known triggers and medical treatment are important for managing the condition and for reducing the potential for increase in severity. Skin care products for sensitive skin are recommended as the skin is very sensitive and irritated, and may be painful.

Couperose

Couperose appears as small, dilated, winding, bright red blood vessels on the cheeks, around the nose and sometimes on the chin. It occurs as a result of poor elasticity of the capillary wall and gives the appearance of diffuse or local redness. It is most obvious on fair skin.

It is aggravated by extremes of temperature, by the use of excessively cold or hot water, nervous disorders, digestive disorders, poor nutrition, saunas, exercise that causes the face to turn very red, drinking very hot liquids, eating spicy foods, blushing, smoking, alcohol, and harsh and aggressive use of products such as scrubs and alcohol-based toners.

Devitalised skin

Devitalised skin takes on a dull cast. This type of skin can handle a lot of massage and stimulation to increase blood circulation. If not looked after, it can become very tired looking.

Cleansers

The most important part of caring for your skin is cleansing it properly. Without careful cleansing, the skin can look dull and various skin conditions may develop or be made worse. If you are in good health and live in idyllic pollution-free conditions, a rinse with warm water may be sufficient.

A cleanser will remove excess oil, perspiration, dirt, dust, pollution, make-up and naturally loosened dead skin cells from the surface of your skin, and to a certain extent, from your skin's pores.

It will help to dislodge blockages, such as blackheads, and can begin to treat a skin problem (for example, rehydrating a dry skin or reducing excess sebum in the case of an oily skin).

Your cleanser should not cause the removal of too much oil or moisture or upset your skin's pH balance significantly. Furthermore, it should not be irritating.

A cleanser is formulated from a choice of the following basic ingredients:

- **water** for moisture and fluidity and to allow any dissolved or dispersed impurities to be rinsed off or removed easily. It also serves as a solvent for water-soluble active ingredients
- **emollients**, such as vegetable oils, to soften and lubricate the skin and to help dissolve impurities for removal
- **emulsifiers** to hold together any water- and oil-based ingredients that have been emulsified and to help lift impurities from the skin into the cleanser. For this reason, cleansers may contain more emulsifier than moisturisers. Additional waxes and gums may be added to assist in stabilising the emulsion
- **surfactants** to produce foam, which dissolves and lifts impurities from the skin. They are most often found in cleansing gels and foaming washes for combination and oily skin
- **active ingredients**, such as plant extracts and essential oils, to help treat a particular skin type or condition. However, as a cleansing preparation remains on the skin only a short time, more expensive active ingredients may be better incorporated into preparations that remain on the skin, such as moisturisers, serums and oils
- **preservatives** to reduce contamination and rapid deterioration of preparations that contain water due to the growth of yeasts, moulds and bacteria, and to protect the user.

Use your cleanser twice daily, in the morning and at the end of the day. Your skin should be cleansed in the morning because your skin excretes waste onto the surface throughout the night. At the end of the day, your skin should be cleansed twice: once to remove surface impurities, such as pollutants and make-up, and again to better cleanse the pores.

If you are wearing eye make-up, remove it first before cleansing the rest of your face.

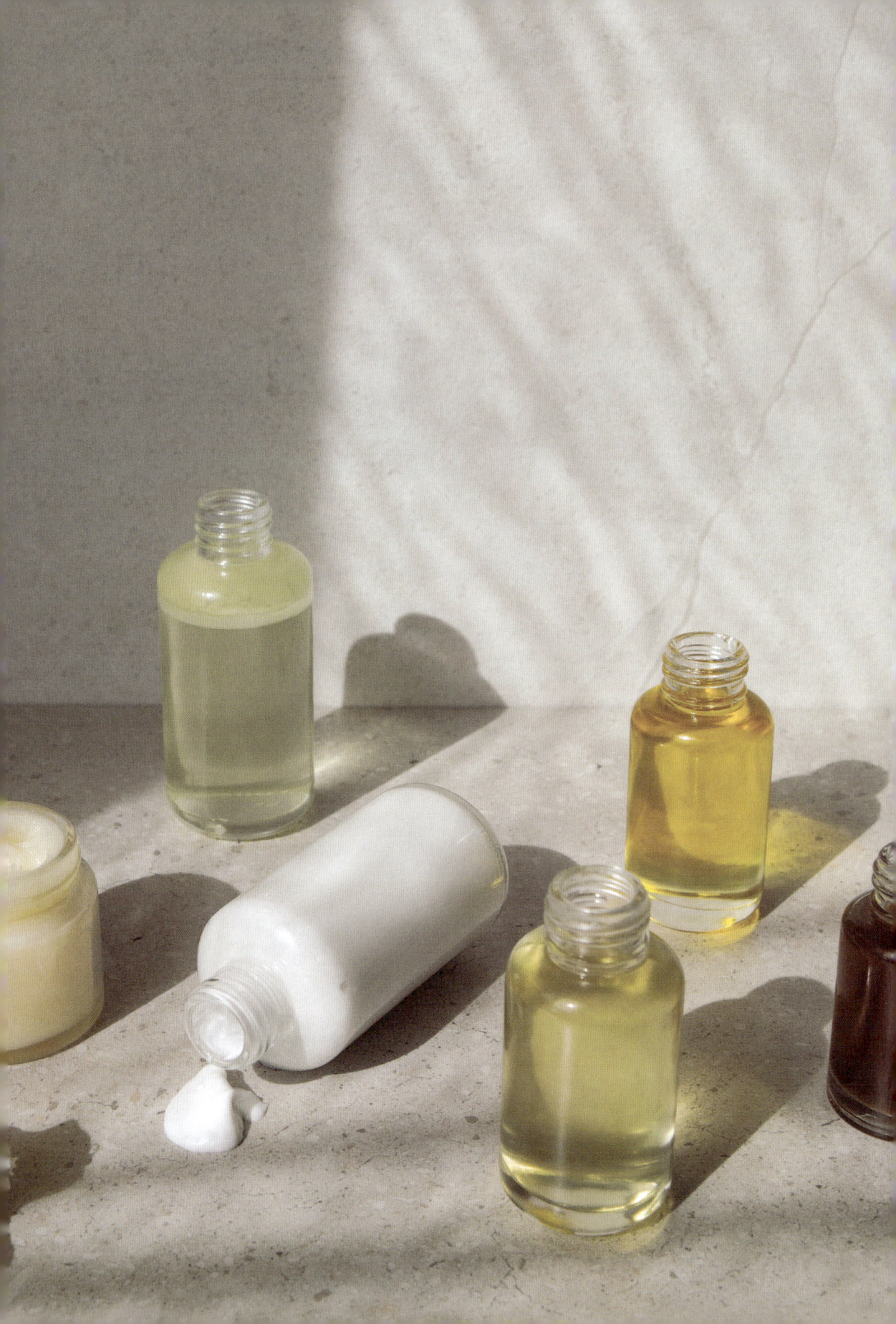

Massage your cleanser thoroughly over your entire face, especially over any areas of blocked pores. Then remove it completely with a damp sponge or cloth, and rinse. Your skin will feel clean, soft and hydrated. Follow with a skin toner or freshener such as a floral water.

Cleansing Oils

As it is the oil in a cleansing cream that helps dissolve impurities, it is often used on its own to remove heavy, oil-based make-up or waterproof mascara. An oil cleanser is especially suitable for very dry skin that is lacking in oil and for delicate, sensitive skin.

A cleansing oil can be used by massaging the oil over your face using circular movements. Ensure you use enough oil to cover your skin well. Then, wet the palms of your hands with warm water and massage over your face. Soak a clean face cloth in warm water, wring out the excess water, place it over your face and press it into your skin. Then, using the cloth, wipe away the cleansing oil. Follow by thoroughly wiping over your face with a cotton pad dampened with a toner or floral water suited to your skin type, ensuring no traces of make-up are left on your skin.

Jojoba oil is a superb choice as a simple cleansing oil as it has a fine texture. Otherwise, apricot kernel oil or sweet almond oil, which have a slightly heavier feel, are good choices.

Jojoba oil can be used to carefully remove eye make-up. Add a few drops of jojoba oil to a cotton pad dampened with warm water and gently wipe the make-up from your

eyelids and lashes. Be careful not to wipe into your eyes. Use jojoba oil without any added essential oils to avoid eye irritation.

Neroli cleansing oil
Skin type: normal to dry

A calming cleansing oil that is also suitable for make-up removal.

95 mL jojoba oil
5 mL sweet almond oil
5 drops neroli essential oil

Simply add the drops of neroli essential oil to the jojoba oil and sweet almond oil in a glass bottle and shake well.

Find more cleansing oil recipes on page 103.

Cleansing Balms

Cleansing balms provide a rich, convenient medium for cleansing dry skin. They are used in the same way a cleansing oil is used to cleanse the skin.

Luxe cleansing balm
Skin type: dry skin

Especially good for dry skin and skin that is constantly exposed to dry environments. It is suitable for make-up removal.

15 g beeswax
75 g apricot kernel oil
10 g coconut oil
9 drops mandarin essential oil
3 drops geranium essential oil
3 drops Roman chamomile essential oil

Make this cleansing balm by following the *Aromatherapy balm method 1* on page 63.

Find *Rose cleansing balm* made with vegan ingredients on page 112.

Cleansing Creams and Lotions

Skin that is dry, dehydrated or sensitive benefits most from cleansing creams and lotions. The removal of make-up is most effectively achieved with a cleansing cream or lotion. Cleansing creams and lotions range from thick, oily creams through to light, water-soluble lotions.

Galen's original cold cream
Skin type: dry

A cold cream is a very rich, water-in-oil emulsion or water-in-oil wax suspension. It contains a large amount of oil and a relatively small amount of water. When applied to the skin, the water quickly evaporates causing a cooling effect, hence the name 'cold' cream. It separates easily allowing this to happen. The oil left on the skin mixes with impurities on the skin. The oil containing the impurities is then removed with warm water and a cleansing sponge or cloth.

It was in the second century AD that the Greek physician Galen made a crude cream by mixing water into a blend of molten beeswax and olive oil — the first cold cream. By the 19th century, borax was added to stabilise the mixture.

Cold creams are useful for make-up removal and are suitable cleansers for very dry skin. The same cream can also be used as a rich moisturiser.

Oil phase
20 g beeswax
90 g olive oil

Water phase
90 g rosewater

This cold cream does not have a preservative. It will need to be stored in the refrigerator and used within a couple of weeks.

Make *Galen's original cold cream* by following the *Method for making an emulsion with beeswax* on page 86.

Rich cleansing cream
Skin type: dry and sensitive

This rich, thick cream is based on a traditional cold cream formula. It is suitable for make-up removal and for cleansing dry, sensitive skin.

Oil phase
10 g plant-derived emulsifying wax
124 g sweet almond oil
1 g antioxidant

Water phase
63 g purified water
2 g preservative

Add at 40°C
1 g (approx. 20 drops) essential oil

pH adjustment
qs citric acid + purified water

Choose an essential oil or essential oil composition for your skin type from pages 39—48 and make this cleanser by following the *Method for making an emulsion with emulsifying wax* on page 79.

Light cleansing cream
Skin type: normal to dry, sensitive

This skin-softening cleansing cream is suitable for dry skin and removing make-up. However, it is lighter and easier to remove than the *Rich cleansing cream* above.

Oil phase
10 g plant-derived emulsifying wax
35 g sweet almond oil
1 g antioxidant

Water phase
152 g purified water
2 g preservative

Add at 40°C
1 g (approx. 20 drops) essential oil

pH adjustment
qs citric acid + purified water

Choose an essential oil or essential oil composition for your skin type from pages 39—48 and make this cleanser by following the *Method for making an emulsion with emulsifying wax* on page 79.

Ultra-light water-soluble cleansing cream
Skin type: most skin types

This cleanser is suitable for use on most skin types as it removes impurities without leaving the skin feeling dry. It is lighter than the previous cleansers and is also suitable for removing make-up. The oil will dissolve the impurities, and the emulsifier will allow the oil and impurities to be lifted off the skin and be mixed with water to be rinsed away.

Oil phase
10 g plant-derived emulsifying wax
19 g apricot kernel oil
1 g antioxidant

Water phase
168 g purified water
2 g preservative

Add at 40°C
1 g (approx. 20 drops) essential oil

pH adjustment
qs citric acid + purified water

Choose an essential oil or essential oil composition for your skin type from pages 39—48 and make this cleanser by following the *Method for making an emulsion with emulsifying wax* on page 79.

Foaming Cleansers

This type of cleanser is especially suitable for oily skin as no oil is left behind to exacerbate blocked pores or pimples. The addition of ingredients such as vegetable oils can reduce the amount of foam produced and the drying effects on the skin.

The following foaming cleansers are based on Castile liquid soap, a skin cleansing liquid soap traditionally made with olive oil.

Simple Castile liquid soap may be used to cleanse oily skin. Only a small quantity needs to be used. Massage it over a damp face and remove it by rinsing or removing it with a damp face cloth or sponge. The addition of the appropriate essential oils will help to improve your skin's condition.

Salt solution for thickening

A salt solution can be added to your Castile liquid soap recipes to thicken them. It is a simple solution of ordinary table salt (sodium chloride) dissolved into purified water.

1. Make a salt solution with 5 g of table salt dissolved into 25 g of purified water.
2. Add drops of the salt solution slowly while stirring into the Castile liquid soap/essential oil mixture. You will need to watch the mixture for the point at which it starts to thicken. Do not add too much salt solution as it will turn into a lumpy gel.

For more recipes based on Castile liquid soap, see page 101.

Castile cleansing wash
Skin type: normal to oily

100 mL Castile liquid soap
20 drops essential oil

1. Choose an essential oil or essential oil composition for your skin type from pages 39–48, add to the Castile liquid soap and shake well.
2. **Optional:** Add up to 60 drops of salt solution for thickening following the instructions above.

Soft almond Castile cleanser
Skin type: normal to dry

A mild cleansing wash for drier skin may be made by adding a small quantity of vegetable oil to the Castile liquid soap.

80 mL Castile liquid soap
20 mL sweet almond oil
20 drops essential oil

1. Choose an essential oil or essential oil composition for your skin type from pages 39–48 and add to the sweet almond oil.

2. Stir the Castile liquid soap into the sweet almond oil mixture, continuing to stir until the mixture is homogenous.
3. Store in a bottle and shake each time before use.

Soapwort gentle skin cleanser
Skin type: sensitive

A particularly gentle cleansing decoction for sensitive, irritated or inflamed skin. It is also suitable for use as a gentle body wash and hair cleanser.

10 g soapwort root
250 mL purified water

1. Boil and simmer the soapwort root in the water for 20–30 minutes.
2. Remove from the heat and allow to cool.
3. Strain the liquid.
4. Massage the liquid over your skin and rinse. Be careful not to get it in your eyes.
5. Store in the refrigerator and use within a couple of days.

Shaving Products

These shaving products can be used on the face or anywhere else on the body you would like to shave.

Lime emollient shaving cream

A hair and skin softening shaving cream that provides glide for a smooth shave. This shaving cream does not lather but provides a smooth surface for shaving.

<u>Oil phase</u>
16 g plant-derived emulsifying wax
31 g macadamia oil
1 g antioxidant

<u>Water phase</u>
150 g purified water
2 g preservative

<u>Add at 40°C</u>
1 g (approx.) 20 drops lime essential oil

<u>pH adjustment</u>
qs citric acid + purified water

1. Make this shaving cream by following the *Method for making an emulsion with emulsifying wax* on page 79 and store in a jar.

2. Before shaving, wet the beard area or area of hair you would like to shave, then smooth on the *Lime emollient shaving cream*.

Patchouli shaving gel

This lathering shaving gel is easy to make and use.

100 mL Castile liquid soap
up to 60 drops salt solution
20 drops patchouli essential oil

1. Add the essential oil to the Castile liquid soap and stir in.

2. Add up to 60 drops of salt solution for thickening following the instructions on page 125.

3. Store in a bottle.

4. Before shaving, wet the beard area or area of hair you would like to shave, then lather up with this shaving gel.

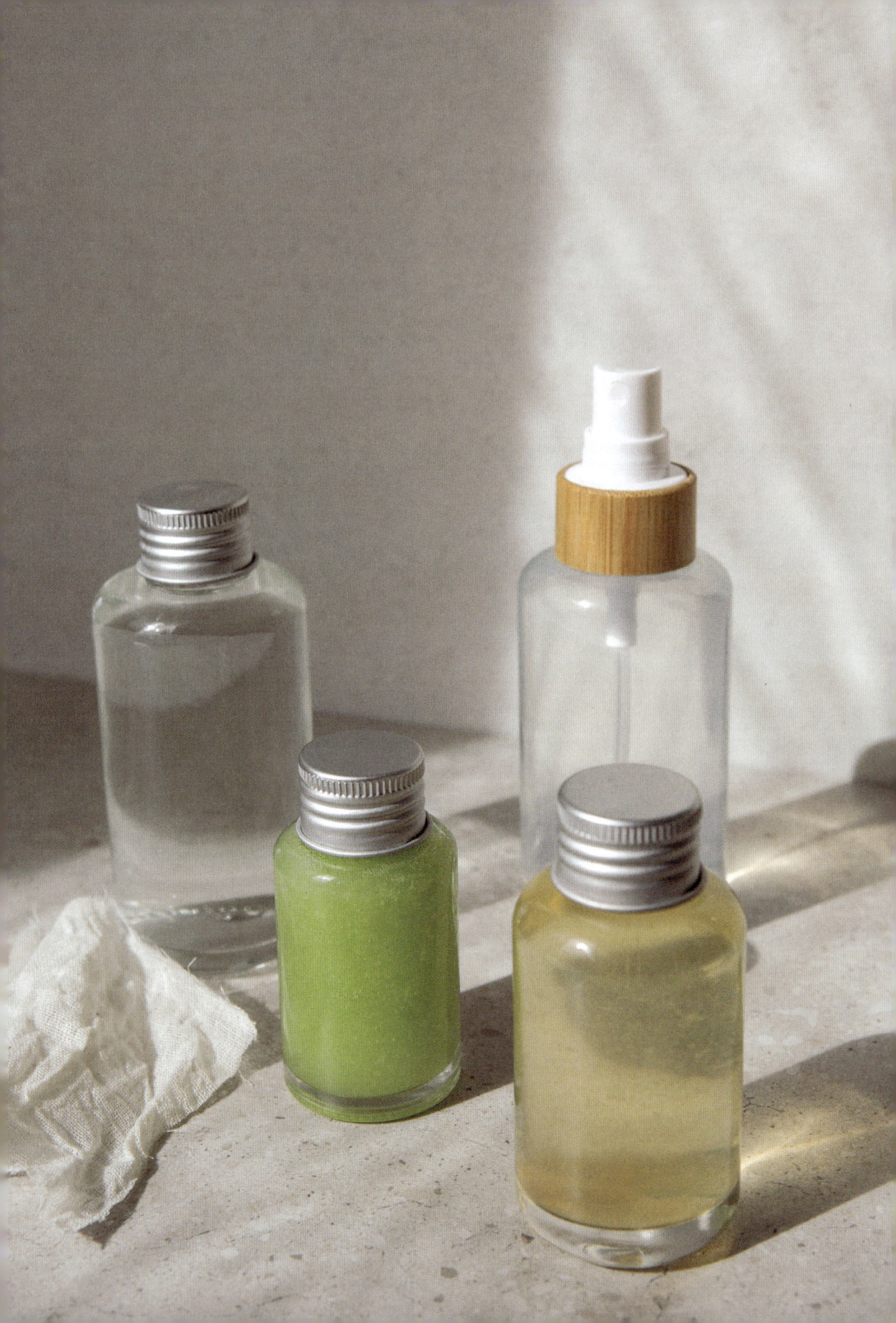

Toners

A toner, also known as a skin freshener or toning lotion, is an aqueous liquid used after cleansing.

Toners are used to:

- remove any traces of cleanser still left on the skin as well as any tap water used to rinse the skin
- cool, soothe and refresh the skin
- help redress the skin's pH balance (the skin does this naturally after a period of time)
- help treat a skin condition due to the content of active ingredients
- minimise pore size temporarily. This happens when the skin is either cooled or restored to its slightly acidic pH. This causes the salt-type cross linkages between the molecules of keratin to reform.

Use your toner by applying it to damp cotton wool and wiping it over your face or misting it over your face.

It is the first step in adding moisture to the skin's surface, as it remains on the skin, and is applied to the skin just before the application of a moisturiser. Do not allow your skin to dry out completely before applying your moisturiser.

Formulate your own toner by using the following active plant ingredients.

Hydrosols/Floral Waters

Distilled floral or herb waters, also known as hydrosols and hydrolats, applied by themselves or in combination with other ingredients, make excellent healing and soothing toning lotions. Refer to page 29 to choose a floral water that is suitable for your skin type.

Herbal Infusions

Herbal infusions that have been allowed to cool can be used as healing toning lotions. Refer to the section starting at page 14 to choose herbs that are suitable for your skin type and follow the *Method for making herbal infusions* on page 49. Alternatively, try one of the suggested mixes from *Clean & Minimal — Beauty Infusions* on page 91. Infusions should be stored in the refrigerator and used within 2 or 3 days as they provide a medium for microbial growth.

Aloe vera juice can be used on its own for its soothing, healing benefits, or added as an ingredient to floral waters or infusions.

Herbal Vinegars

Herbal vinegars make excellent skin toners. Apple cider vinegar helps redress the skin's pH while the herbs add other healing properties. However, apple cider vinegar should be carefully diluted before application to the skin.

Make a herbal vinegar by following the *Method for making herbal vinegars* on page 54 and choose one for your skin type from the *Clean & Minimal — Beauty Vinegars* on page 108.

To make a skin toner, dilute 1 teaspoon of the herbal vinegar in 100 mL of purified water, floral water or herbal infusion. Once diluted, a herbal vinegar toner should be used within 2 or 3 days as the solution provides a medium for microbial growth.

Simple apple cider vinegar toner
Skin type: all skin types

100 mL purified water
1 tsp apple cider vinegar

Add the apple cider vinegar to the purified water and store in a bottle. Keep in the refrigerator and use within 2 or 3 days.

Honey water
Skin type: oily and blemished

A soothing toner for oily and blemished skin.

100 mL purified water
1 tsp honey
1 tsp apple cider vinegar

Dissolve the honey in warmed purified water, stir in the apple cider vinegar and store in a bottle. Keep in the refrigerator and use within 2 or 3 days.

Lavender and myrrh healing toner
Skin type: oily and blemished

A healing, antiseptic and gentle astringent for oily and blemished skin.

100 mL lavender water
20 drops myrrh tincture

Add the myrrh tincture to the lavender water and store in a bottle.

Chamomile and calendula soothing mist
Skin type: sensitive

A calming, soothing skin freshener for sensitive and irritated skins.

1. Make a chamomile and calendula infusion by following the *Method for making herbal infusions* on page 49.
2. Pour the infusion into a spray bottle and mist over your face or apply to cotton wool pads and wipe over your face.
3. Store the liquid in a bottle and keep in the refrigerator. Use within 2 or 3 days.

Aloe vera skin toner
Skin type: all skin types, including sensitive

A very soothing, cooling and hydrating skin toner.

1. Make your aloe vera liquid by chopping off an aloe vera leaf from the plant, then slicing off the outer skin revealing the gel inside. Rinse the gel, then place into a blender and blend until it liquefies.
2. Store the liquid in a bottle and keep in the refrigerator. Use within 2 or 3 days.

Chilled cucumber tonic
Skin type: normal, combination and sensitive

A cool, refreshing skin toner for normal, combination and sensitive skin.

½ cucumber

Peel the cucumber, juice and strain. Store the liquid in a bottle in the refrigerator and use within 2 or 3 days.

Aromatic facial mist
Skin type: all skin types

Imagine misting your face with notes of rose, sandalwood or neroli. To make this a wonderfully refreshing mist, keep in the refrigerator in summer and mist over you to cool and calm your skin.

**100 g purified water or floral water
0.5 g (approx. 10 drops) essential oil
1 g essential oil solubiliser
1 g preservative**

pH adjustment
qs citric acid + purified water

1. Choose an essential oil or essential oil composition for your skin type from pages 39–48.
2. In a glass jug or beaker, mix your chosen essential oil or essential oil composition with the essential oil solubiliser.
3. Add the water or floral water to this mixture and stir well.
4. Add the preservative and stir well.
5. Check the pH and adjust following the instructions on page 74.
6. Store in a bottle.

Alternatively, follow steps 1 to 3, then store the mist in the refrigerator and use within 2 weeks.

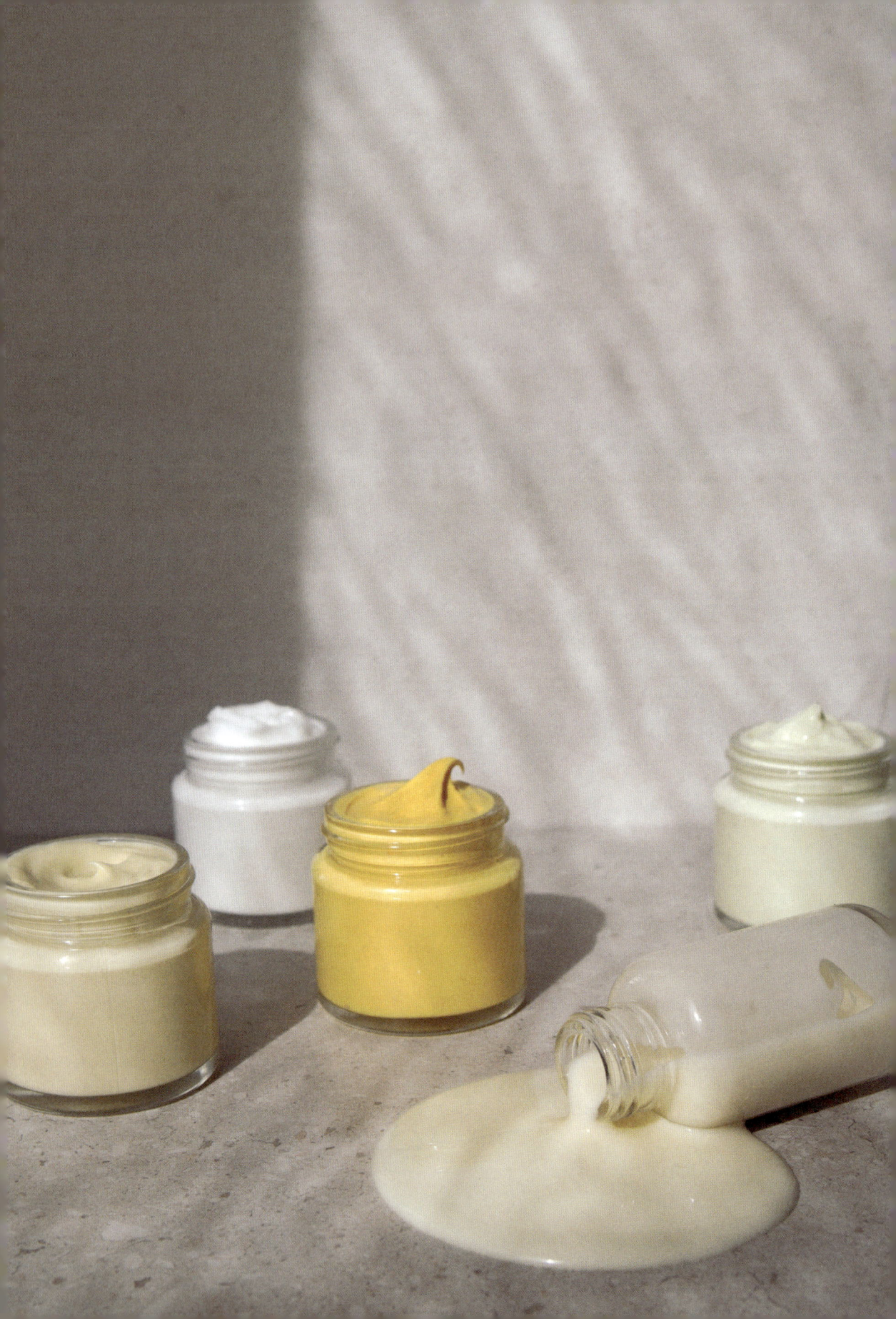

Moisturisers

A moisturiser, as the name implies, will provide moisture to the surface layers of the skin and will prevent dehydration and dryness. It keeps your skin smooth and supple.

A moisturiser is formulated with a selection of the following ingredients:

- **water** to add moisture to your skin and fluidity to your moisturiser. Choose from distilled water, purified water, floral waters or aloe vera juice for the water component of your skin moisturisers. Moisturisers for oilier skin types will tend to have a higher water content than moisturisers for drier skin

- **emollients and occlusives** to soften and lubricate the skin and prevent moisture/water evaporation. Cold-pressed vegetable oils and natural plant butters, such as cocoa butter and shea butter, have these properties. Moisturisers for dry skin will have a higher emollient content than moisturisers for oilier skin

- **emulsifiers** to hold together any water and oil components in the form of a cream or lotion

- **waxes** to thicken and give the product structure. Depending on the quantity used, the wax may provide a useful barrier on the skin

- **gums**, such as xanthan gum, which may be added in small amounts to assist in thickening and stabilising the emulsion

- **humectants** to bind water. They hold moisture in your cream and onto your skin. Vegetable glycerin is often used for this purpose

- **active ingredients** chosen to help treat a particular skin type or condition. These include essential oils, herbal extracts and antioxidants

- **preservatives** to prevent and reduce the growth of mould, yeast and bacteria.

A moisturiser is applied after toning and before make-up application. Massage it over and into the skin with firm upward strokes and then press into the skin.

A selection of moisturising creams follows. Once you feel confident with your emulsion-making skills, you may like to create recipes of your own by substituting the specified vegetable oils, infused oils, floral waters and essential oils with alternatives you decide are suitable.

When using the creams on your face, remove them from jars with a clean spatula or spoon to avoid contaminating them with microbes.

Cocoa butter rich moisture cream
Skin type: very dry

A rich, moisturising cream for very dry skin. It may also be used as a night cream.

Oil phase
10 g cocoa butter
10 g plant-derived emulsifying wax
40 g avocado oil
1 g antioxidant

Water phase
127 g purified water
10 g vegetable glycerin
2 g preservative

Add at 40°C
1 g (approx. 20 drops) sandalwood essential oil
or dry skin composition on page 48

pH adjustment
qs citric acid + purified water

Make this cream by following the *Method for making an emulsion with emulsifying wax* on page 79.

Rosehip vital essence cream
Skin type: dry and mature

A rich, nourishing cream for mature skin that has become dry, damaged and lacking in tone.

Oil phase
9 g plant-derived emulsifying wax
8 g shea butter
12 g apricot kernel oil
8 g evening primrose oil
8 g rosehip oil
4 g carrot infused oil
1 g antioxidant

Water phase
142 g rosewater
6 g vegetable glycerin
2 g preservative

Add at 40°C
1 g (approx. 20 drops) frankincense essential oil
or mature skin composition on page 48

pH adjustment
qs citric acid + purified water

Make this cream by following the *Method for making an emulsion with emulsifying wax* on page 79.

Add the evening primrose oil and rosehip oil, which are very heat sensitive, to the oil phase just as it reaches the correct temperature to ensure they are not exposed to a high temperature for too long.

Calendula caring cream
Skin type: sensitive

A wonderfully soothing and healing cream for sensitive skin, including skin with eczema, psoriasis and dermatitis.

Oil phase
9 g plant-derived emulsifying wax
40 g calendula infused oil
1 g antioxidant

Water phase
142 g purified water
6 g vegetable glycerin
2 g preservative

Add at 40°C
0.5 g (approx. 10 drops) everlasting essential oil
or sensitive skin composition on page 48

pH adjustment

qs citric acid + purified water

Make this cream by following the *Method for making an emulsion with emulsifying wax* on page 79.

Soothing lavender face cream
Skin type: dry and sensitive

A soothing, hydrating cream for dry and sensitive skin.

Oil phase

**8 g shea butter
8 g plant-derived emulsifying wax
15 g sweet almond oil
10 g calendula infused oil
1 g antioxidant**

Water phase

**150 g purified water
6 g vegetable glycerin
2 g preservative**

Add at 40°C

**0.5 g (approx. 10 drops) lavender essential oil
or sensitive skin composition on page 48**

pH adjustment

qs citric acid + purified water

Make this cream by following the *Method for making an emulsion with emulsifying wax* on page 79.

Pure plant moisturising cream
Skin type: normal

This cream is suitable for normal skin, that is, skin that is relatively balanced in its oil and moisture content. It will help maintain the skin's hydration level and protect it from dryness.

Oil phase

**8 g plant-derived emulsifying wax
20 g jojoba oil
12 g apricot kernel oil
1 g antioxidant**

Water phase

**151 g purified water
6 g vegetable glycerin
2 g preservative**

Add at 40°C

**1 g (approx. 20 drops) ylang ylang essential oil
or normal skin composition on page 48**

pH adjustment

qs citric acid + purified water

Make this cream by following the *Method for making an emulsion with emulsifying wax* on page 79.

Rare roses moisture cream
Skin type: most skin types

The feel and smell of preparations containing pure rose extracts are a divine treat for the skin and soul. The *Rare roses moisture cream* is a beautiful, light moisture cream for most skin types, except for very oily skins.

Oil phase

**8 g plant-derived emulsifying wax
30 g sweet almond oil
1 g antioxidant**

Water phase

153 g rosewater
6 g vegetable glycerin
2 g preservative

Add at 40°C

0.5 g (approx. 10 drops) rose absolute or
rose otto

pH adjustment

qs citric acid + purified water

Make this cream by following the *Method for making an emulsion with emulsifying wax* on page 79.

Jojoba fine moisture cream
Skin type: combination

A beautiful cream for skin requiring a lighter moisturiser. Combination skin as well as skin that is both oily and dehydrated will benefit from using this cream.

Oil phase

7 g plant-derived emulsifying wax
22 g jojoba oil
1 g antioxidant

Water phase

162 g purified water
6 g vegetable glycerin
2 g preservative

Add at 40°C

1 g (approx. 20 drops) geranium essential oil or combination skin composition on page 48

pH adjustment

qs citric acid + purified water

Make this cream by following the *Method for making an emulsion with emulsifying wax* on page 79.

Hydration emulsion
Skin type: oily and combination

This is a lightweight hydrating emulsion for oily and combination skin.

Oil phase

30 g jojoba oil
1 g antioxidant

Water phase

8 g lecithin granules
149 g purified water
2 g xanthan gum
8 g vegetable glycerin
2 g preservative

Add at 40°C

1 g (approx. 20 drops) mandarin or combination skin composition on page 48

pH adjustment

qs citric acid + purified water

Make this emulsion by following the *Hot-process method for making an emulsion with lecithin* on page 84.

Oil-regulating moisture gel
Skin type: oily

An oil-free moisturiser for very oily skin that may block and break out when products containing oil are applied.

1 g xanthan gum
189 g purified water (or floral water)
8 g vegetable glycerin
2 g preservative
10 drops lemon essential oil
4 drops geranium essential oil
4 drops juniper essential oil

pH adjustment

qs citric acid + purified water solution

Make this gel by following the *Method for making gel bases* on page 67.

Blemish gel

This gel is an antiseptic healing gel for pimples and spots. It should be applied directly to the pimple or spot only, not spread over the face, as the concentration of essential oils is high. Apply twice a day after cleansing and avoid the area with moisturiser.

1 g xanthan gum
191 g lavender water
6 g vegetable glycerin
2 g preservative
50 drops lavender essential oil
20 drops geranium essential oil
20 drops tea tree essential oil
10 drops German chamomile essential oil

pH adjustment
qs citric acid + purified water solution

Make this gel by following the *Method for making gel bases* on page 67. Shake each time before use.

Pick-me-up gel

A great pick-me-up gel that cools and refreshes all skin types. It may be applied before putting on your regular moisturiser or throughout the day whenever you need a refreshing pick-me-up!

1 g xanthan gum
191 g rosewater
6 g vegetable glycerin
2 g preservative
11 drops sweet orange essential oil
4 drops ylang ylang essential oil

pH adjustment
qs citric acid + water solution

Make this gel by following the *Method for making gel bases* on page 67.

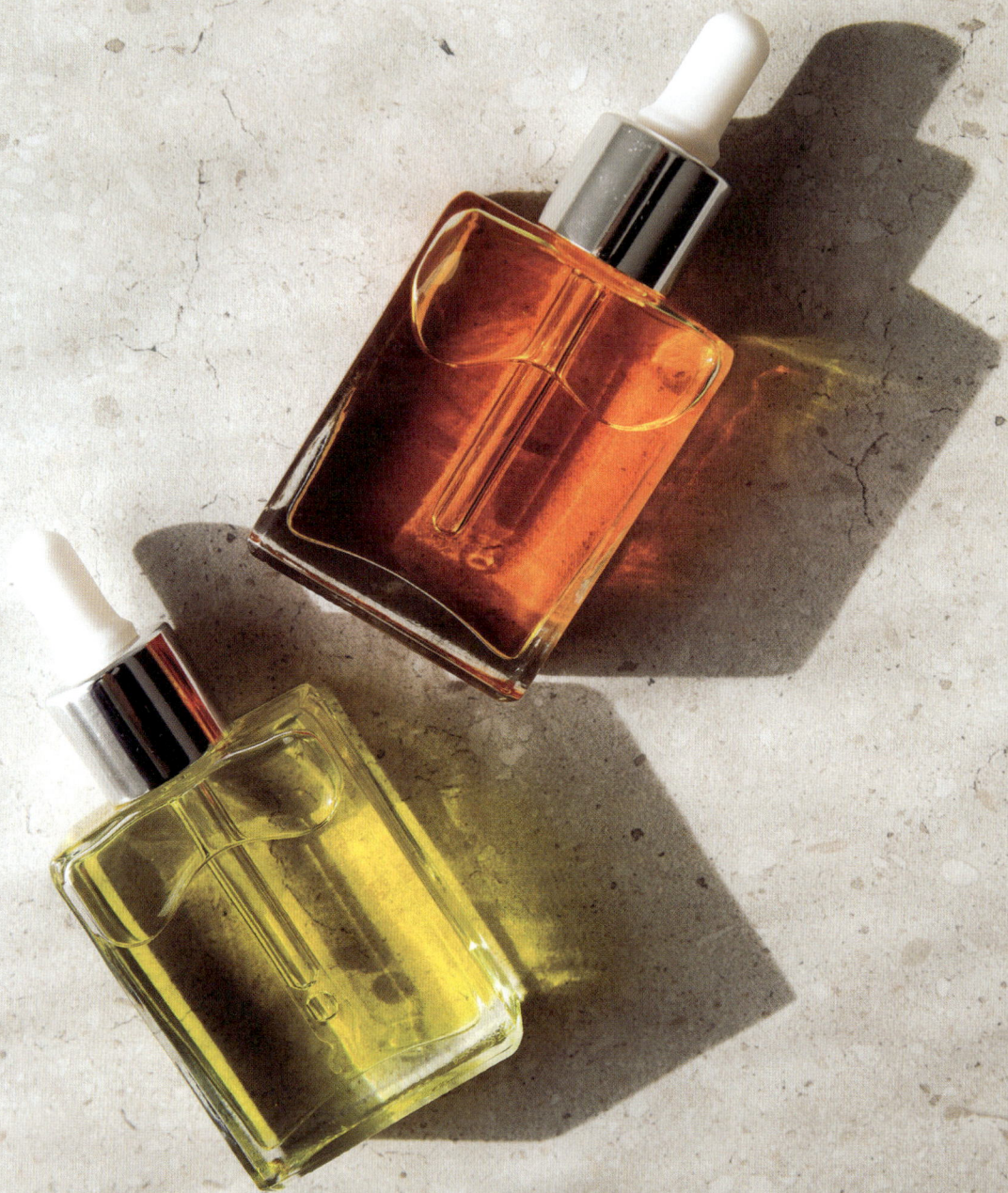

Facial Treatment Oils

Facial treatment oils are also known as oil serums and elixirs. They are combinations of cold-pressed vegetable oils, infused oils and essential oils blended together. They are rich in essential fatty acids, oil-soluble vitamins and the beneficial properties of essential oils.

Facial treatment oils may be applied to your skin as a moisturiser or just before the application of a moisturiser. You may prefer to use a facial treatment oil at night instead of a night cream or under a night cream. They may also be used during a facial treatment as a massage oil.

To make your own personalised facial treatment oil, choose suitable cold-pressed vegetable oils, infused oils and essential oils for your skin type. Make sure you follow the directions for diluting essential oils on page 36.

The following blends make superb facial treatment oils. 1% or 0.5 g of antioxidant (mixed tocopherols) are added to reduce the occurrence of rancidity and to benefit the skin.

The following recipes will make around 100 mL of facial oil. Add the ingredients to a glass bottle and shake well.

Dry skin treatment oil

30 g avocado oil
29.5 g evening primrose oil
20 g macadamia oil
20 g rosehip oil
0.5 g antioxidant
10 drops sandalwood essential oil
6 drops rose otto or absolute
4 drops neroli essential oil

Dehydrated skin treatment oil

60 g apricot kernel oil
39.5 g jojoba oil
0.5 g antioxidant
10 drops sandalwood essential oil
6 drops lavender essential oil
4 drops ylang ylang essential oil

Mature skin treatment oil

57.5 g apricot kernel oil
40 g rosehip oil
2 g carrot infused oil
0.5 g antioxidant
12 drops rose otto or absolute
6 drops frankincense essential oil
2 drops patchouli essential oil

Scar treatment oil

40 g rosehip oil
40 g wheatgerm oil
19.5 g calendula infused oil
0.5 g antioxidant
8 drops lavender essential oil
6 drops frankincense essential oil
6 drops patchouli essential oil

Combination/oily skin treatment oil

60 g jojoba oil
39.5 g argan oil
0.5 g antioxidant
12 drops lemon essential oil
4 drops geranium essential oil
4 drops juniper essential oil

Sensitive skin treatment oil

50 g apricot kernel oil
49.5 g calendula infused oil
0.5 g antioxidant
6 drops sandalwood essential oil
2 drops German chamomile essential oil
2 drops everlasting essential oil

Devitalised skin treatment oil

76 g apricot kernel oil
20 g wheatgerm oil
3.5 g carrot infused oil
0.5 g antioxidant
16 drops lemon essential oil
4 drops vetiver essential oil

Broken capillary/couperose treatment oil

99.5 g calendula infused oil
0.5 g antioxidant
10 drops cypress essential oil
6 drops geranium essential oil
4 drops German chamomile essential oil

Australian skin recovery elixir

A simple and beautifully absorbed oil to relieve dry, irritated skin made entirely from Australian ingredients.

100 g macadamia oil
20 drops kunzea essential oil

Pimple treatment oil

Apply lavender or tea tree essential oil, with a cotton bud, directly to a pimple 3 times a day. Do not wipe the essential oil onto the surrounding skin to avoid irritation. If you have sensitive skin, this treatment may not be suitable.

Lip Balms and Scrubs

Lip Balms

Lip balms soften and protect the skin on your lips, reduce dryness, and can encourage healing and repair. Natural lip balms are made from vegetable oils, waxes and butters rather than petrolatum and mineral oils.

Essential oils may be included in your lip balm to add delicious flavours or for their healing and antiseptic properties. As the lips have especially sensitive skin and anything applied to them may be ingested, care must be taken in choosing essential oils and ingredients for lip products. Essential oils should be non-toxic, and they should not photosensitise the skin. A maximum dilution of 1% essential oil may be added to your lip balms and scrubs (approximately 20 drops to every 100 g of lip balm).

Choose from the following essential oils to add to your lip balm:

> aniseed, lavender, lime, mandarin, myrrh, sweet orange, peppermint, rose otto, sandalwood and spearmint

Include healing infused oils such as calendula and carrot in your lip balm too.

Find more lip balm recipes on page 111.

Bush remedy lip balm

Protects your lips and helps them repair.

45 g macadamia oil
10 g beeswax
5 g raw honey
3 drops lemon myrtle essential oil

1. Melt the beeswax, macadamia oil and raw honey together in a *bain-marie*.
2. Once all ingredients have melted, remove from the heat and add the drops of lemon myrtle essential oil.
3. Continue to stir the mixture as it cools to ensure the honey does not drop to the bottom of the mixture.
4. Once it begins to thicken, scoop into a jar.
5. Allow to cool to room temperature before adding lids. The jars of balm can be put in the freezer for 2 hours to speed up solidification time, but allow to come back to room temperature before adding lids.

Fat chocolate lip balm

For lovers of chocolate. Smells and tastes wonderful.

15 g beeswax
5 g cocoa butter
5 g raw honey
65 g jojoba oil
10 g vanilla essence

1. Melt the beeswax, cocoa butter, jojoba oil and raw honey together in a *bain-marie*.
2. Once all ingredients have melted, remove from the heat and add the vanilla essence.

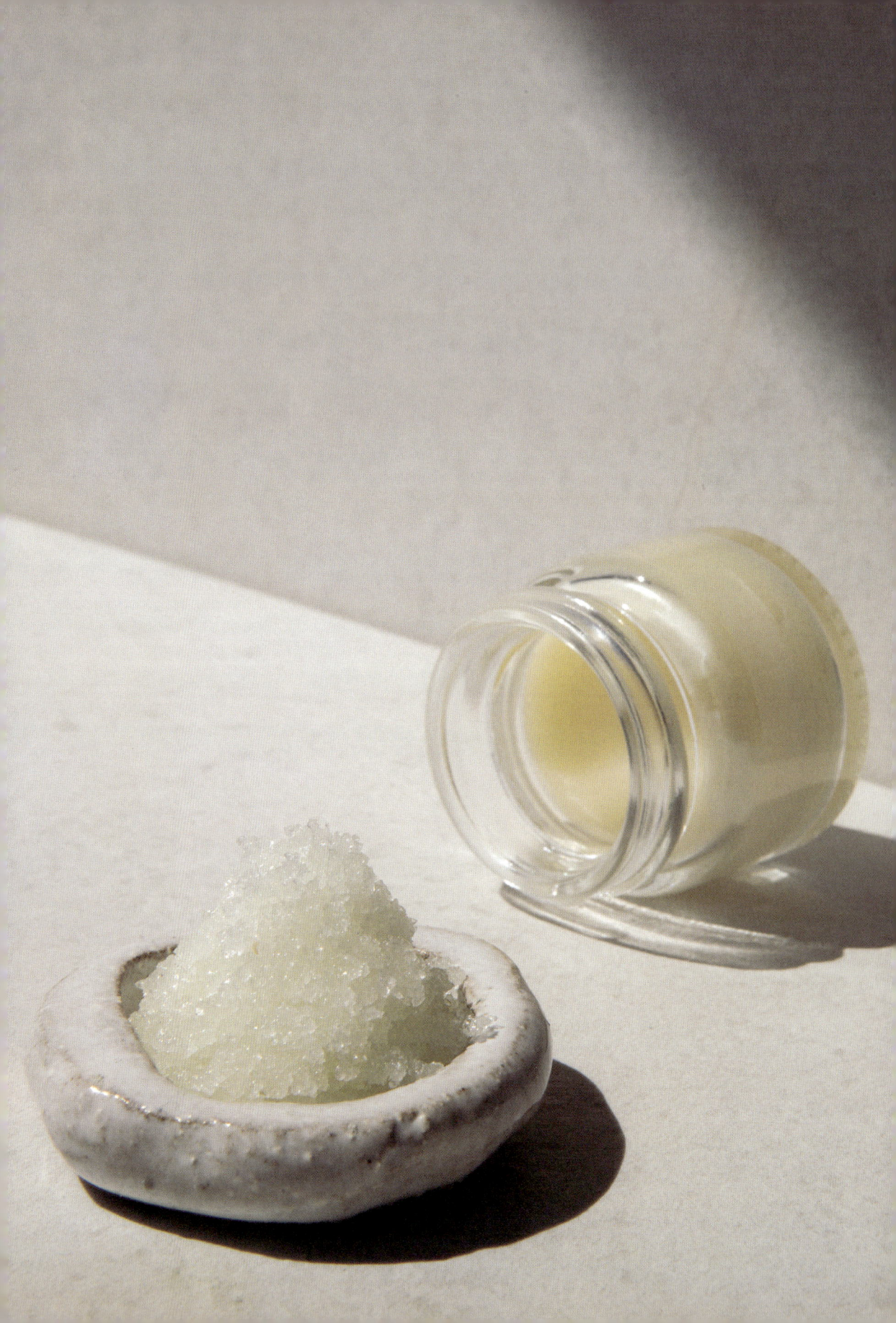

3. Continue to stir the mixture as it cools to ensure the honey and vanilla do not drop to the bottom of the mixture or separate out from the mixture.

4. Once it begins to thicken, scoop into a jar.

5. Allow to cool to room temperature before adding lids. The jars of balm can be put in the freezer for 2 hours to speed up solidification time, but allow to come back to room temperature before adding lids.

Healing lip balm

This lip balm is wonderful for healing dry, cracked, sore lips.

10 g beeswax
5 g cocoa butter
5 g shea butter
70 g jojoba oil
5 g calendula infused oil
4.5 g carrot infused oil
0.5 g antioxidant
3 drops sandalwood essential oil
2 drops myrrh essential oil

Make this lip balm by following *Aromatherapy balm method 1* on page 63.

Pure shea butter may be used as a softening and protective lip balm by itself. Otherwise, essential oils, vegetable oils, infused oils and honey may be stirred into it.

Luscious lime lip balm

A delicious, fun, natural lip balm for keeping your lips soft and moisturised.

15 g shea butter
5 drops lime essential oil

Simply soften the shea butter in a small dish by working it with a spoon and stir in the drops of lime essential oil.

Creamy honey lip balm

It will be tempting to lick your lips.

13 g shea butter
2 g honey

Simply soften the shea butter in a small dish by working it with a spoon and stir in the honey.

Cocoa coco lip balm

60 g cocoa butter
25 g coconut oil
15 g shea butter

Make this lip balm by following *Aromatherapy balm method 1* on page 63.

Lip Scrubs

These tasty natural lip scrubs buff away dry, flaky skin with sugar crystals and leave them feeling soft and smooth with vegetable oils. Perfect for when your lips are braving the cold, dry weather and before applying a lip balm or lip colour. Simply make these lip scrubs by stirring all ingredients together and storing in a jar.

Chocolips lip scrub

4 tsp caster sugar
½ tsp cacao powder
1 tsp coconut oil
1 tsp jojoba oil

Mojito lip scrub

4 tsp caster sugar
1½ tsp apricot kernel oil
5 drops lime essential oil
1 drop peppermint essential oil

Cold sore healing preparation

Cold sores are a result of having been infected with the *Herpes simplex* virus. Stress compromises the immune system and this is when a cold sore may rear its ugly head. Melissa (*Melissa officinalis*) essential oil applied neat to the cold sore at regular intervals throughout the day will help clear it quickly. However, as it is a very expensive essential oil and cheaper versions are often adulterated, this tincture is an alternative option.

15 drops tea tree essential oil
10 drops geranium essential oil
3 drops thyme ct. linalool essential oil
25 mL myrrh tincture

Mix the essential oils into the myrrh tincture in a bottle, and using a cotton bud, apply the tincture to the cold sore at regular intervals throughout the day.

Facial Compresses

Facial compresses can be used daily after cleansing or once or twice a week after the application of a mask.

They are especially useful for acne and dehydrated skin depending on the essential oils chosen for use in the compress.

Facial compresses benefit your skin in the following ways:

- soften sebum build-up and loosen dead skin cells
- improve skin hydration
- improve circulation
- allow for the better absorption of preparations such as moisturisers.

1. Choose a herb for your skin type from pages 14–18 or an essential oil for your skin type from pages 39–48.
2. Cleanse your face first.
3. Prepare a herbal infusion or add five drops of essential oil to very warm water and stir through rapidly.
4. While the water is still quite warm (and before the essential oil rises to the top), place a cloth onto the surface of the water and then wring out any excess.
5. Press the cloth over your freshly cleansed face. Hold it onto your face for 10 seconds or so.
6. Once the cloth feels cool, repeat the procedure. Do this about 5 times.
7. Follow with a toner, moisturiser or facial treatment oil.

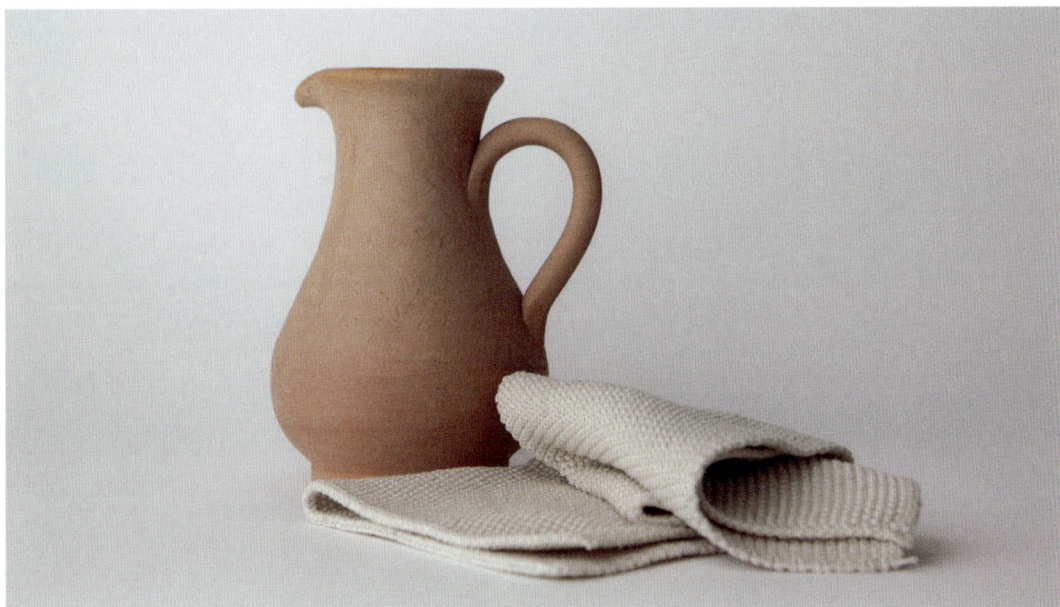

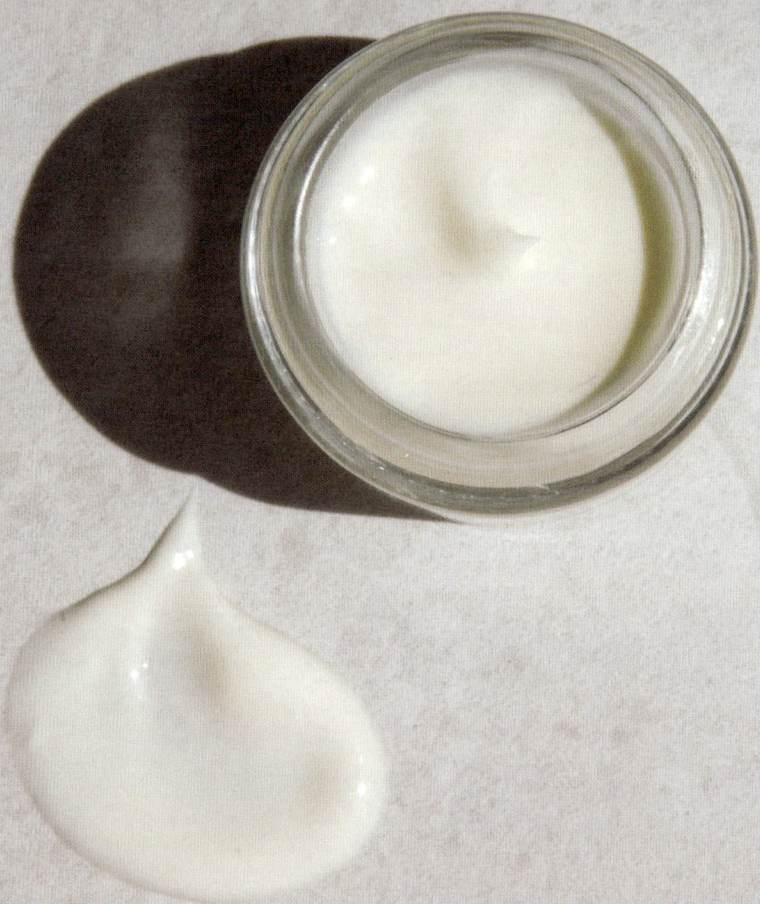

Eye Creams and Gels

The skin around the eyes is very thin and has fewer oil glands than the rest of the face. It is also wrinkled up and stretched out many times during our day, as we talk and express ourselves, squint to protect our eyes from the sun and bright lights, and blink to keep our eyes lubricated.

It is important to keep the skin around the eyes moisturised and protected without weighing it down with heavy creams.

Light eye cream

This is a light moisturising cream for the skin around the eyes. It is suitable for most skin types, including sensitive.

Oil phase
7 g plant-derived emulsifying wax
20 g apricot kernel oil
10 g calendula infused oil
1 g antioxidant

Water phase
154 g purified water
6 g vegetable glycerin
2 g preservative

pH adjustment
qs citric acid + water solution

Make this eye cream by following the *Method for making an emulsion with emulsifying wax* on page 79.

Nourishing eye cream

This eye cream is a rich moisturiser for dry, wrinkled skin around the eyes. Use sparingly.

Oil phase
10 g shea butter
8 g plant-derived emulsifying wax
10 g avocado oil
10 g macadamia oil
2 g carrot infused oil
1 g antioxidant

Water phase
151 g rosewater
6 g vegetable glycerin
2 g preservative

pH adjustment
qs citric acid + water solution

Make this eye cream by following the *Method for making an emulsion with emulsifying wax* on page 79.

Revitalising eye gel

This is a soothing, revitalising eye gel for tired and puffy eyes.
1 g xanthan gum
6 g vegetable glycerin
191 g rosewater
2 g preservative

pH adjustment
qs citric acid + water solution

Make this eye gel by following the *Method for making gel bases* on page 67.

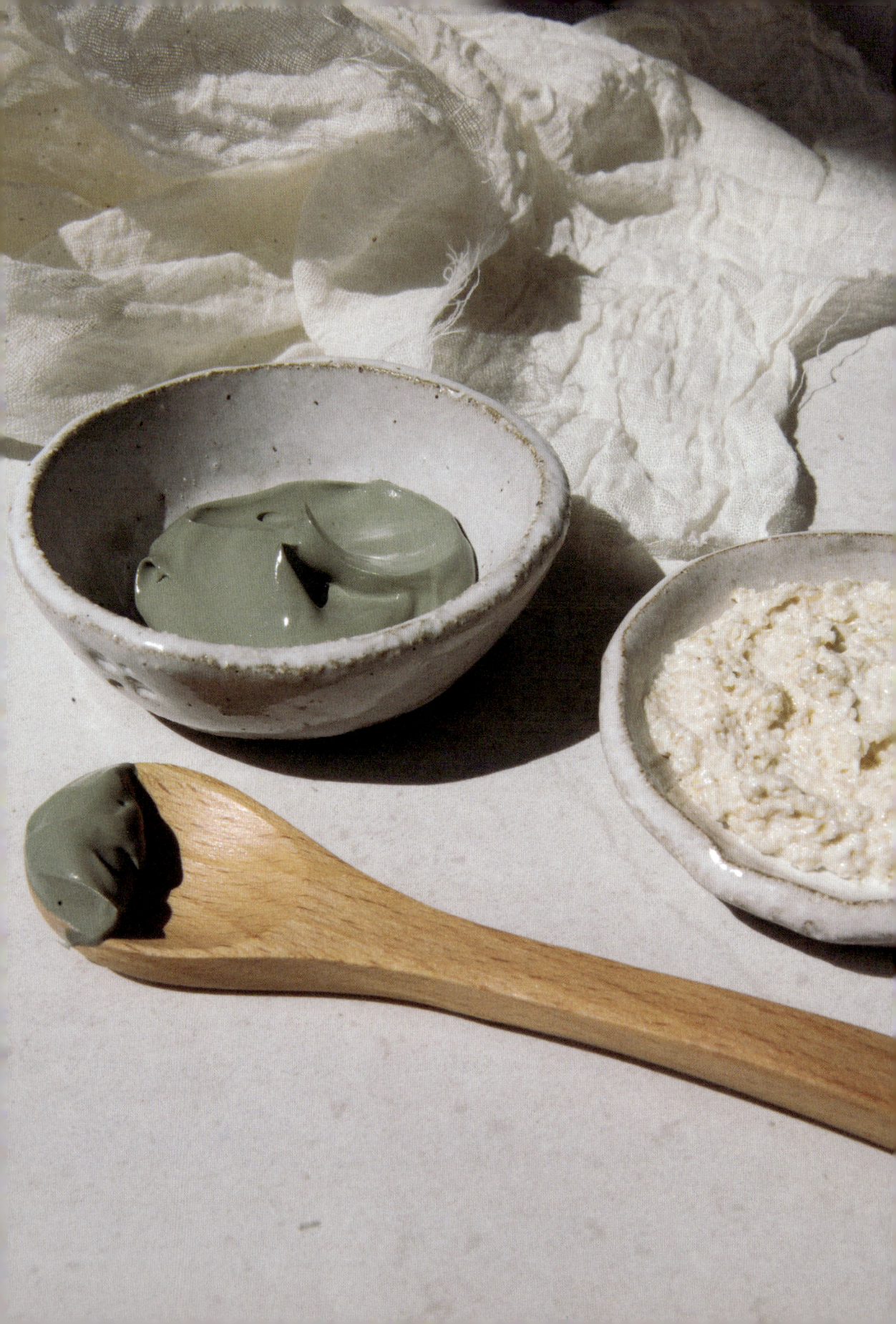

Masks

Use a mask regularly to revitalise your skin. Masks are used to cleanse the skin, absorb excess oil, remove dead skin cells, soften blackheads, heal damaged or blemished skin, stimulate the circulation in the skin and promote healthy cell regeneration, nourish, moisturise, hydrate and soothe your skin, and improve skin tone — all depending on the ingredients used to make your mask.

There are two basic types of masks:

- **Setting masks** — these kinds of masks dry and set on the skin. They are generally cleansing, drawing, toning and stimulating and may contain healing ingredients. Clays form the bases of these kinds of masks.
- **Non-setting** — these kinds of masks will infuse active ingredients into the skin, hydrate, soothe and calm, heal and freshen the skin. They tend to remain moist on the skin and may be cream or gel-based or made from plants, fruits, vegetables, herbs, honey or eggs. Clays may also be added to these masks if they remain moist or are contained in a cream type base.

Different types of masks may be applied to your face at the same time to treat different skin types and conditions. For example, your skin may be oily and blocked in your T-zone and on this area you would use a clay mask, whereas your cheeks may be dry and sensitive and here a cream mask may be more suitable.

A mask is usually applied after the skin has been cleansed. If you are giving yourself a facial, use a mask after cleansing and exfoliating. Leave your mask on for approximately 5–15 minutes, depending on your skin and type of mask, before removing it. Always follow with a toner and moisturiser.

Freshly Cooked Masks

When you're making your dinner, save some of your cooked vegetables for later. Use them in your face masks to soothe and soften your skin. Potatoes, sweet potatoes, carrots and pumpkin can be mashed and mixed into a smooth paste with a small amount of vegetable oil and milk. Apply this to your face and leave it on for 10–15 minutes before removing it. Great for hydrating and softening dry and sensitive skins.

Gel Masks

Gel masks are hydrating, refreshing, cooling and soothing to the skin. Xanthan gum, guar gum and linseeds are some of the gelling agents that can be used to make your gel masks. You can make gel masks using the *Gel base 2* recipe and following the *Method for making gel bases* on page 67. Gel masks can be made with floral waters or herbal infusions in place of water. To make an aromatherapy gel mask, add 2 drops of essential oil to every 50 g of gel.

Clay Masks

Clay masks are absorbent and adsorbent, cleansing, toning and healing. Clays are available in different colours depending on their mineral content. They have various healing properties on the skin.

Argiletz clays (green, pink, red, yellow, white), Australian clays, kaolin and bentonite are all suitable clays for face masks. See page 18 for more information on clays and how to choose clays suitable for your skin.

Making a clay mask

When making a clay mask, use glass, porcelain or stainless-steel utensils (avoid corrosive metals).

To make a clay face mask, mix approximately 2 teaspoons of clay with 1–2 teaspoons of water and mix into a smooth paste. Floral waters, fruit and vegetable juices, herbal infusions, aloe vera juice, milk or yoghurt may be used in place of water.

To use a clay mask, first cleanse and exfoliate the skin. Then while the skin is still damp, apply the clay mask with your fingers or a brush. The mask can be applied in layers to allow for a thick application of clay. For oily and acne skin, leave the mask on for approximately 10 minutes and allow the mask to dry but not completely dry out. For dry, dehydrated and sensitive skin, leave the mask on for 5 minutes, ensuring the mask remains damp. The mask can be misted with water or floral water while it is on to ensure it does not dehydrate the skin. A small amount of vegetable oil may be added to the mask to help prevent it from drying out.

Remove the clay mask by dampening it well with a wet face cloth or sponge, then removing it well and flush the skin with water, for example, while showering. Inspect the skin carefully to ensure it has all been removed. Follow with a toner and moisturiser. Use clay masks once or twice a week.

Clay masks are easily made up fresh each time you would like to use one.

Deep cleansing green clay mask
Skin type: oily and combination

A cleansing and healing mask for oily, combination and clogged skins.

2 tsp green Argiletz clay
2 tsp neroli water
1 drop juniper essential oil
1 drop lemon essential oil

Revitalising yellow clay mask
Skin type: dull and devitalised

A cleansing and stimulating mask for skin that needs a refreshing pick-me-up.

2 tsp yellow Argiletz clay
2 tsp yoghurt
1 drop sweet orange essential oil
1 drop sage essential oil

Tonifying red clay mask
Skin type: dry and mature

A gently cleansing and tonifying mask.

2 tsp red Argiletz clay
1 tsp rosewater
1 tsp yoghurt

Find more masks making use of the benefits of clay and botanicals on page 95.

Fresh From the Fridge

Open your refrigerator door to find the ingredients to make fresh facial masks for your skin. Make them up in small quantities and store them in the refrigerator, using them within a day or two.

Tahini

To soften and moisturise dry skin, cleanse your skin and spread tahini over your face. Leave on for 10–15 minutes before wiping away and rinsing.

Yoghurt

To hydrate, cool and soothe your skin, spread a couple of teaspoons of natural yoghurt over your face and leave on for 10 minutes before rinsing.

Fresh fruit and vegetable masks

Strawberries, cucumbers, bananas, grapes, tomatoes, watermelons, apples, citrus fruits and juice, passionfruits, peaches, pears, potatoes, rockmelons, pineapples and paw paws ... Whether they're straight from your garden, your local organic food supplier or supermarket, fresh fruit and vegetables make superb face masks, full of enzymes, vitamins, minerals, sugars, proteins and more. For more detailed information on the properties of each of these fresh fruits and vegetables, and which ones are suitable for your skin, see page 7.

Mash, grate or juice the fruit or vegetable and apply to your face after cleansing. Otherwise, mix with clay or flour such as wheat, corn, potato or lentil, or a gum such as xanthan gum or guar gum, into a paste so that the fruit can be easily applied to your face. Remember to wash your fruit thoroughly before making your masks.

Here are a few fresh fruit and vegetable mask recipes to get your imagination going. They are all made fresh and in small quantities, enough for one application. Apply to your face, neck and décolletage. If not using your mask immediately, store it in the refrigerator and use it within 2 days.

Fruit crush mask
Skin type: oily and blemished

This mask gently cleanses and exfoliates the skin; the pineapple and paw paw enzymes dissolve the surface skin cells and the kaolin absorbs impurities.

2 tsp kaolin clay
1 tsp paw paw
1 tsp pineapple

Finely chop the paw paw and pineapple, then mash with the back of a spoon into a pulp. Mix into a smooth paste with the kaolin. Apply to a freshly cleansed face and leave on for 10 minutes.

Grape hydration mask
Skin type: all skin types

A cooling, hydrating mask for the skin.

6 grapes
1/8 tsp guar gum

Peel the grapes and remove the seeds. Crush the grapes into a liquid. Slowly sprinkle the powder into the liquefied pulp while stirring well. Allow to thicken and apply to your freshly cleansed face. Leave on for 10 minutes.

Avocado moisturising mask
Skin type: dry and mature

A moisturising and skin-softening mask for dry and mature skin.

**¼ ripe avocado
½ tsp avocado oil
2 tsp cream**

Mix the ingredients together into a smooth paste and apply to a freshly cleansed, damp face. Leave on for 10–15 minutes.

Cucumber cooling mask
Skin type: all skin types

This mask is hydrating and toning. Slice a cool cucumber that has been in the refrigerator into very thin slices. Lie on the bed or couch and using a mirror to see what you are doing, apply to your face. Relax for 15 minutes before removing.

Seaweed mask
Skin type: dehydrated

A calming, hydrating and healing mask for all skin types.

**1 tsp seaweed or kelp powder
2 tsp water or yoghurt**

Mix the ingredients together into a smooth paste and apply to a freshly cleansed, damp face. Leave on for 10 minutes before removing and rinsing.

Calming oat mask
Skin type: sensitive and inflamed

Soothes irritated and inflamed skin.

**1 tsp oat flour or oat bran
2 tsp yoghurt**

Mix the ingredients together into a smooth paste and apply to a freshly cleansed, damp face. Leave on for 10 minutes before removing and rinsing.

Healthy herb masks

The number of herbal masks you can make is limited only to what you can wild harvest, grow in your garden, or buy from a greengrocer or local market.

Fresh parsley and mint face mask
Skin type: dull and devitalised

A great pick-me-up for your skin. Blend a handful of finely chopped parsley and mint together with 1 tablespoon of yoghurt. Smooth this mask over your face to stimulate a dull, sluggish skin. Leave on for 10 minutes before removing and rinsing. If not using your mask immediately, store it in the refrigerator and use it within 2 days.

Marshmallow and comfrey mask
Skin type: sensitive

This mask is particularly healing and soothing to sensitive skin.

**2 tsp dried marshmallow root
2 tsp dried comfrey leaves
½ cup purified water
3 tsp vegetable glycerin
1 tsp guar gum**

1. Soak the marshmallow root and comfrey leaves in the purified water overnight to create an infusion.
2. Strain the plant matter from the water the next day.
3. In a separate container, mix and disperse the guar gum into the glycerin.
4. While stirring, slowly pour the glycerin and guar gum into the infusion.
5. Allow the mixture to thicken.
6. Apply the gel mask to clean, damp skin.
7. Leave on for 10–15 minutes to calm and hydrate the skin.
8. Gently remove with a damp face cloth and rinse with warm water.
9. If not using your mask immediately, store it in the refrigerator and use it within 2 days.

Cream masks

Cream masks are softening and nourishing to the skin. They act as intensive moisturisers to the skin.

Regenerative cream mask
Skin type: dry and mature

This mask is very nourishing to dry and mature skin. It is rich in antioxidants such as beta-carotene and vitamin E. The *Regenerative cream mask* may be applied as a mask first, left on for 15 minutes, then any excess massaged into the skin. It is a great mask to apply before going to bed. As this mask contains a preservative, it can be stored for at least 6 months in cool, hygienic conditions.

Oil phase
14 g plant-derived emulsifying wax
62 g avocado oil
15 g rosehip oil

10 g carrot infused oil
1 g antioxidant

Water phase
90 g rosewater
6 g vegetable glycerin
2 g preservative
qs citric acid + water solution

Add at 40°C
20 drops patchouli essential oil
or mature skin composition on page 48

Make this cream mask by following the *Method for making an emulsion with emulsifying wax* on page 79.

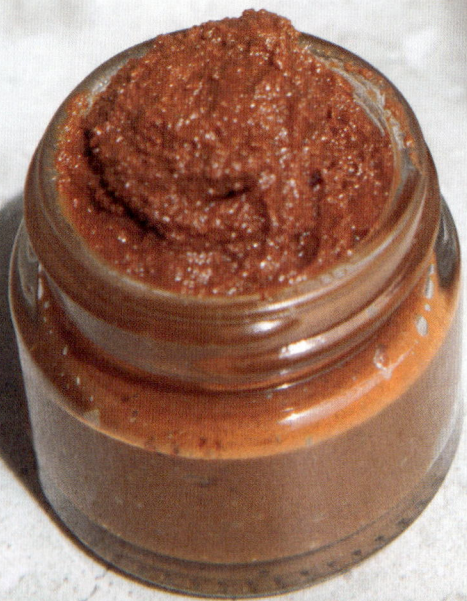

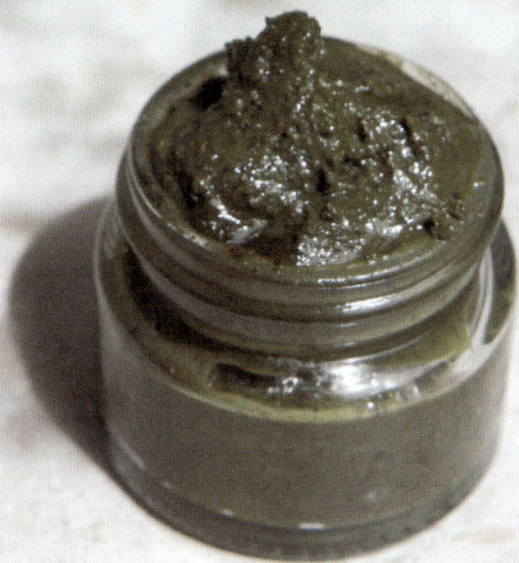

Scrubs and Exfoliants

Scrubs, exfoliants and peels are used to remove dead skin cells from the surface of the skin and help dislodge clogging of the skin, including blackheads and whiteheads.

The removal of surface skin cells and the stimulation of circulation will encourage cellular renewal and allow for the better absorption of active ingredients in masks, moisturisers, serums and oils.

How often you need to exfoliate will depend on the type of exfoliant used and on your skin type and condition. This could be once a fortnight on extremely fine and sensitive skin or up to 3 times a week on oily skin at times when it is prone to breaking out. Overuse and using preparations with sharp granules can cause problems such as rough skin due to damage and dehydration of the new cells that are forming in the germinative layer of the skin. Skin irritation, disturbance of the skin's pH and broken capillaries can be other adverse effects.

Exfoliants are available in the following forms.

- **Granular:** Granular exfoliants are creamy preparations containing granules that, when massaged over the surface of the skin, mechanically lift the dead skin cells off the surface of the skin and, to a certain extent, cleanse the pores. The granules can be made from ground and polished nuts, seeds, grains and pulses, including almond meal, oatmeal, oat flakes, ground lentils, adzuki beans, rice, semolina and bran. This type of exfoliant is of special benefit to oily skin with blocked pores. Care must be taken not to aggravate the skin through excessive pressure or overuse.

- **Enzymatic:** Enzymatic exfoliants contain enzymes that dissolve and digest the protein of dead skin cells and help dissolve build-up in pores. Paw paw and pineapple contain natural plant enzymes, papain and bromelain, which have this action.

- **Fruit acids:** Alpha-hydroxy acids (AHAs) occur naturally in fruits such as citrus (citric acid), apples (malic acid) and tomatoes (lactic acid). When AHAs are used in low dilution, they act as moisturisers, but in higher concentrations they cause skin exfoliation. The AHAs in masks made from fresh fruits are buffered by other constituents such as fruit sugars. Caution should be exercised if considering using fruit with a high acid content on the skin.

- **Gommage:** A gommage exfoliant is creamy and is applied to the skin and allowed to dry. Dead skin cells adhere to the gommage, which is then removed by friction — gentle rubbing with the pads of the fingers while supporting the skin. Fine, sensitive and dehydrated skin benefits from this type of exfoliant.

Fresh From the Fridge

The following facial scrubs and exfoliants are made fresh. They are delicious and very effective. Make them up in small quantities and store them in the refrigerator, using them within 2 days. The following quantities will give you one to 2 applications.

For more facial exfoliant recipes, see page 96.

Gentle fruit acid and enzyme mask
Skin type: all skin types with blocked pores

A wonderful skin smoothing, softening and cleansing exfoliant that makes use of the natural acids and enzymes in fruit.

1 tsp grated green apple
1 tsp mashed paw paw
1 tsp mashed strawberry
1 tsp green Argiletz clay
1 tsp oat flour
1 tsp natural yoghurt

1. Grate the green apple on a fine grater and mash the strawberry and paw paw.
2. Mix and mash the fruit together.
3. Add the oat flour, green clay and natural yoghurt and mix together.
4. Smooth and pat over your face and leave on for 10–15 minutes.

Banana peel
Skin type: normal to dry, sensitive

A scrumptious mask and peel for normal to dry and sensitive skin.

2 tsp mashed banana
1 tsp almond meal
1 tsp oat flour

1. Mix all ingredients into a smooth paste.
2. Apply as a face mask first and leave on for 15 minutes or until it has just dried.
3. Massage over your face while supporting the skin. It will ball up into small balls and function as a gentle peel.
4. Gently rub off as much as possible.
5. Rinse with warm water.

Exfoliant Pastes

The following exfoliants make use of natural granules such as almond meal, rice flour and wattle seeds.

Rose dual action facial paste
Skin type: dry and mature

This fine rose scrub is suitable for dry and mature skin. It exfoliates, softens and hydrates the skin. It can be kept for at least 6 months if stored out of the heat and uncontaminated. Do not allow moisture to enter the jar.

2½ tsp pink Argiletz clay
2 tsp almond meal
2 tsp oat flour
1 tsp white rice flour
1 tsp rose petal powder
3 tsp glycerin
1 tsp honey
1 tsp jojoba oil
2 drops rose otto

1. Sieve the almond meal through a mesh tea strainer to remove larger particles. Use the smaller sieved particles.
2. Mix the dry ingredients — the pink clay, almond meal, oat flour, white rice flour and rose powder — together in a small bowl.
3. Add the liquid ingredients — glycerin, honey, jojoba oil and rose otto.
4. Stir the mixture thoroughly.
5. Scoop into a glass jar for storage.
6. Massage a small quantity over a damp face to exfoliate. Then, leave on for up to 5 minutes as a mask before rinsing with warm water.

Green dual action facial paste
Skin type: oily and combination

This green scrub is suitable for oily and combination skin. It can be kept for at least 6 months if stored out of the heat and uncontaminated. Do not allow moisture to enter the jar.

2½ tsp green Argiletz clay
2 tsp oat flour
1 tsp almond meal
1 tsp hemp flour
1 tsp matcha powder
1 tsp white rice flour
3 tsp glycerin
2 tsp honey
2 drops geranium essential oil

1. Sieve the almond meal through a mesh tea strainer to remove larger particles. Use the smaller sieved particles.

2. Mix the dry ingredients — green clay, oat flour, almond meal, hemp flour, matcha powder and white rice flour — together in a small bowl.

3. Add the liquid ingredients — glycerin, honey and geranium essential oil.

4. Stir the mixture thoroughly.

5. Scoop into a glass jar for storage.

6. Massage a small quantity over a damp face to exfoliate. Then, leave on for up to 5 minutes as a mask before rinsing with warm water.

Outback elements face mask and scrub

An exfoliating, deep cleansing and rejuvenating clay mask and scrub for normal, combination and oily skin made from entirely Australian ingredients.

2 tsp Australian olive green clay
2 tsp ground wattle seeds
1 tsp Kakadu plum powder

1. Mix the ingredients together and store in a glass jar.

2. To use, mix one heaped teaspoon with one teaspoon of water or yoghurt into a smooth paste.

3. Smooth over your face and leave on for 10 minutes or until just dry.

4. Once the mask has dried, jump in the shower and wet the mask.

5. Gently massage it over your face and rinse well.

6. Follow with a floral water or skin freshener and moisturiser for your skin type.

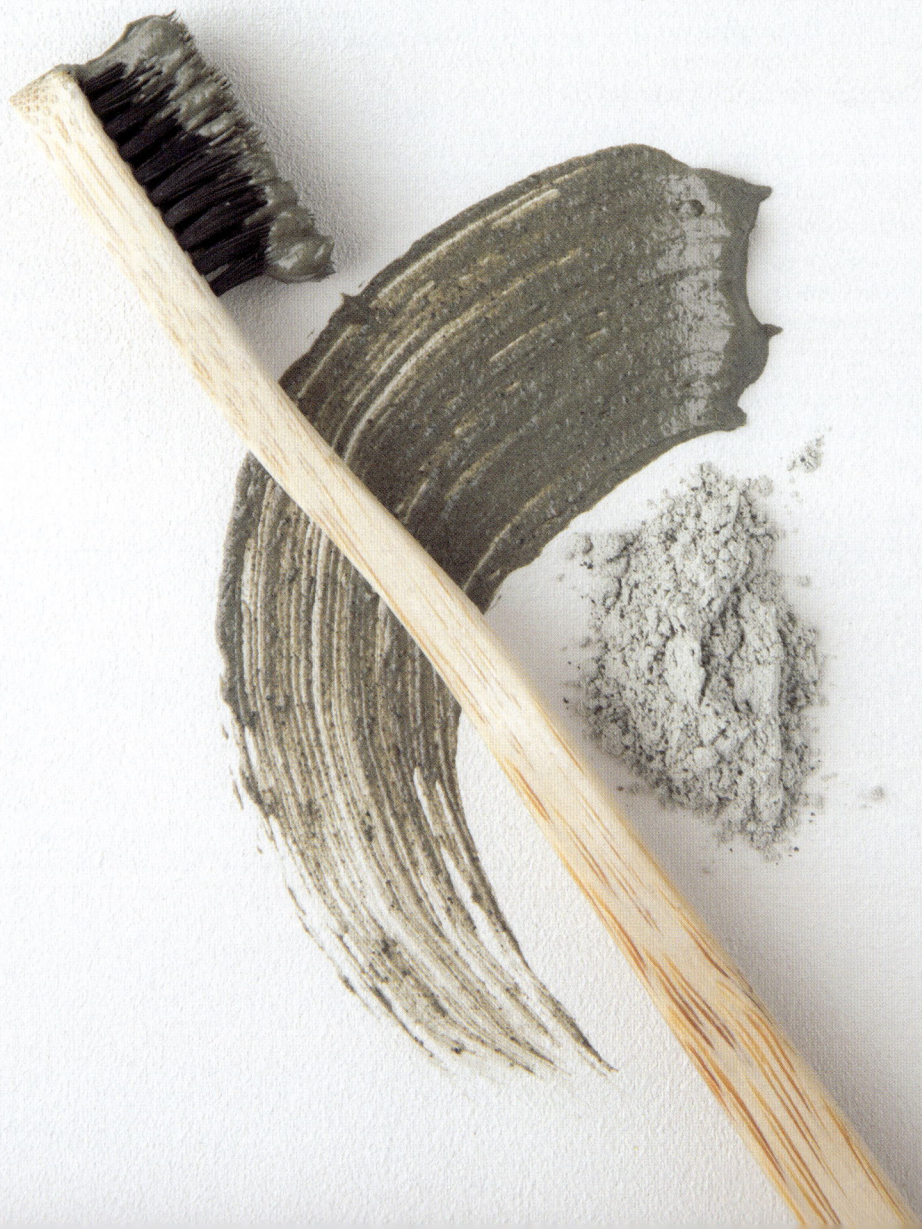

Teeth Powders and Pastes

We clean our teeth to remove plaque and anything else stuck to our teeth. We clean them to prevent them from developing cavities, to freshen our breath and to keep our gums healthy. These teeth cleaning powders contain gentle abrasives to gently clean and polish your teeth, herbs to encourage gum health and a small amount of essential oil to freshen your breath. Check with your dentist before using this teeth cleaning powder to ensure it is suitable for you if you have teeth or gum problems.

Teeth cleaning powder

Part A

90 g bentonite clay
5 g stevia powder
2 g sodium bicarbonate

Part B

3 g herbal powders — choose one or a combination of the following ground or powdered plants: neem, aloe vera, turmeric, clove, sage, activated charcoal
1 g (approx. 20 drops) essential oil — choose from essential oils that will taste good, freshen the breath and are non-sensitising and non-toxic — such as peppermint, spearmint, lime, sweet orange, lemon

1. Finely grind any dried herbs in a coffee grinder.
2. Sieve through a fine mesh tea strainer and remove any large pieces.
3. Stir all dry ingredients together in a bowl.
4. Add the drops of essential oil, ensuring you sprinkle them uniformly over the mixture, then stir them in.
5. Sieve the mixture several times to ensure any lumps are broken down and the essential oils are evenly distributed throughout the mixture.
6. Store in an airtight glass jar.
7. Use by removing ½ teaspoon of powder with a clean spoon, then dipping your wet toothbrush into it and brushing your teeth.
8. Do not dip your wet toothbrush into the jar of powder as the addition of moisture into the powder will provide an environment for microbes to grow.

Sage and clove teeth cleaning powder

Add to Part A of the *Teeth cleaning powder* recipe:

2 g sage powder
1 g clove powder
20 drops peppermint essential oil

Turmeric and activated charcoal teeth cleaning powder

Add to Part A of the *Teeth cleaning powder* recipe:

2 g activated charcoal powder
1 g turmeric powder
20 drops lemon essential oil

Teeth cleaning paste

To make a paste, make the *Teeth cleaning powder above* and add an equal quantity of vegetable oil to make a paste. The vegetable oil quantity should be half coconut oil, which will be solid in winter, and half liquid vegetable oil, such as macadamia oil or sweet almond oil so that the paste won't be completely solid in winter.

**50 g teeth cleaning powder
(recipe above)
25 g coconut oil
25 g macadamia or sweet almond oil**

1. Mix all ingredients together.
2. Store in a glass jar.
3. Use by removing ½ teaspoon of the paste with a clean spoon, and applying to your wet toothbrush and brushing your teeth.
4. Do not dip your wet toothbrush into the jar as the addition of moisture will provide an environment for microbes to grow.

Colour Cosmetics

Adding a hint of colour to your cheeks, lips and eyes can add freshness and a healthy glow to your appearance. The decoration of our faces and bodies also speaks to our creative nature and desire to transform the physical representation of ourselves.

The following equipment and method can be used to make these colour cosmetics: face powders, blush and eyebrow powder.

Equipment

- 2 small glass or ceramic bowls
- teaspoon
- mesh tea strainer
- jar
- label

Method for making colour cosmetic powders

1. Stir all the dry ingredients together in a bowl.
2. Sieve the mixture into another bowl and sieve again several times to break down any lumps and ensure even colour distribution.
3. Store in an airtight jar.
4. Apply to your face with a powder brush.

Face Powders

Gorgeous goddess face powder

This gorgeous powder can be used over foundation or applied to the skin directly to add some colour and give a matte finish to the skin. The ratio of ingredients can be changed to alter the shade of the powder. Suitable powders include cacao powder, kaolin clay and tapioca flour or arrowroot flour. Darker shades can be achieved by increasing the amount of cacao powder and reducing the amount of white powders.

Light beige colour
4 g cacao powder
4 g kaolin clay

Mid beige colour
6 g cacao powder
2 g kaolin clay

Mid-dark brown colour
cacao powder

Blush

Various natural powders can be applied to the cheeks to give the face a natural healthy blush. Powders that work well to colour the cheeks include finely powdered rose petals, red clay and combinations of these. They can be combined with kaolin for a lighter colour or with cacao powder for subtle warm brown hues.

Cheeky goddess blush

Finely powdered red rose petals give a soft pink colour to the cheeks.

red rose petal powder

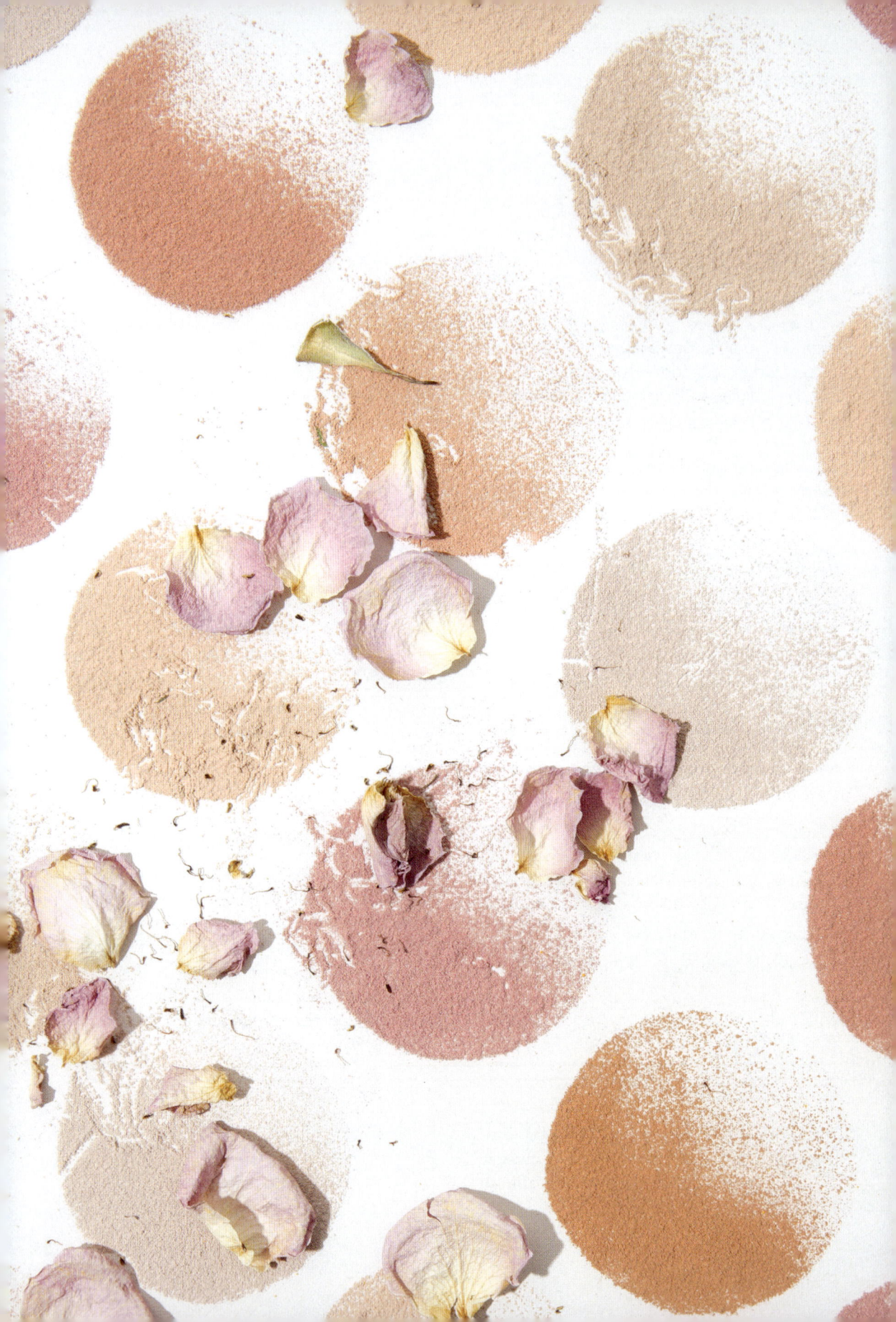

Warm goddess blush

This powder imparts a warm rust, pink colour to the cheeks.

6 g red rose petal powder
1 g red Argiletz clay

Earth goddess blush

Red clay applied to the cheeks imparts an intense orange, rust colour to the cheeks.

red Argiletz clay

Peachy goddess blush

This powder gives a soft peach colour to the cheeks.

4 g red Argiletz clay
1 g kaolin clay

Solar goddess blush

This powder gives a soft, warm, tan colour to the cheeks and can be dusted lightly over the face to provide a touch of 'weekend at the beach' tan on paler skin.

3 g red Argiletz clay
2 g cacao powder

Eyebrow Powder

Eyebrow colourant can be made using cacao powder for brown or lighter coloured eyebrows, or activated charcoal for black or darker eyebrows. A mixture of the two can also be used. Apply using an eyebrow brush.

Eye Colour

A multi-purpose eye colour product can be created using natural pigments incorporated into a balm base.

Solid eye colour

This eye colour product is suitable for use as an eyebrow colour, eyeliner or eyeshadow.

Cacao powder and activated charcoal powder can be added to a waxy balm base to create a solid product. Cacao powder gives a warm brown colour, whereas activated charcoal gives a soft, dark grey, charcoal colour.

The following recipe can be applied as an eyebrow colour using a short, stiff-bristled eyebrow brush. It can be applied as eyeliner using a thin, stiff-bristled brush, and as eyeshadow using your finger or an eyeshadow brush.

10 g cacao powder or activated charcoal
powder
9 g jojoba oil
1 g candelilla wax

1. Sieve the powder into a small bowl using a fine mesh tea strainer to break down any lumps.
2. Melt the jojoba oil and candelilla wax in a small heat-resistant jug in a *bain-marie*.
3. Stir the powders into the melted oil and wax mixture.
4. Spoon into a small glass jar.
5. Allow to cool to room temperature before adding lids. It can be put in the freezer for 2 hours to speed up solidification time, but allow to come back to room temperature before adding lids.
6. Apply using an eyebrow brush, eyeliner brush or eyeshadow brush.

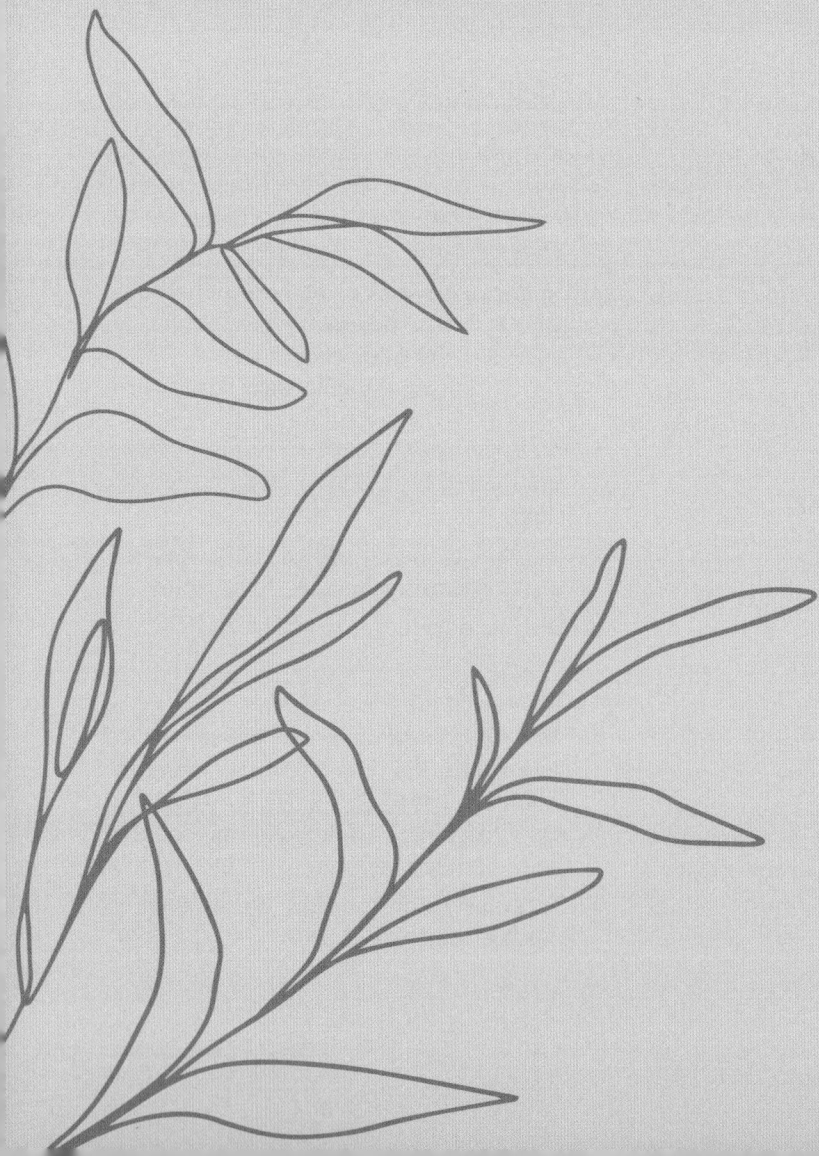

Soap

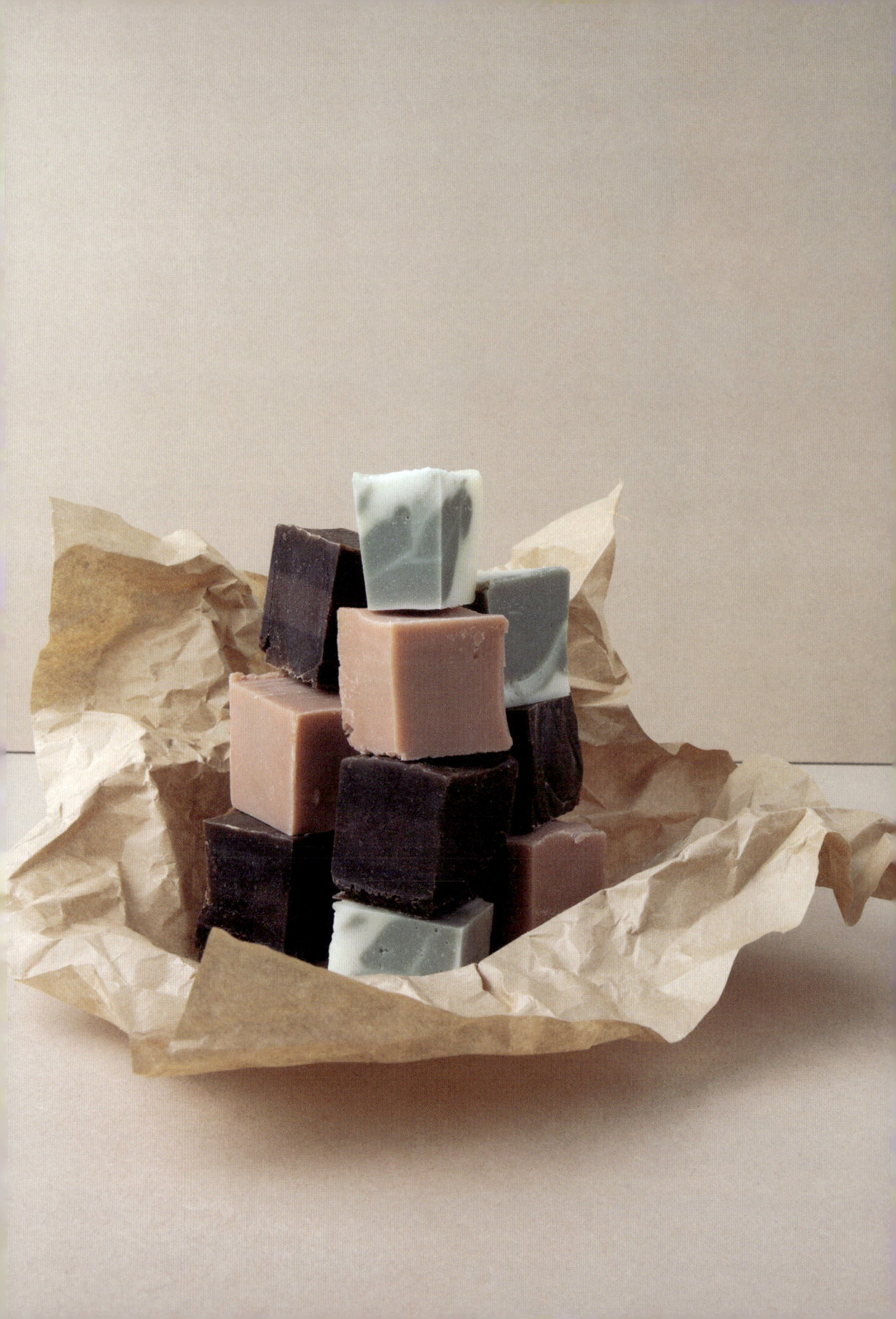

Introduction to Soap Making

The Beginnings of Soap Making

One myth has it that the word 'soap' was derived from Mount Sapo, which was a location for animal sacrifice. Melted animal fats and plant ashes would be washed down from the mountain and, in the clay along the banks of the River Tiber, a crude soap would form. People found that washing their clothes in this water would result in cleaner clothes. However, the earliest records of the production of a type of soap appear to be on a clay tablet from ancient Babylon (modern-day Iraq).

The Chemistry of Soap Making

Soap is made by reacting fats and oils together with lye. The fats and oils may be animal or vegetable in origin, and the lye may be an alkaline solution of caustic soda (sodium hydroxide) or caustic potash (potassium hydroxide) dissolved in water.

The natural fats and oils from nuts and seeds used to make soap are esters of the alcohol glycerol and a variety of fatty acids, for example, stearic acid, oleic acid and palmitic acid. In an example of a soap reaction, coconut oil (mainly stearic acid + glycerol) reacts with caustic soda to produce a mixture of soap (sodium stearate) and glycerol (glycerin). This reaction is called saponification.

In commercial soaps, the glycerol is removed to make the soaps harder and make them last longer. Home-made soaps retain the glycerol, which is emollient to the skin, giving the soap a milder action on the skin.

Making your own soap from scratch can be done using a cold-process or hot-process method. The ingredients and many of the processes in each method are similar except that heat is used to speed up the process of saponification in the hot-process method. One benefit of making soap using the hot-process method is that you can use your soap within a day, whereas you will need to wait four weeks or so for the soap to harden using the cold-process method. Soap made using the hot-process method looks rougher in appearance, whereas cold-process soap looks smoother and allows for the introduction of some interesting effects such as swirls. The soap recipes in this book are made using the cold-process method.

Basic Soap Making

Basic Soap Ingredients

Lye

Lye is a constant ingredient in all soaps. It is a strong alkaline solution of caustic soda (sodium hydroxide) or caustic potash (potassium hydroxide) and water. Caustic soda yields hard soaps and caustic potash yields soft or liquid soaps. In the past, people 'leached' their own lye by running water through wood or plant ashes. The soaps made were often harsh on the skin and soft in texture. Caustic soda, which is readily available, is now most commonly used in soap making. It is available in most supermarkets and hardware stores among the cleaning supplies.

Water

Water is used to make the lye solution. The caustic soda is dissolved into the water. The water used should be clean, unpolluted rainwater, purified water or bottled spring water. Tap water or 'hard' water contains minerals and impurities, which can interfere with the action of the lye and result in a failed batch of soap.

The quantity of lye solution required to form soap varies depending on the vegetable oils and fats used. Lye calculators are available on several websites if you would like to create your own soap formula with a particular choice of vegetable oils. The recipes in this book have already had the quantities calculated.

Cautions when using lye

- Caustic soda and potash are strongly alkaline and corrosive substances.
- Protect your skin, eyes and work area. Wear rubber gloves and protective eyewear. Wear long sleeves, long pants and covered shoes.
- If you get any caustic soda or potash on your skin, rinse if off immediately, within 5–10 seconds, under running water. Vinegar will help neutralise its alkaline effects.
- If you get caustic soda or potash in your eyes, rinse for several minutes with water. Do not put vinegar in your eyes. Seek professional help quickly.
- Don't breathe in the fumes.
- If swallowed, drink water. Don't induce vomiting. Seek professional help quickly.
- Cover your benches with paper.
- Making soap with lye is not an activity for children. Keep children and pets away.
- Caustic soda and potash must be added to water. If water is added to caustic soda or potash, the situation could potentially be dangerous as the temperature rises very quickly.
- Never put caustic soda or potash, or soap solutions containing unsaponified caustic soda or potash, into aluminium, tin, iron or Teflon as it corrodes these materials.
- Read the information and cautions on containers of caustic soda or potash.

Fats and oils

As your main fat or oil component in the saponification process, use coconut oil or olive oil, as they saponify readily to give you a relatively hard soap that lathers well, and they are inexpensive. Other vegetable oils and fats (such as apricot kernel, sweet almond, jojoba, evening primrose, hemp, wheatgerm, avocado, shea butter and cocoa butter) can be added for their emollient and skin-softening properties.

The term 'superfatting' means the quantity of oil and fat is higher than the lye can possibly saponify, and therefore a portion of the oil and fat remain in the soap unaltered, making it less drying, softer, creamier and more emollient on the skin.

Additives

Emollients, exfoliants, colourants and essential oils may be added to your soaps to benefit your skin or delight your senses. Emollients such as vegetable oils, infused oils and vegetable butters can be included as part of the total vegetable oil content at the start of the recipe, whereas exfoliants and colourants are added once the soap thickens. If they are added too early, the caustic soda may affect them or they may interfere with the saponification process.

Emollients

Emollients make a soap milder and gentler on the skin. They include the following skin softening and smoothing ingredients:

> vegetable oils, infused oils, vegetable butters such as cocoa butter and shea butter, honey, lecithin, glycerin

Exfoliants

Exfoliating ingredients are added to soaps to help slough off dead skin cells, keeping the skin smooth. Some of these include:

> ground oats, bran, almond meal, cinnamon, cornmeal, poppy seeds, pumice and sand

Colourants

Natural colourants such as dried, powdered botanicals and clays give soaps lovely earthy colours. However, be mindful that some botanical colourants will change colour and fade radically in the presence of lye.

The following herbs, spices and clays make excellent natural soap colouring agents:

- **Paprika** or **annatto** will produce light to deep apricot shades.
- **Madder root** gives natural reddish, pink colours.
- **Turmeric** will produce beige to yellow/orange colours.
- **Spirulina** and **chlorophyll** give green colours.
- **Cloves**, **cinnamon** and **cacao powder** will produce beige to chocolate colours.
- **Green clay**, **red clay**, **pink clay** and **yellow clay** will add their respective colours to the soap, with yellow tending towards a beige colour rather than yellow.
- **Carrot infused oil** will add a rich yellow colour to the soap.
- **Charcoal powder** will produce grey to black colours.

The quantity added will affect the final intensity of colour produced, from pastel shades through to richer colours.

Dried botanicals

Dried flowers are best added to the tops of soaps where they can be seen and make the soap look beautiful. They can be stirred throughout the soap, but be prepared for them to turn brown and lose their appeal. Calendula petals are relatively good at retaining their colour when mixed into soap. Flecks of dried, ground leaves and spices can look attractive stirred throughout soaps.

Essential oils

Essential oils may constitute up to 3% of the total vegetable oil/fat quantity of the soap recipe, depending on their odour intensity and your skin sensitivity. Citrus essential oils are generally not recommended for use as the main fragrance in a soap as their odour intensity is low and their scent fades quickly. Fresh smelling essential oils such as lemongrass, may chang or lemon myrtle will be better options.

Odour intense essential oils are especially suitable for use in soap. Some of these include cedarwood, eucalyptus, geranium, lavender, lemongrass, lemon myrtle, patchouli, peppermint, petitgrain, rosemary, spearmint, tea tree, vetiver and ylang ylang.

See Precautions on page 38 before choosing essential oils to ensure their suitability for use on the skin.

Equipment

- 2 cooking thermometers (they must register temperatures as low as 20°C and as high as 100°C)
- digital scales
- 2 large heat-resistant jugs or bowls
- 1 heat-resistant jug
- 2 stainless-steel saucepans
- silicon spatula
- wooden or stainless-steel mixing spoon
- electric stick mixer
- rubber gloves
- protective safety glasses
- long-sleeved shirt and trousers
- covered shoes
- paper to cover benches
- old blankets or towels
- moulds

Moulds

The best moulds to use with the Basic soap recipe are plastic, silicon or lined wooden moulds in box, loaf or slab styles. Alternatively, cardboard boxes, such as shoe boxes lined with compostable baking paper, ice cream containers and milk cartons also make suitable moulds. If a mould is somewhat flexible, the soap is more easily removed. Specialised moulds can be purchased from soap making suppliers.

Basic soap recipe

This Basic soap recipe is a simple vegetable-based soap with a creamy, gentle lather. It is superfatted with vegetable oils, ensuring it is kind and less drying to the skin. You can choose to add exfoliants, colourants or essential oils and tailor-make your own soap, or leave them out if you prefer a simple soap.

Ingredients

350 g olive oil
330 g coconut oil
220 g purified water
100 g caustic soda

———————————

up to 20 g colourants
up to 20 g exfoliants
10 g to 20 g essential oils

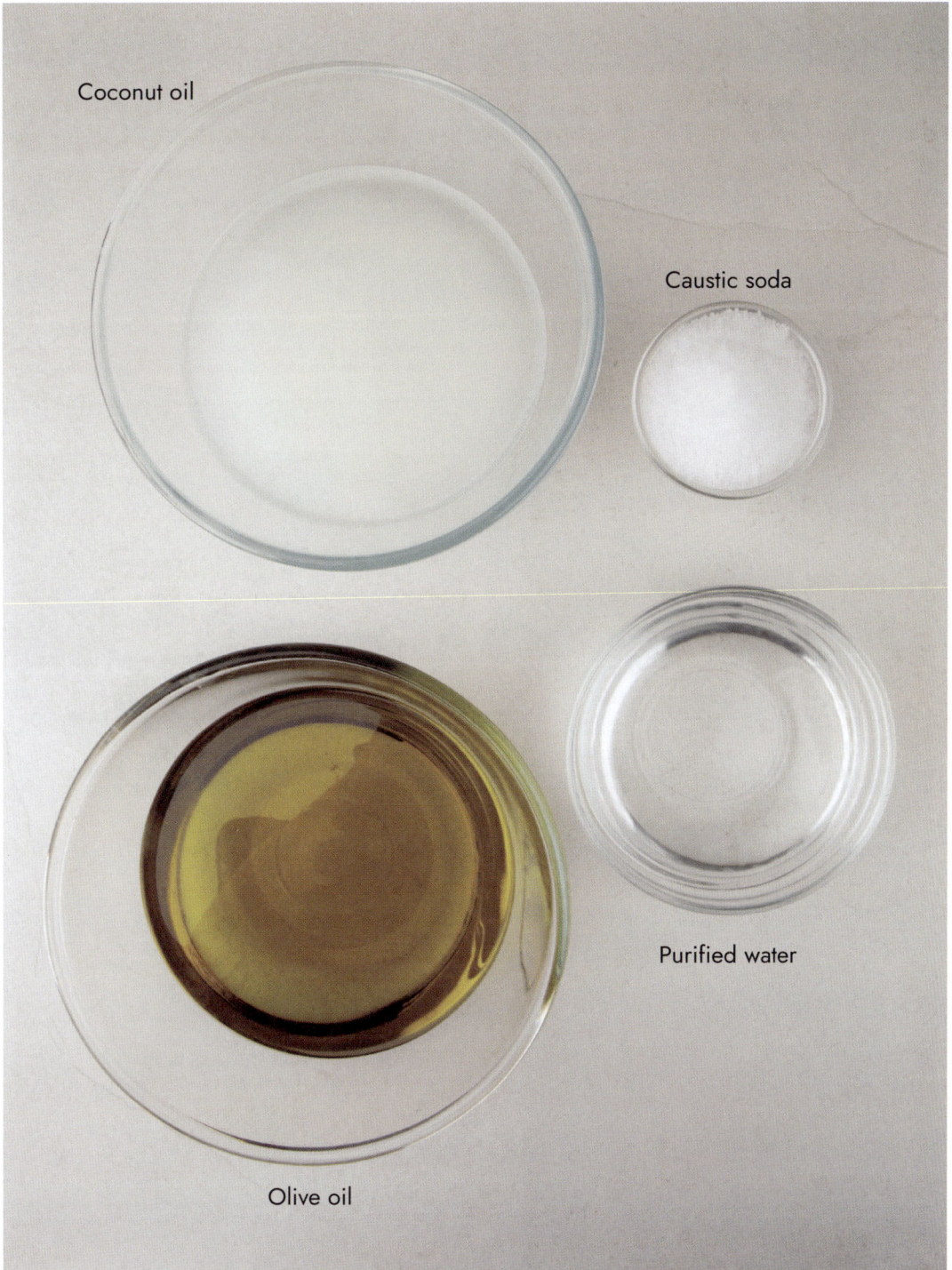

Coconut oil

Caustic soda

Olive oil

Purified water

Basic soap recipe ingredients

Cold-process method for making soap

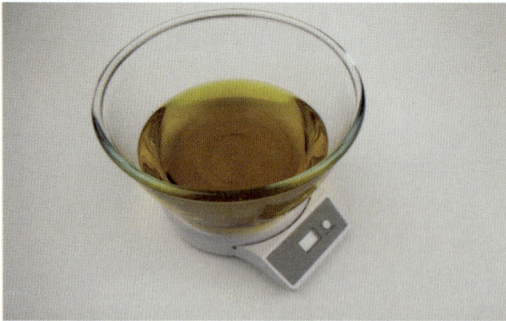

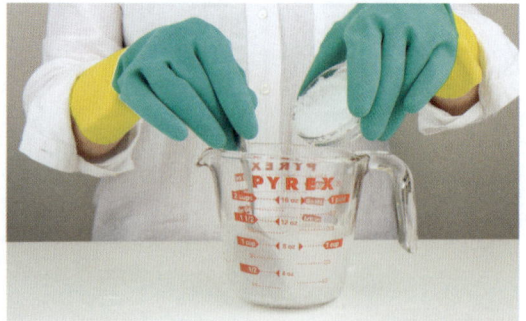

1. Read 'Cautions when using lye' on page 168 first or the label on the caustic soda container.
2. Weigh out the ingredients.

3. Pour the purified water into a heat-resistant glass jug.
4. Wearing gloves, protective safety glasses and protective clothing, slowly add the caustic soda into the water as you stir. It will increase in temperature to around 70°C without heat being applied. Ensure that it has dissolved properly. This solution is now called 'lye'.

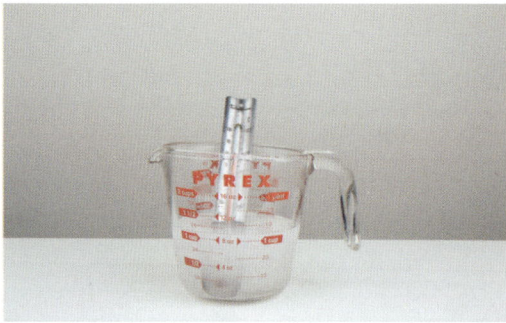

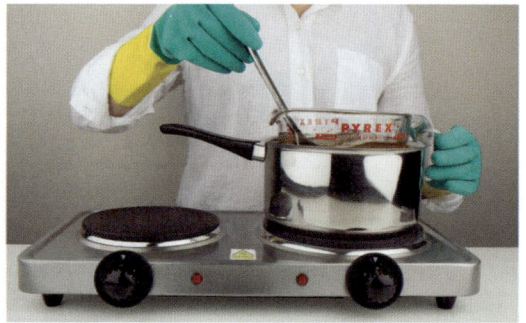

5. Leave the lye to cool until the temperature is 35–38°C. Otherwise, stand the jug of hot lye in cold water in the sink to speed up the cooling process. It can be heated back up to the correct temperature in a *bain-marie* if necessary.

6. Melt the oils and fats in the heat-resistant glass bowl in a *bain-marie* and heat to 35–38°C. Once again, place the bowl in a sink of cold water to lower the temperature if required.

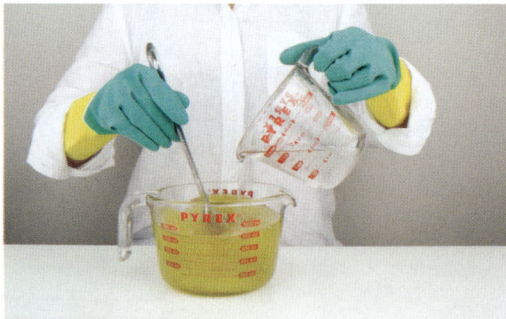

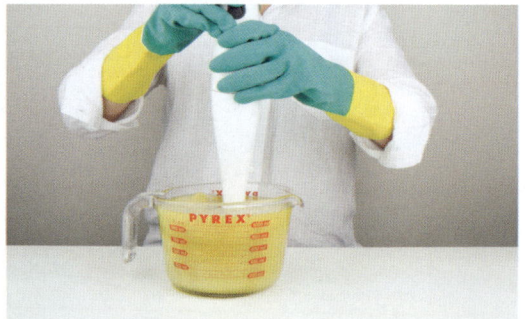

7. Once both mixtures reach 35–38°C, pour the lye in a slow constant stream into the oils and fats while stirring constantly and smoothly at a medium pace. The correct temperature is important to ensure the saponification reaction occurs properly. If you see too much lye floating on the surface of the fats and oils while you are pouring the lye solution, stop pouring until the lye has been incorporated. Continue pouring and stirring.

8. Once all the lye has been incorporated, use an electric stick mixer to fully emulsify the mixture. If you stir by hand, the process can take a lot longer. Do not emulsify too long with the stick mixer as the mixture may become too thick to add the additional ingredients easily.

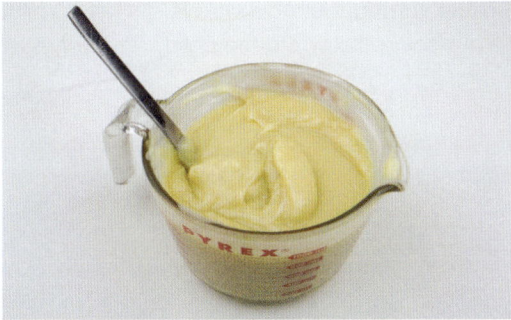

9. The mixture will now become opaque and thicken. Using a spoon, drizzle some of the soap mixture across the surface of the soap. When the soap is thick enough to momentarily hold the drizzle on the surface of the mixture (this is known as '**tracing**'), it is ready to pour into a mould or have any additives incorporated into it. See page 174.

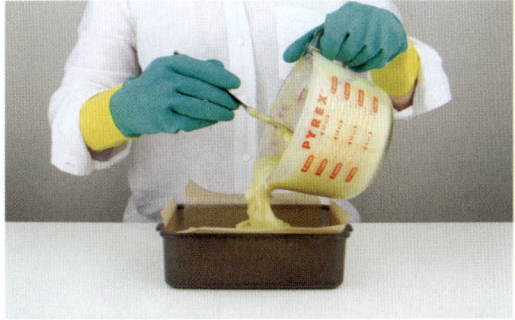

10. Pour the finished soap mixture into a mould.

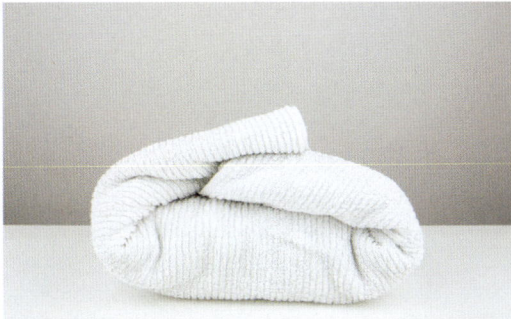

11. Place a lid or cover on top of the mould and wrap it in several thick blankets to keep the soap warm, and leave your soap to solidify. This takes around 24–48 hours. Do not interfere with your soap during this time.

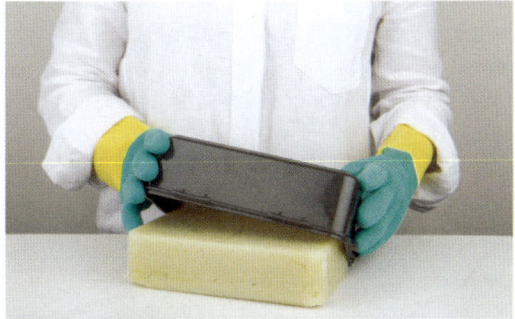

12. After 24–48 hours, remove the blankets from around the mould and check on your soap. Your soap should be firm but will still be a little soft. If it is too soft, leave it in the mould unwrapped for a day or so to dry and harden. You will then be less likely to damage your soap when trying to remove it.

13. Wearing rubber gloves, gently remove it from the mould.

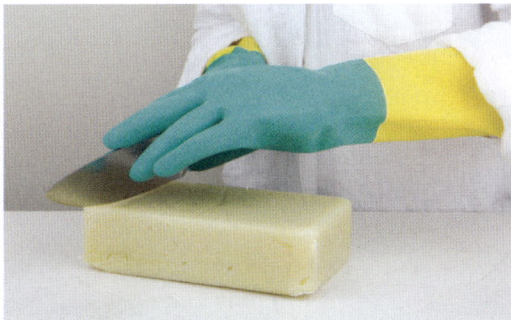

14. Place the block of soap on a clean surface. The soap will become reasonably firm over the next 7 days. Leave your soap to harden and finish curing for about 4 weeks. A reaction is still going on, although considerably slower. You may notice a slightly powdery layer on your soap. This is sodium carbonate, also known as 'soda ash', and is a reaction of the lye with carbon dioxide in the air. Slice this off once you have allowed your soap to finish curing or wipe it off carefully with a damp cloth.

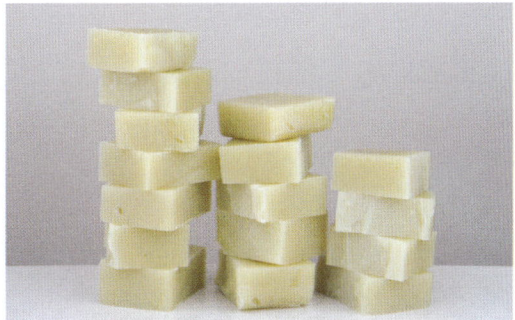

15. Cut into bars. Voila! You now have ready-to-use bars of soap.

16. Wrap soaps that you will not be using immediately in cellophane or waxed paper or store in a container. This reduces the evaporation of any essential oils and keeps the soap fresh.

Basic Soap Making **173**

Adding colours, fragrances, emollients and exfoliants

Add any colours, fragrances, emollients and exfoliants in step 9. Pour or spoon out a small amount of the soap mixture from the main bowl or jug into a smaller jug. Mix your additives into this small amount of soap mixture before incorporating it back into the main soap mixture. Ensure the additives are mixed in thoroughly. Add it back into the main soap mixture and use an electric hand mixer to ensure it is mixed in homogeneously, or hand stir for a more rustic look.

Soap Making Problems

Problems which occur when making soap are usually due to:

- incorrect measurement of ingredients
- incorrect temperature
- poor quality ingredients.

Separation

If your mixture is separating in the bowl, heat the mixture again, stirring as it melts. Remove from the heat and blend with an electric stick mixer. Once it thickens, pour into the mould.

Not thickening

If your mixture isn't thickening, reheat it, then remove it from the heat and blend with an electric stick mixer.

If your mixture won't trace but looks thick, pour it into your mould and cover it more thoroughly with blankets to keep it warm.

Caustic bubbles

Except for a thin coating of soda ash on the surface, your soap should look much the same throughout. If pockets of lye form in your soap, throw out the batch, as the lye will cause skin irritation.

Soap Recipes

To get yourself started and to build your confidence in soap making, try one of these gorgeous recipes, using the *Method for making cold-process soap* on page 172.

Chocolate cake soap

Looks just like chocolate cake and contains many similar ingredients. Absolutely delicious to use!

60 g cocoa butter
320 g olive oil
300 g coconut oil
220 g purified water
100 g caustic soda
20 g cacao powder

Add the cacao powder at the end of step 9.

French angel soap

A gorgeous pink soap with a fragrance that lifts the spirits.

60 g shea butter
320 g olive oil
300 g coconut oil
220 g purified water
100 g caustic soda
20 g pink clay
5 g geranium essential oil
5 g ylang ylang essential oil

Add the pink clay and essential oils at the end of step 9.

Peppermint twist soap

Smells fresh and delicious and looks great.

320 g olive oil
300 g coconut oil
60 g sweet almond oil
220 g purified water
100 g caustic soda
20 g green clay
10 g peppermint essential oil

1. Add the essential oil to the soap mixture as per the instructions at the end of step 9.

2. Once the peppermint essential oil has been added back into the soap mixture and stirred in well, remove another small quantity of the soap mixture and add the green clay to it and stir through it.

3. Pour the rest of the soap mixture into the soap mould.

4. Then add the green clay soap mixture back into the rest of the soap, swirling it through with a long-handled spoon to create twists throughout the soap.

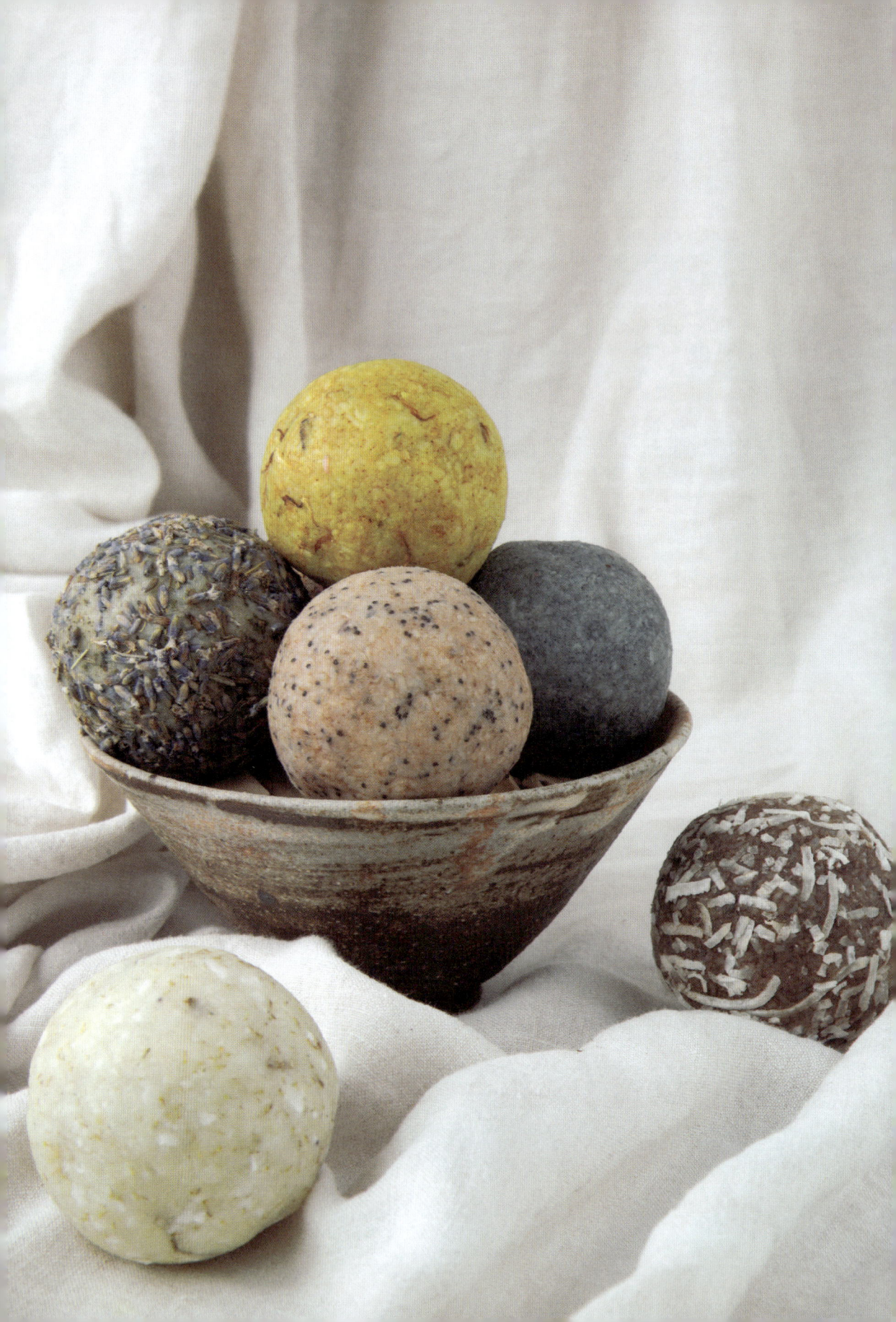

Soap Balls

Eye-catching soap balls and other shapes can be made using this easy method.

Basic soap ball recipe

Ingredients

250 g grated soap base
up to 20 g colourants
up to 20 g emollients
up to 20 g exfoliants
dried herbs and petals
2–3 g essential oil or essential oil blend
20–50 mL purified water

Method for making soap balls

1. Make the *Basic soap recipe* on page 170.

2. Once the soap has cured, grate it down finely, ready for mixing with other ingredients.

3. Weigh out the ingredients.

4. Mix the dry additives together in a bowl.

5. Then, mix the dry additives through the grated soap base.

6. Drizzle and mix through any liquid ingredients into the soap base, except for water.

7. Finally, add the water, small amounts at a time, and mix through until moist. It is important not to add all the water specified as you may only need a small amount of water if your soap base is especially moist.

8. Working quickly, knead the ingredients together into a dough.

9. Your soap mixture can now be formed into various shapes. You can roll the mixture into balls the size of a plum or you can also get creative and form other shapes. Otherwise, you can press the mixture firmly into moulds (such as chocolate moulds). Ensure there are no air bubbles.

10. Leave to dry and set properly in a warm, dry, airy spot. The soap balls will dry in about 3 days up to a week. The soap pressed into moulds may take a week before it can be removed from the moulds. Alternatively, it can be placed in the freezer until hard, then removed from the moulds and left to dry.

Choose one of the recipes below and follow the steps above to make some gorgeous soap balls.

Daydream soap balls

Sweet and gentle on the skin.

250 g grated soap base
2 tbsp cocoa butter (chopped finely)
1 tbsp crumbled dried chamomile flowers
30 drops ylang ylang essential oil
20–50 mL purified water

Choc bliss soap balls

Deliciously chocolatey. Roll the damp balls in the desiccated coconut to finish your choc bliss soap balls.

250 g grated soap base
2 tbsp cacao powder
1 tbsp desiccated coconut
20 mL vanilla essence
5–30 mL purified water

Good vibrations soap balls

Earthy pink balls with tiny poppy seed speckles.

250 g grated soap base
4 tsp poppy seeds
2 tsp kaolin clay
1 tsp pink Argiletz clay
40 drops patchouli essential oil
20–50 mL purified water

Medieval herbal soap balls

A fresh, herbaceous soap. Roll the damp balls in the lavender flowers to finish your medieval soap balls rather than add them to the soap mixture.

250 g grated soap base
2 tbsp sage powder
2 tbsp lavender flowers
1 tbsp elderflowers
30 drops lavender essential oil
20 drops rosemary essential oil
10 drops sage essential oil
20–50mL purified water

Calendula petal soap balls

A yellow soap ball that smells of delicious oranges.

250 g grated soap base
2 tbsp calendula flowers
1 tsp turmeric
70 drops sweet orange essential oil
20–50mL purified water

Persian love soap balls

A sweet, spicy soap. Roll the damp balls in the crumbled rose petals to finish your soap balls rather than add them to the soap mixture.

250 g grated soap base
4 tsp kaolin clay
1 tsp cinnamon powder
1 tsp pink Argiletz clay
50 drops mandarin essential oil
25–50 mL rosewater
2 tbsp crumbled dried rose petals

Charcoal shave soap

A creamy shaving soap. The added sweet almond oil gives you a smooth surface to shave.

250 g soap base
20 mL sweet almond oil
½ tsp activated charcoal
60 drops Atlas cedarwood essential oil
25–50 mL purified water

Multi-coloured soap balls

Create fun coloured soap balls by making soap from scratch in two different colours then mixing them together when you follow the steps for the *Basic soap ball recipe*. For example, the *Chocolate cake soap* and the *French angel soap* can both be grated down and then mixed together to create a pink and brown motley soap. Add more colours if you have other soap available.

Body

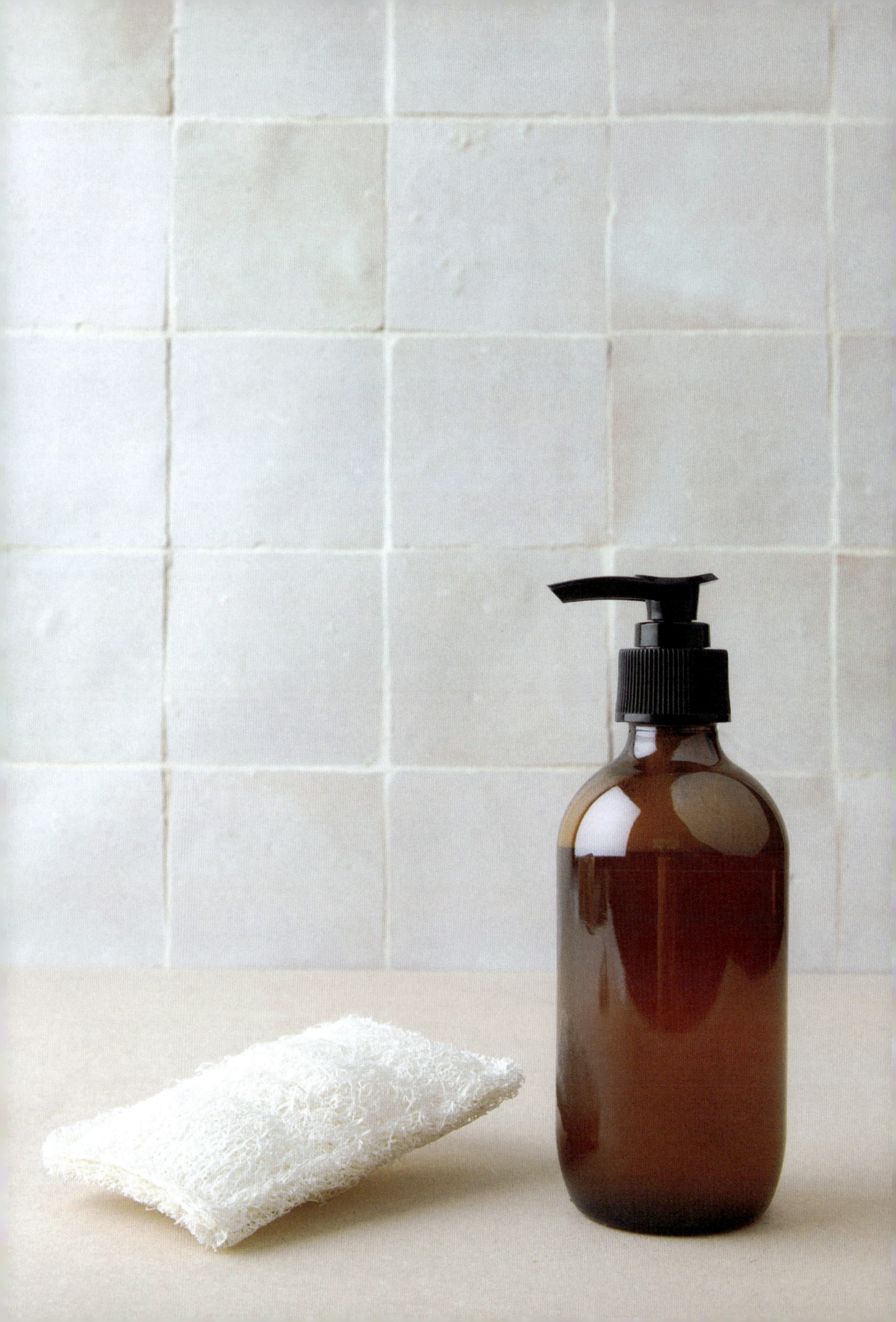

Body Washes

Body washes are liquid preparations that can be used to cleanse your skin and are an alternative to using bars of soap.

Soapwort body wash

A particularly gentle cleansing decoction for sensitive, irritated or inflamed skins.

10 g soapwort root
250 mL purified water

1. Boil and simmer the soapwort root in the water for 20–30 minutes.
2. Remove from the heat and allow to cool.
3. Strain the liquid.
4. Pour over your body and gently massage to cleanse the skin.
5. Store any unused liquid in the refrigerator and use it within a couple of days.

Castile liquid soap body wash

Castile liquid soap is made on pure olive oil and, oftentimes, in combination with coconut oil. It is a gentle body wash and is generally suitable for sensitive skin. Add approximately 20 drops of your favourite essential oil/oils to every 100 mL of Castile liquid soap.

Plain Castile liquid soap can be purchased readily from aromatherapy suppliers, bulk food shops and health food stores.

Add salt solution for thickening

A salt solution can be added to your Castile liquid soap recipes to thicken them. It is a simple solution of ordinary table salt (sodium chloride) dissolved into purified water.

1. Make a salt solution with 5 g of table salt dissolved into 25 g of purified water.
2. Add drops of the salt solution slowly, while stirring into the Castile liquid soap/ essential oil mixture. You will need to watch the mixture for the point at which it starts to thicken. Do not add too much salt solution as it will turn into a lumpy gel. Add approximately 30–60 drops to each 100 mL of Castile liquid soap.

Add vegetable oil to reduce dryness

To reduce the drying effects of Castile liquid soap, add 20 mL of vegetable oil to each 100 mL of Castile liquid soap. Shake the bottle to mix the vegetable oil throughout the Castile liquid soap then shake each time before use.

Adding both salt solution and vegetable oil

If you have thickened Castile liquid soap with salt solution, adding vegetable oil to the mixture will thin it out again. You will only be able to add a small amount of vegetable oil, approximately 1%, i.e. around 1 mL to each 100 mL of thickened Castile liquid soap.

For more recipes based on Castile liquid soap see page 101.

Body wash base

A body wash base made from plant-derived surfactants can oftentimes be purchased from aromatherapy suppliers. It allows you to easily customise your body wash by adding your favourite essential oils. Add approximately 20 drops of your favourite essential oil/s to each 100 g or mL of body wash base.

You may like to choose one of these essential oil compositions to add to Castile liquid soap or body wash base. The quantities specified here are to be added to each 100 g or mL of base.

Essential oil compositions for body washes

Alive composition	Citrus juice composition	Relaxing composition
Fresh and exuberant	*Deliciously fruity*	*Uplifting and relaxing*
8 drops pine	8 drops bergamot	8 drops sandalwood
7 drops lemongrass	8 drops sweet orange	6 drops bergamot
5 drops Atlas cedarwood	4 drops lemon	6 drops lavender

Body Scrubs

Smooth and polish your skin with a body scrub. Wash your skin first, then massage one of these mouth-watering body scrubs all over your body. Rinse, then follow with a beautiful body moisturiser.

Sugar and Salt Scrubs

The following scrubs make use of sugar to exfoliate the skin. However, salt could be substituted for sugar. As the sugar and salt granules exfoliate the skin, they gradually dissolve in the bath or shower water. The emollient ingredients remain on the skin to soften, protect and keep the freshly revealed skin moisturised.

Orange marmalade body scrub

This delicious body scrub is suitable for smoothing and moisturising dry skins.

4 tbsp granulated raw sugar
2 tbsp sweet almond oil
zest of one orange

1. Grate the skin of the orange to obtain the zest.
2. Mix the zest with the sugar and oil in a bowl.
3. Store the scrub in a jar.
4. Massage over your body before rinsing in the shower.

Lime body smoother

Smooth your skin and be revived with this wonderful body scrub. Suitable for most skin types.

4 tbsp granulated raw sugar
2 tsp poppy seeds
⅛ tsp green tea powder
⅛ tsp turmeric powder
2 tbsp macadamia oil
20 drops lime essential oil

1. Mix all the dry ingredients together in a bowl.
2. Add the oils and mix well.
3. Store the scrub in a jar.
4. Massage over your body before rinsing in the shower.

River revitalisation body scrub

Refreshes your senses and leaves your skin feeling silky smooth. This scrub is made entirely from Australian ingredients.

70 g Murray River salt flakes
30 g macadamia oil
1 tsp dried quandong powder
20 drops rosalina essential oil

1. Break down the salt flakes in a mortar and pestle or coffee grinder to a smaller granule size suitable for exfoliating the skin.
2. Mix together with the dried quandong powder.
3. Add the macadamia oil and rosalina essential oil and mix well.
4. Store the mixture in a jar.
5. Massage over your body before rinsing in the shower.

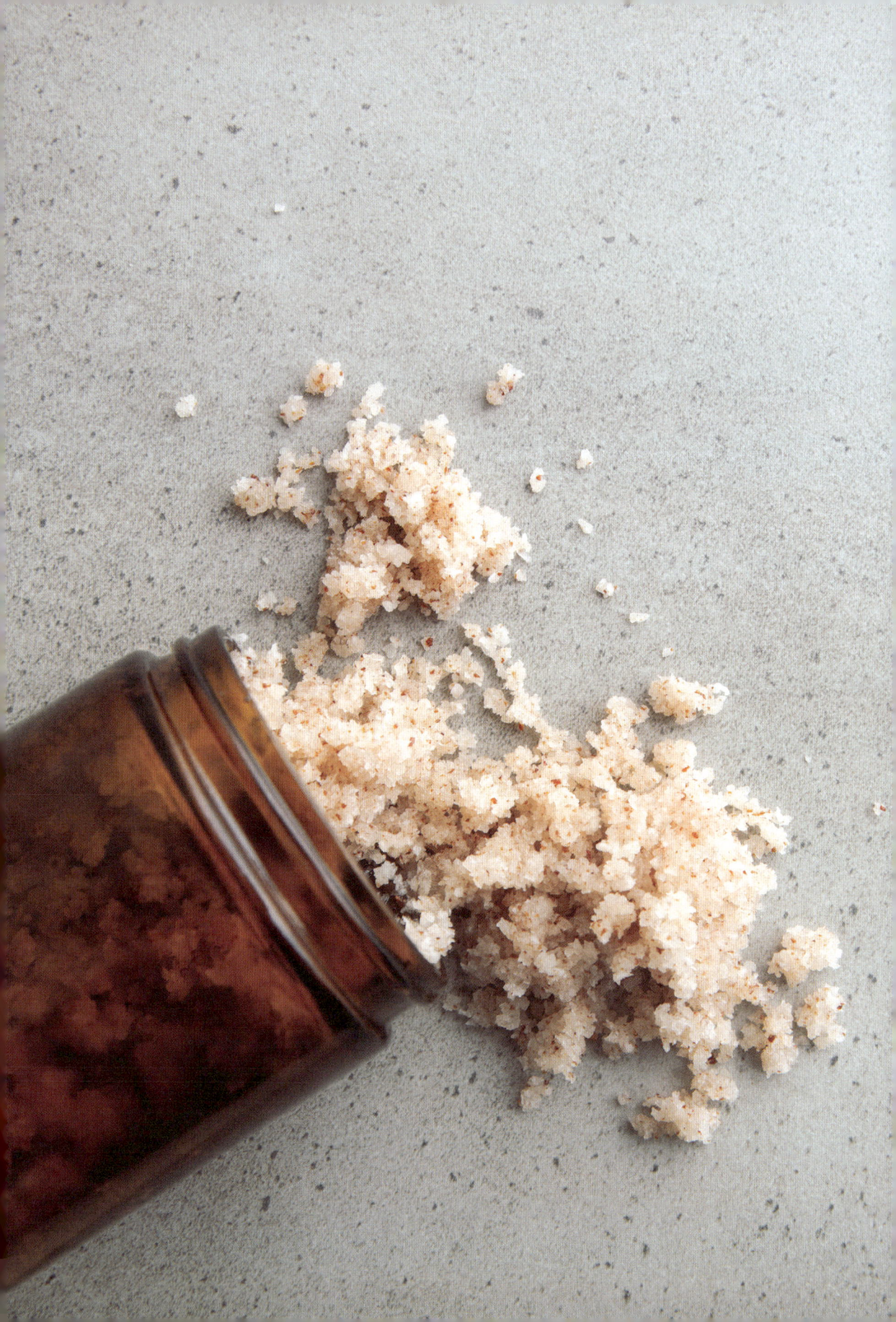

Exfoliating Body Bars

Exfoliating bars are solid salt and sugar scrubs. Cocoa butter is the ingredient that makes the bars hard. It also assists in moisturising as it melts into the skin.

Lemon myrtle exfoliating bar

A refreshing solid exfoliating bar.

80 g cocoa butter
20 g shea butter
100 g granulated raw sugar
1 tsp lemon myrtle powder
30 drops lemon myrtle essential oil

1. Mix the sugar and lemon myrtle powder together in a bowl.
2. Melt the cocoa butter and shea butter in a *bain-marie*.
3. Remove from the heat and stir in the essential oil, sugar and lemon myrtle powder.
4. Pour into moulds such as a muffin tray.
5. Place in the refrigerator or freezer and once set, remove from the moulds.
6. In hot weather, store the bars in a container in the refrigerator to prevent melting.
7. Massage over your skin in the shower or bath.

Coffee buff bar

Wakes you up and smooths your skin.

80 g cocoa butter
20 g shea butter
100 g granulated raw sugar
50 g coffee granules

1. Mix the sugar and coffee granules together in a bowl.
2. Melt the cocoa butter and shea butter in a *bain-marie*.
3. Remove from the heat and stir in the sugar and coffee granules.
4. Pour into moulds such as a muffin tray.
5. Place in the refrigerator or freezer and once set, remove from the moulds.
6. In hot weather, store the bars in a container in the refrigerator to prevent melting.
7. Massage over your skin in the shower or bath.

Fresh Body Scrubs

Fresh creamy body scrubs to reveal fresh smooth skin.

Green grapefruit body scrub

This body scrub is superb for cleansing and smoothing oily and blemished skins. This scrub may be applied as a body mask first and left on for 10 minutes or so before using it as a scrub. If the mask has dried, pat on a small amount of water before massaging it over your body as a scrub.

Part A
4 tbsp green Argiletz clay
4 tbsp white rice flour
15 drops grapefruit essential oil
10 drops juniper berry essential oil

Part B
water or natural yoghurt

1. Mix the green clay and white rice flour together in a bowl.
2. Sieve to break down any lumps in the powder.

3. Add the drops of essential oils, ensuring you sprinkle them uniformly over the mixture, then stir them in.

4. Sieve again a couple of times to ensure any lumps are broken down and the essential oils are evenly distributed throughout the mixture.

5. Store in a jar until ready to use.

6. To use, spoon 2 tablespoonfuls of Part A (dry ingredients) into a small bowl and stir in 1½ tablespoons of Part B (water or yoghurt.) Mix together to form a paste and massage over your skin before showering.

3. To use, spoon 2 tablespoons into a small bowl and stir in 1½ tablespoons of water. Mix together to form a fizzy, creamy mousse. Massage over damp skin and leave on for up to 5 minutes.

4. Remove by massaging and rinsing well in the shower.

Banana smoothie body scrub

A gentle, creamy body scrub for dry, sensitive skin. Use this body scrub fresh.

1 tbsp mashed banana
1 tsp oat flour
2 tbsp almond meal
2 tsp honey

1. Mash the banana, then mix together in a bowl with the other ingredients.

2. Massage over your skin while bathing.

Vitamin cacao body smoother

A delicious, fizzy, creamy, mousse exfoliant that leaves your skin feeling silky smooth.

1 tbsp cacao powder
1 tsp cinnamon powder
1 tbsp kaolin clay
1 tbsp rhassoul clay
1 tsp L-ascorbic acid (vitamin C)
2 tsp sodium bicarbonate

1. Mix all the ingredients together in a bowl.

2. Store in a jar until ready to use.

Body Masks

Revive and renew your skin with a fresh body mask made especially for you. Body masks may be used all over the body or on problem areas such as the upper back, shoulders and chest, where there can be pimples, or on areas where there is inflammation or dryness. Masks for the face may also be used as body masks.

To use a body mask, wash your skin first and exfoliate with a body scrub if necessary. Apply your body mask to those areas of skin you desire. Leave the mask on for 15–20 minutes or the time specified in the recipes, then rinse off under the shower. Follow with a body moisturiser.

Paw paw (papaya) and clay body mask

A cleansing body mask for oily and blemished skin. Especially good for chests, upper backs and where pimples appear. Use this body mask fresh.

2 tbsp green Argiletz clay
1 tbsp kaolin clay
1 tbsp mashed paw paw (papaya)
1 tbsp natural yoghurt
4 drops grapefruit essential oil

1. Mash the paw paw and mix it well with the yoghurt, green clay, kaolin and grapefruit essential oil until you have a smooth consistency.
2. Smooth over your skin and leave on for 15–20 minutes.
3. Remove with a damp sponge or cloth and rinse well in the shower.

Soft and soothing body mask

A soothing, calming body mask for sensitive skin. Especially good for soothing itchy, dry, irritated skin. It may also be used on the face. Use this mask fresh.

1 tbsp oat flour
1 tbsp potato starch
1 tbsp coconut milk powder
1 tbsp aloe vera juice

1. Mix the oat flour, potato starch and coconut milk powder together in a bowl and sieve to break down any lumps.
2. Mix with 1 tablespoon of aloe vera juice into a smooth paste.
3. Smooth over clean skin and leave on for 10 minutes.
4. Remove with a damp sponge or cloth and rinse well in the shower.

Seaweed body mask

A hydrating and healing mask for dry skin. It may also be used on the face. Use this mask fresh.

20 g kelp powder
80 g purified water

1. Add enough water to the kelp powder to form a paste.
2. Smooth over damp skin and leave on for 10–15 minutes.
3. Remove with a damp sponge or cloth and rinse well in the shower.

187

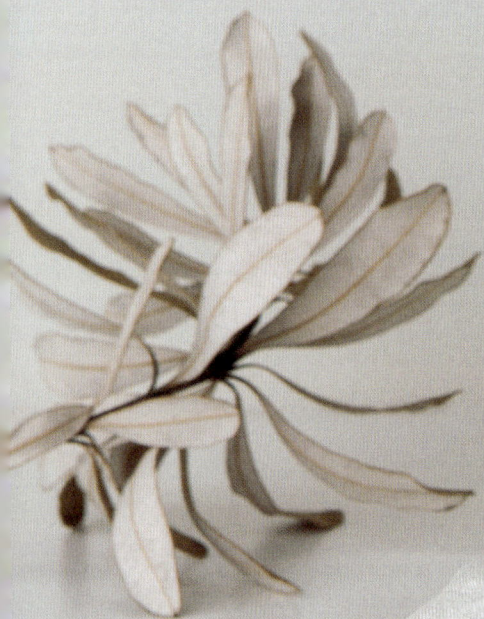

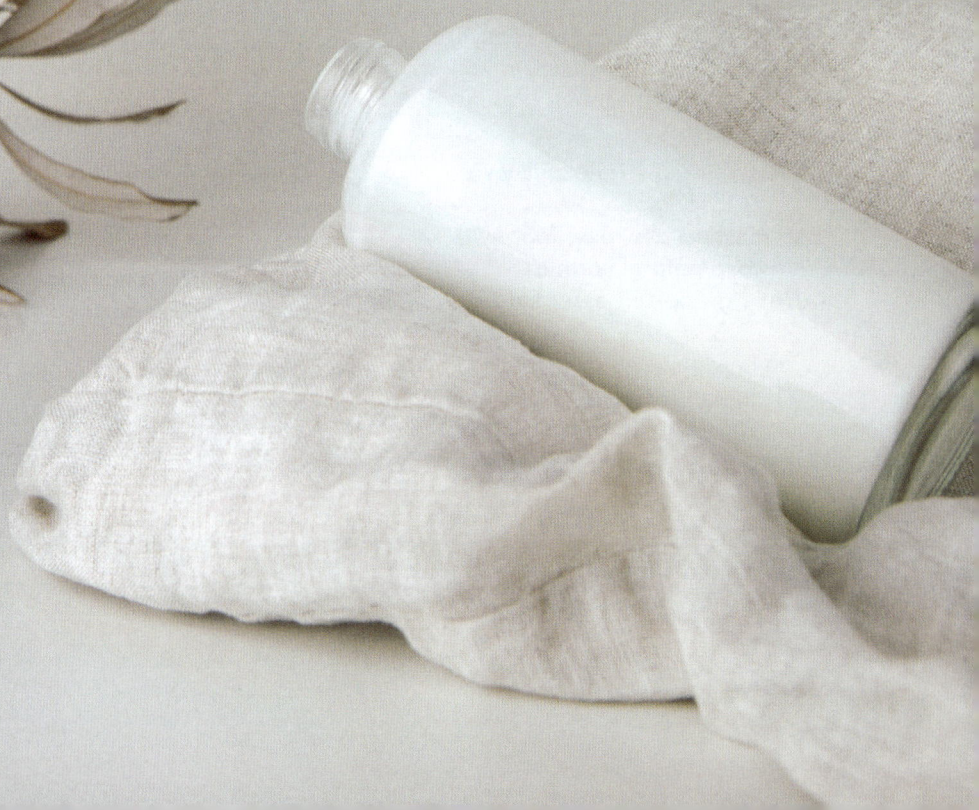

Body Moisturisers

Keep your skin soft and hydrated with these beautiful skin creams.

Jojoba light body lotion

This body lotion is instantly absorbed by your skin and doesn't feel greasy. It leaves your skin feeling lightly moisturised. Suitable for all skin types.

Oil phase
> 7 g plant-derived emulsifying wax
> 20 g jojoba oil

Water phase
> 164.5 g purified water
> 6 g vegetable glycerin
> 0.5 g xanthan gum
> 2 g preservative

Add at 40°C
> 2 g (approx. 40 drops) essential oil

pH adjustment
> qs citric acid + purified water

Choose an essential oil from pages 39–48 or essential oil composition for your skin type from page 48 and make this body lotion by following the *Method for making an emulsion with emulsifying wax* on page 79.

Avocado nourishing body cream

If you like a body lotion that is nourishing and protective, this one is beautifully rich. Suitable for dry skin.

Oil phase
> 11 g plant-derived emulsifying wax
> 40 g avocado oil
> 20 g macadamia oil
> 1 g antioxidant

Water phase
> 120 g purified water
> 6 g vegetable glycerin
> 2 g preservative

Add at 40°C
> 2 g (approx. 40 drops) essential oil

pH adjustment
> qs citric acid + purified water

Choose an essential oil from pages 39–48 or essential oil composition for your skin type from page 48 and make this cream by following the *Method for making an emulsion with emulsifying* wax on page 79.

Ultra-rich body cream

This cream is an incredibly rich, thick moisturiser for very dry skin.

Oil phase
> 14 g plant-derived emulsifying wax
> 67 g avocado oil
> 15 g wheatgerm oil
> 5 g carrot infused oil
> 1 g antioxidant

Water phase
> 90 g purified water
> 6 g vegetable glycerin
> 2 g preservative

Add at 40°C
> 2 g (approx. 40 drops) essential oil

<u>pH adjustment</u>
qs citric acid + purified water

Choose an essential oil from pages 39–48 or essential oil composition for your skin type from page 48 and make this cream by following the *Method for making an emulsion with emulsifying wax* on page 79.

Body Massage Preparations

Body oils, balms and bars lubricate your skin, giving you a smooth surface to massage. When applied after bathing or showering, they reduce moisture loss and keep the skin feeling soft, smooth and supple.

Using cold-pressed vegetable oils infused with herbs or blended with essential oils will fragrance your skin, lift your spirits and provide therapeutic benefits to your skin and body.

Cold-pressed vegetable oils enhance the absorption of the essential oils into your skin and give you the lubrication you need for a smooth, soothing massage. They contain vitamins and essential fatty acids which, along with the essential oils, soften, smooth and nurture your skin.

Vegetable oils such as apricot kernel oil, sweet almond oil and macadamia oil make superb massage oils and body oil bases as they provide enough lubrication and are eventually absorbed into the surface of the skin.

Herbal Infused Massage and Body Oils

You can use herbal infused oils made with cold-pressed vegetable oils, herbs and flowers as massage or body oils. Follow the methods for making herbal infused oils on page 52.

- **Pine needles, rosemary** and **ginger** are excellent choices to infuse for sore, aching muscles.
- Infuse **lavender** and **chamomile** flowers to make a relaxing massage or body oil.
- **Jasmine**, **honeysuckle** and **frangipani** flowers make a truly luxurious and sensual massage or body oil.

Aromatherapy Massage and Body Oils

Aromatherapy massage and body oils are simple to make. Choose your essential oils according to their properties. Enjoy their diverse and enticing aromas as well as their health-giving benefits. However, it is important to check for any contraindications and safety issues on page 38 before using your choice of essential oils.

To make an aromatherapy massage oil, add up to a maximum of 2.5% essential oil to a cold-pressed vegetable oil, that is, approximately 50 drops of essential oil to 100 mL of cold-pressed vegetable oil. Sweet almond oil, apricot kernel oil or macadamia oil can be used as a simple base for a massage oil.

To make an aromatherapy body oil to use on a daily basis, reduce the amount of essential oil added to around 1%, which is approximately 20 drops of essential oil to 100 mL of cold-pressed vegetable oil.

Massage oil base

This blend of cold-pressed vegetable oils may be used unscented or blended with a favourite essential oil or essential oil composition suitable for your skin type. It will help protect and keep your skin moisturised.

50 mL macadamia oil
25 mL avocado oil
25 mL rosehip oil
20–50 drops essential oil

Choose an essential oil from pages 39–48 or an essential oil composition for body and massage preparations from page 196. Add the essential oils to the vegetable oils in a glass bottle and shake well.

Scar treatment oil

This blend of oils is rich in vitamins and essential oils to encourage skin repair and address redness.

15 mL rosehip oil
5 mL calendula infused oil
5 mL carrot infused oil
5 drops lavender essential oil
3 drops frankincense essential oil
2 drops everlasting essential oil

Add the essential oils to the vegetable oils in a glass bottle and shake well. Initially, apply the blend to the area around the wound. Once the skin has formed over the top of the wound, massage the blend gently into the healing skin twice daily.

Skin soothing body oil

This massage oil is a combination of skin soothing oils to calm red, irritated, dry skin.

80 mL jojoba oil
20 mL calendula infused oil
6 drops sandalwood essential oil
5 drops lavender essential oil
3 drops yarrow essential oil
1 drop German chamomile essential oil

Add the essential oils to the vegetable oils in a glass bottle and shake well. Apply twice daily, especially after washing.

Gorgeous goddess body elixir

A nourishing and rejuvenating body oil for the skin or to be enjoyed as an exquisite massage oil.

85 mL macadamia oil
15 mL rosehip oil
10 drops rose absolute
6 drops geranium essential oil
5 drops ylang ylang essential oil
4 drops frankincense essential oil

Add the essential oils to the vegetable oils in a glass bottle and shake well. Smooth over your body after bathing or showering.

For more body oil recipes, see page 104.

Aromatherapy Massage and Body Balms

Balms are convenient to use. Unlike massage or body oils, balms won't spill. Just dip your fingers into your jar of balm and apply it to your skin for a massage. Alternatively, after your bath or shower, smooth a little over your skin to keep it feeling soft and smooth.

To make a balm, follow the *Methods for making aromatherapy balms* on page 63 and add your choice of essential oils or an essential oil composition for body and massage preparations from page 196.

For more balm recipes, see page 111.

Bush sanctuary hand and body balm

An uplifting and skin smoothing balm to protect and soften dry skin. Smooth over the skin after a shower to seal in moisture.

80 g macadamia oil
20 g beeswax
20 drops Australian sandalwood essential oil
5 drops rosalina essential oil

Create an easy-to-use and portable massage balm with one of these recipes. Rub into your temples, neck and shoulders or into those muscles that need tension released.

Calm balm

A calming, relaxing massage balm.

15 g candelilla wax
85 g sweet almond oil
20 drops lavender essential oil
15 drops sandalwood essential oil
5 drops Roman chamomile essential oil

Loosen-up massage balm

Releases muscle tension.

15 g beeswax
85 g apricot kernel oil
20 drops lavender essential oil
20 drops rosemary essential oil
10 drops ginger essential oil

Positive energy massage balm

Brightens your spirit.

15 g candelilla wax
85 g sweet almond oil
15 drops sweet orange essential oil
10 drops petitgrain essential oil
5 drops neroli essential oil

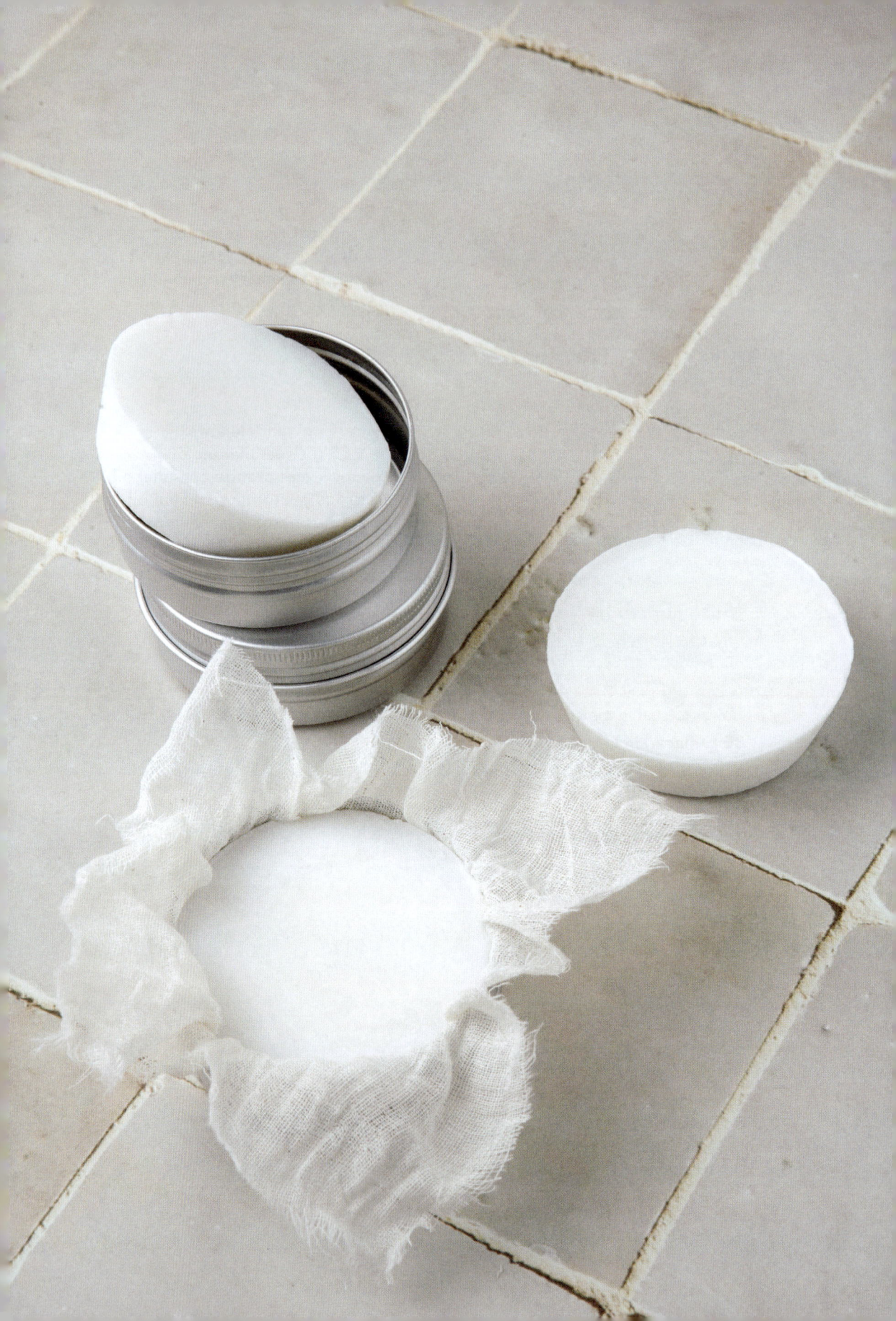

Solid Body Bars

Solid massage and body moisturising bars are made mostly from cocoa butter, and when massaged over the skin, they melt (cocoa butter melts at skin temperature). This provides excellent lubrication for a great massage and keeps your skin feeling soft and smooth. They are especially good for dry skin when smoothed over the skin straight after a shower or bath.

Pour the following mixtures into chocolate moulds or muffin tray moulds to create shapes that make them functional and look enticing.

Cocoa butter body bar base recipe

80 g cocoa butter
20 g vegetable oil or shea butter
1 g (approx. 20 drops) essential oil

1. Choose an essential oil from pages 39–48 or an essential oil composition for body and massage preparations from page 196.
2. Melt the cocoa butter with the vegetable oil or shea butter in a *bain-marie*.
3. Remove from the heat and add the drops of an essential oil or essential oil composition.
4. Pour into moulds.
5. Place into the refrigerator or freezer and once set, remove from the moulds.
6. In hot weather, store your massage and body bars in the refrigerator.
7. Massage over your skin after a bath or shower.

Coconut massage and body moisturising bar

A rich, delicious coconut treat for dry skin. Especially good in winter and dry climates.

80 g cocoa butter
20 g coconut oil
1 g (approx. 20 drops) essential oil

To make this body bar, follow the directions above.

You may like to choose one of these essential oil compositions to add to your massage or body care preparation. The quantities specified here are to be added to each 100 g or mL of base. If you are using the product every day, reduce the amount of essential oils to approximately half.

Essential oil compositions
for body and massage preparations

Relaxing composition
Induces relaxation
25 drops sweet orange
17 drops lavender
8 drops sweet marjoram

Joyous composition
Positive and uplifting
25 drops bergamot
15 drops geranium
10 drops clary sage

Sensual composition
Rich and seductive
30 drops sweet orange
12 drops ylang ylang
8 drops patchouli

Sore muscle composition
Relieves aching muscles
21 drops lavender
16 drops rosemary
13 drops ginger

Dream composition
For sweet dreams
26 drops mandarin
16 drops geranium
8 drops frankincense

Detoxifying composition
Enhances lymphatic drainage
23 drops lemon
13 drops juniper
9 drops peppermint
5 drops cypress

Floral composition
Sweet and fresh
10 drops lavender
6 drops geranium
4 drops ylang ylang

Precious patchouli composition
Warm and earthy
12 drops bergamot
8 drops Atlas cedarwood
6 drops patchouli

Deodorants

Essential oils added to a range of natural bases may be used to keep your underarms smelling sweet.

Unlike antiperspirants, deodorants do not interfere with your body's natural secretion of perspiration. What they do, for the most part, is mask body odour. Some deodorants may actually create an environment in which the bacteria that cause the odour (as they feed off your secretions) find it difficult to live. Sodium bicarbonate and magnesium hydroxide do this by creating an alkaline environment in which bacteria cannot live.

When choosing essential oils to use in your deodorant, remember that the skin in your armpits can be sensitive. This means that, not only do they need to deodorise, they need to be non-sensitising too.

Choose from the following essential oils to make a deodorant you would like to wear:

clary sage, cypress, eucalyptus, frankincense, geranium, juniper, lavender, manuka, patchouli, sage, sandalwood, tea tree, ylang ylang

IMPORTANT

Sodium bicarbonate is very effective when it comes to combatting body odour. However, some people are sensitive to sodium bicarbonate. It is recommended that you use only a small amount of product on a tiny area of your armpit to test for sensitivity. Some people develop sensitivity over time. If you develop sensitivity at any stage, discontinue use. Do not use it directly after shaving your underarms. Wait at least overnight before using.

Deodorant Pastes

Deodorant pastes are easy to make and effective. Sodium bicarbonate and magnesium hydroxide are often used as the main active ingredients.

High performance deodorant paste

30 g shea butter
20 g coconut oil
25 g arrowroot flour
15 g sodium bicarbonate
10 g bentonite clay
1 g (approx. 20 drops) essential oil

1. Choose an essential oil from pages 39–48 or an essential oil composition for deodorants from page 201.
2. In a bowl, stir together and sieve the dry ingredients: sodium bicarbonate (or magnesium hydroxide if following the recipe on page 198), arrowroot and bentonite clay.
3. Melt the shea butter and coconut oil in a *bain-marie*.
4. Remove from the heat and add the dry ingredients, mixing them together well.
5. Add and stir in the essential oils.
6. Scoop the mixture into a jar and allow it to cool to room temperature before adding the lid.
7. Massage a small amount over your armpits to prevent body odour.

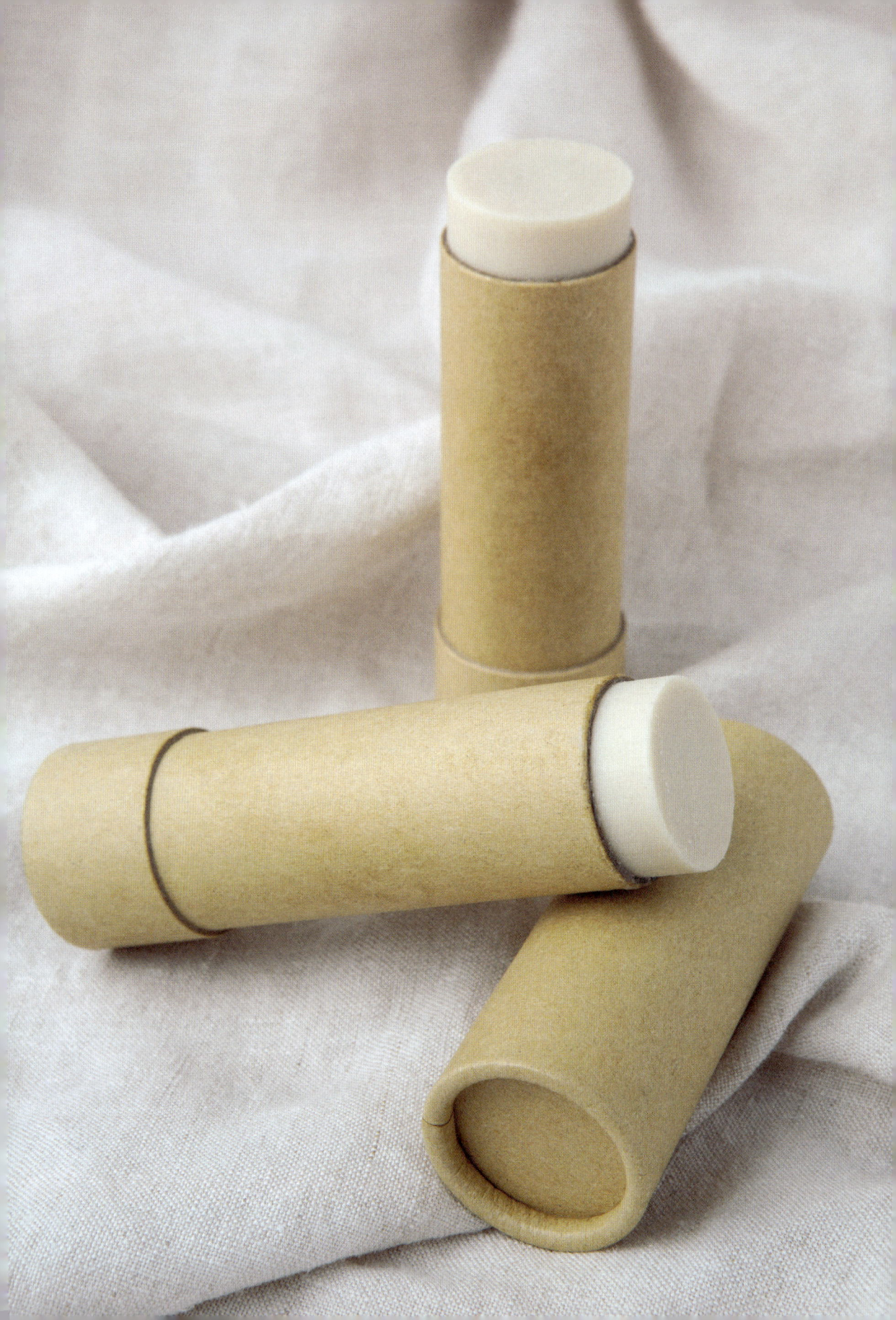

Sensitive skin deodorant paste

Magnesium hydroxide can be substituted for sodium hydroxide for people with sensitive skin. However, it is not quite as effective as sodium bicarbonate in reducing body odour and needs to be used at a higher proportion. Follow the instructions above to make this paste.

30 g shea butter
20 g coconut oil
25 g magnesium hydroxide
15 g arrowroot flour
10 g bentonite clay
1 g (approx. 20 drops) essential oil

Deodorant block

Smooth this deodorant block over your armpits to keep them fresh.

45 g cocoa butter
15 g candelilla wax
5 g coconut oil
15 g sodium bicarbonate
10 g arrowroot flour
10 g kaolin clay
1 g (approx. 20 drops) essential oil

1. Choose an essential oil from pages 39–48 or an essential oil composition for deodorants from page 201.

2. In one bowl, stir together and sieve the dry ingredients — the sodium bicarbonate (or magnesium hydroxide if following the recipe below), arrowroot flour and kaolin.

3. To a heat-resistant jug, add the cocoa butter, candelilla wax and coconut oil, and sit in a *bain-marie*.

4. Heat the mixture until all ingredients have melted.

5. Remove the jug from the heat and add the dry ingredients. Stir in well.

6. Add the essential oils and stir well.

7. Continue stirring until the mixture begins to thicken.

8. Scoop the mixture into a mould such as a muffin tray or, alternatively, a cardboard push-up tube, and place it in the refrigerator or freezer to solidify.

9. When your deodorant block has set, remove it from the mould.

10. You may need to store it in the refrigerator in very hot weather.

Delicate skin deodorant block

45 g cocoa butter
10 g candelilla wax
5 g coconut oil
25 g magnesium hydroxide
10 g kaolin clay
5 g arrowroot flour
1 g (approx. 20 drops) essential oil

Make this deodorant block by following the directions above.

Deodorant Vinegar

Aromatic vinegar deodorant

85 g purified water
15 g apple cider vinegar
0.5 g (approx. 10 drops) essential oil

1. Choose an essential oil from pages 39–48 or an essential oil composition for deodorants from page 201.
2. Shake the apple cider vinegar together with the water and essential oils in a spray bottle. It is now ready for use at any time.
3. Shake well prior to use each time.

Herbal vinegar deodorant

85 g purified water
15 g herbal vinegar

1. Make a fragrant herbal vinegar by following the *Method for making herbal vinegars* on page 54.
2. Shake the herb vinegar together with the water in a spray bottle. It is now ready for use at any time.

Deodorant Powder

Use these deodorant powders to absorb excess perspiration and to add the fragrance of essential oils to your body.

Fresh skin deodorant powder

50 g corn starch
35 g kaolin clay
15 g sodium bicarbonate
1 g (approx. 20 drops) essential oil

1. Choose an essential oil from pages 39–48 or an essential oil composition for deodorants from page 201.
2. Mix the sodium bicarbonate (or magnesium hydroxide if following the recipe below), corn starch and kaolin together in a bowl.
3. Sieve to break down any lumps in the powder.
4. Add the essential oils, ensuring you sprinkle them uniformly over the mixture, then stir them in.
5. Sieve again a couple of times to ensure any lumps are broken down and the essential oils are evenly distributed throughout the mixture.
6. Store the mixture in a shaker bottle or container such as an icing sugar or parmesan cheese shaker. Alternatively, using a funnel, pour the mixture into a bottle. This way a small amount can be decanted for use each time.

Mild skin deodorant powder

45 g corn starch
30 g kaolin clay
25 g magnesium hydroxide
1 g (approx. 20 drops) essential oil

Make this soothing deodorant powder by following the instructions above.

You may like to choose one of these essential oil compositions to use in your deodorant. The quantities specified here are to be added to each 100 g or mL of base.

Essential oil compositions for deodorants

Fresh composition
Fresh and clean
10 drops bergamot
7 drops geranium
3 drops cypress

Deep forest composition
Fresh and woody
10 drops lime
6 drops pine
4 drops Virginian
cedarwood

Soft composition
Soft and gentle
10 drops lavender
6 drops patchouli
4 drops ylang ylang

Insect Repellents

Citronella is a well-known insect repellent, with many other essential oils also having varying degrees of insect repellent properties.

The following essential oils can be used in insect repellent blends:

cajeput, Virginian cedarwood, citronella, blue Mallee eucalyptus, lemon-scented eucalyptus, peppermint eucalyptus, geranium, lemon myrtle, niaouli, peppermint, spike lavender, tea tree, lemon scented tea tree

The essential oils are used by blending them with any of the following bases.

Insect repellent body oil
Add 60 drops of citronella essential oil or one of the essential oil compositions for insect repellents on page 203 to 100 mL of vegetable oil such as sweet almond oil or apricot kernel oil in a bottle and shake well.

Insect repellent balm
Add 60 drops of citronella essential oil or one of the essential oil compositions for insect repellents on page 203 to 100 g of balm base. Follow the *Methods for making aromatherapy balms* on page 63.

Insect repellent cream
Add 60 drops of citronella essential oil or one of the essential oil compositions for insect repellents on page 203 to 100 g of *Base cream*. See page 77 for the *Base cream* recipe.

Insect repellent spray
70 mL perfume ethanol
30 mL purified water
3 g (approx. 60 drops) essential oil

1. Choose citronella essential oil or one of the essential oil compositions for insect repellents on page 203.
2. Add the essential oil to the perfume ethanol.
3. Then add the water to this mixture and shake well.
4. Pour into a spray bottle.

Mosquito bite relief oil
Apply pure lavender or tea tree essential oil, with a cotton wool ball, directly to a mosquito bite. Hold the cotton wool ball against the mosquito bite until the itch subsides.

You may like to choose one of these essential oil compositions to use in your insect repellent. The quantities specified here are to be added to each 100 g or mL of base.

Essential oil compositions for insect repellents

Wilderness composition
25 drops citronella
20 drops pine
15 drops lemon-scented tea tree

Summer nights composition
20 drops citronella
20 drops blue Mallee eucalyptus
20 drops geranium

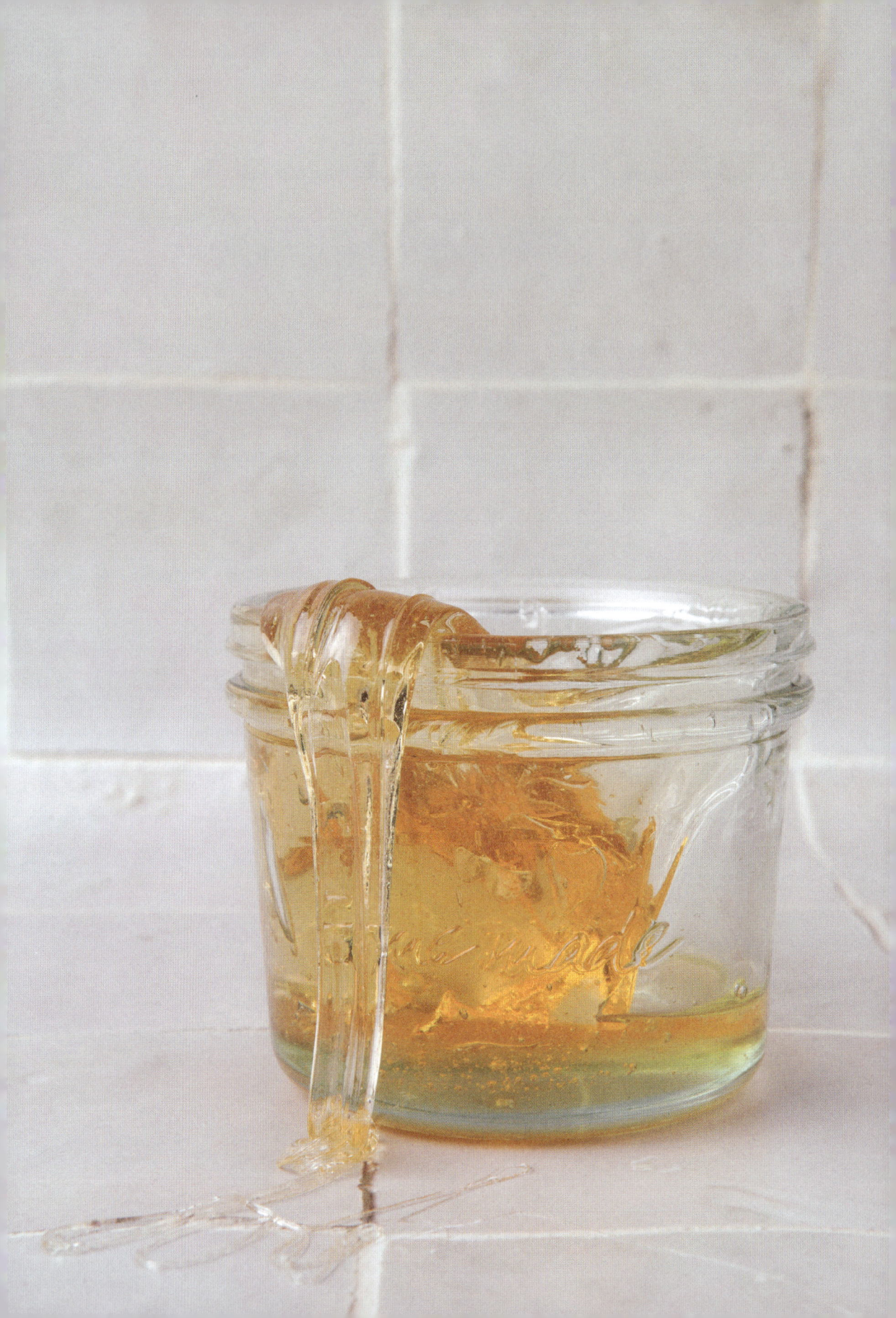

Hair Removal

If you like to have smooth, hairless skin, 'sugaring' is a concoction that is easy to make and very effective at removing hair.

Sugaring

Sugaring is a common longstanding method of hair removal in many cultures. It is like waxing your body with a toffee-like mixture. A very simple recipe is made up whenever it is needed, or stored in a heatproof container and melted down when required.

The recipe below was developed in a warm, subtropical climate. It can be adjusted a little if the climate is cool and it becomes too hard to work with. The temperature to which the recipe is heated can be reduced or a little more water may be introduced to adjust the sugaring's consistency accordingly.

It is important to ensure your skin is dry before sugaring. If your skin is moist, the sugaring mixture will not adhere well. Hot humid weather and body heat will affect it too, potentially making it too soft to use. Dust powder such as arrowroot flour or corn starch onto your skin if you need to.

The mixture is water-soluble, which means any drips or spills are easy to clean up.

Traditional sugaring

Traditional sugaring uses a lump of pliable sugar mixture to remove hair. It is pressed into the hair and then rapidly removed. This is then repeated, moving over the area where the hair is to be removed. It can be stored in a heat-proof jar and used as required.

250 g white granulated sugar (made from sugar cane)
35 g lemon juice
35 g purified water

1. Squeeze the lemon juice and strain it through a fine mesh tea strainer.

2. Weigh all ingredients.

3. Add all ingredients to a small saucepan and stir well.

4. Place the saucepan onto a hot plate and heat the mixture.

5. Make sure you use a thermometer, such as a digital thermometer, which shows temperatures above 130°C.

6. Continue heating the mixture until it reaches 130°C.

7. Every so often pick up the saucepan and give it a little swirl to ensure it doesn't burn.

8. Once it reaches 130°C, remove it from the heat immediately. It is important not to overheat it as it may become solid on cooling.

9. Decant directly into a heat-resistant bowl or jar.

10. Allow the mixture to cool down to room temperature. As it cools down it will thicken.

11. Always test a small amount on the inside of your wrist to be sure it's not going to burn your skin.

12. Once cool enough to the touch, but still warm, remove a ball of the mixture.

13. Knead and stretch it several times to make it pliable.

14. Ensure your skin is clean and dry. Dust powder such as arrowroot flour or corn starch onto your skin if you need to.

15. Smooth it firmly over your hair and skin against the direction of the hair growth. Then, flick up the top edge of the sugar. And with a second flick, remove the sugaring in the direction of your hair growth. Ensure you support your skin by holding it taut with your other hand just above where you are removing the hair.

16. In one hair removal session, the same ball of sugaring can continue to be used until it becomes too soft. Simply remove another ball of sugaring to continue removing more hair.

17. Discard the balls when finished. They will be full of hairs and dead skin cells but will be fully biodegradable and compostable.

Sugar strips

This sugaring method is similar to waxing, where the hair is removed with calico strips. The sugaring can be stored in a heatproof jar and warmed up to make it more liquid. Sit the jar in a saucepan of water and warm on a hot plate. It is important not to overheat the sugaring as it will burn the skin. Always test a small amount on the inside of your wrist to be sure it's not going to burn your skin. The calico strips can be cut to approximately 7 cm wide by 20 cm long.

250 g white sugar (made from sugar cane)
40 g lemon juice
40 g purified water
calico strips

1. Squeeze the lemon juice, then strain through a fine mesh tea strainer.

2. Weigh all ingredients.

3. Add all ingredients to a small saucepan and stir well.

4. Place the saucepan onto a hotplate and heat the mixture.

5. Make sure you use a thermometer, such as a digital thermometer, which shows temperatures above 125°C.

6. Continue heating the mixture until it reaches 125°C.

7. Every so often pick up the saucepan and give it a little swirl to ensure it doesn't burn.

8. Once it reaches 125°C, remove it from the heat immediately. It is important not to overheat it as it may become solid on cooling.

9. Decant directly into a heat-resistant bowl or jar.

10. Allow the mixture to cool down to room temperature. As it cools down it will thicken.

11. Ensure your skin is clean and dry. Dust powder such as arrowroot flour or corn starch onto your skin if you need to.

12. Apply the sugaring mixture with a spatula in a strip down your leg, for example, in the direction of hair growth. Make sure the application is as thin as possible.

13. Smooth the calico strip over the strip of sugaring in the direction of hair growth.

14. To remove the hairs and sugaring, grip the bottom edge of the calico strip and rapidly pull off against the direction of hair growth — parallel to your skin. Ensure you support your skin by holding it taut with your other hand just below where you start to pull the strip off.

15. Continue to repeat application and removal until you have removed hair from the areas you wish to remove it from.

16. Re-use the calico strip until the sugaring mixture has built up on it too thickly to be effective. Use fresh strips as needed.

17. When you have finished removing the hair, rinse off any sticky bits left on your hands or legs with water.

18. Apply a soothing oil, lotion or gel.

19. Calico strips can be rinsed, washed and dried for re-use.

20. The sugaring can be stored in a heatproof jar.

21. It can be warmed up to make it more liquid by sitting the jar in a saucepan of water, which is then heated on a hot plate. It is important not to overheat the sugaring as it will burn the skin.

After waxing skin soother

To calm redness after waxing or sugaring, apply this calming massage oil blend to the skin. The essential oils chosen are anti-inflammatory and antiseptic.

75 mL apricot kernel oil
25 mL calendula infused oil
20 drops lavender essential oil
12 drops sandalwood essential oil
8 drops German chamomile essential oil

Alternatively, the essential oils in this recipe may be added to 100 g of the *Base cream* recipe on page 77.

Sun Care

In some circles, a deep tan used to be a sign of wealth and good health because only the rich could afford to lie around in the sun all day. Fortunately, we now realise that a tan indicates little more than damaged skin unless you are lucky enough to be born with naturally melanin-rich skin.

Faking the Tan

Strong black tea is one answer to a natural tan without baking in the sun.

30 g black tea
300 g boiling water

1. Steep for an hour.
2. Strain.
3. Pour into a spray bottle with a fine mist spray.
4. Very lightly spray over your skin. Spraying too much at once will only cause the tea to run.
5. Allow to dry and spray again to enhance the colour. You may want to apply 5–6 layers.
6. Use a handheld fan to speed drying.

Sunburn Treatments

When your skin has been scorched by the sun, cooling and anti-inflammatory preparations are called for.

Aloe vera gel

Slice it fresh from the plant or squeeze it from a bottle if you don't have one of these fabulous succulents in your garden. If purchasing aloe vera gel, look for one that is as pure as possible. Apply the aloe vera gel to your sunburn regularly. As soon as your sunburn heats up again, apply some more. Keep your aloe vera gel in the refrigerator.

Sunburn healing and soothing gel

50 g aloe vera gel
5 drops lavender essential oil

Mix the lavender oil into an aloe vera gel base and apply to the burned area. Reapply the gel each time the area heats up. Keep the gel in the refrigerator for a cooling effect.

Chamomile tea

Make a bowl of chamomile tea and add ice cubes to it or put it in the refrigerator to cool. Use a cloth to dip into the cool chamomile tea and place it over your sunburn. When the cloth heats up from the warmth of the skin, re-dip the cloth into the cool water and reapply to the skin. Repeat several times to reduce the soreness and redness of your sunburn.

Cucumber

Take your cucumber straight from the refrigerator and cut it into thick strips lengthways and rub these over your sunburn. Use as often as necessary to soothe and cool.

Oatmeal

Tie a handful of oatmeal in a square of cloth and use it in a cool bath with you. Squeeze the wet oatmeal bag into the water and over your skin. Great for soothing any irritated skin.

Tea

Pour a cup of boiling water over 4 teaspoons or teabags of black tea. Strain the tea and add several ice cubes. Blot the cooled liquid all over your sunburn with cotton wool pads or an old cloth to soothe the irritation.

Yoghurt

Smooth cool natural yoghurt over your skin to relieve sunburn. Once the yoghurt dries on your skin, rinse with cool water and smooth on more yoghurt.

Soothing essential oil lotion

Add 20 drops of lavender or German chamomile essential oil to 100 mL of the *Body lotion* recipe on page 77 and slather it over your body.

Soothing essential oil bath

Add 20 drops of lavender or German chamomile essential oil to 100 mL of the *Liquid castile dispersing bath oil* recipe on page 224 and pour 1–2 tablespoons into a cool bath to calm and soothe your sunburn.

Body Powders

Applying body powders is another wonderful way to fragrance your body as well as absorb excess moisture.

Corn starch, tapioca flour and kaolin make excellent body powders.

Body dusting powder
80 g tapioca flour or corn starch
20 g kaolin clay
1 gm (approx. 20 drops) essential oil

1. Choose an essential oil from pages 39–48 or an essential oil composition for body powders listed below.
2. Mix the tapioca flour or corn starch and kaolin together in a bowl.
3. Sieve to break down any lumps in the powder.
4. Add the drops of essential oil, ensuring you sprinkle them uniformly over the mixture, then stir them in.
5. Sieve again a couple of times to ensure any lumps are broken down and the essential oils are evenly distributed throughout the mixture.
6. Store the mixture in a shaker bottle or container such as an icing sugar or parmesan cheese shaker. Alternatively, using a funnel, pour the mixture into a bottle. This way a small amount can be decanted for use each time.

You will find a recipe for baby powder on page 237.

You may like to choose one of these essential oil compositions to add to your body dusting powder. The quantities specified here are to be added to each 100 g of base.

Essential oil compositions for body powders

Exotica composition
8 drops sweet orange
4 drops cinnamon bark
4 drops palmarosa
4 drops petitgrain

Heaven composition
9 drops geranium
6 drops jasmine absolute
5 drops ylang ylang

Pleasure composition
9 drops bergamot
7 drops ylang ylang
4 drops vetiver

Hand Care

Soft, clean, warm, caring ... Our hands are exposed to everything including the scorching sun, washing up detergents and soft baby's skin.

Slather your hands with a softening, smoothing, moisturising hand cream and keep them looking and feeling great.

Virgin olive hand cream

Soften and smooth your hands with this moisturising hand cream.

Oil phase

8 g plant-derived emulsifying wax
33 g virgin olive oil
1 g antioxidant

Water phase

150 g rosewater
6 g vegetable glycerin
2 g preservative

Add at 45°C
2 g (approx. 40 drops) geranium essential oil

pH adjustment
qs citric acid + purified water

Make this hand cream by following the *Method for making an emulsion with emulsifying wax* on page 79.

Soothing hand cream

This hand cream contains ingredients to soothe red, irritated and itchy hands and to moisturise dry skin.

Oil phase

10 g cocoa butter
10 g plant-derived emulsifying wax
32 g apricot kernel oil
10 g calendula infused oil
1 g antioxidant

Water phase

129 g purified water
6 g vegetable glycerin
2 g preservative

Add at 45°C
15 drops lavender essential oil
5 drops German chamomile essential oil

pH adjustment
qs citric acid + purified water

Make this hand cream by following the *Method for making an emulsion with emulsifying wax* on page 79.

Healing hand cream

This is a rich emollient cream balm for dry, cracked and damaged hands. It is formulated to leave your hands feeling soft, smooth and enriched.

Oil phase

15 g shea butter
10 g plant-derived emulsifying wax
34 g avocado oil
4 g carrot infused oil
1 g antioxidant

Water phase

128 g purified water
6 g vegetable glycerin
2 g preservative

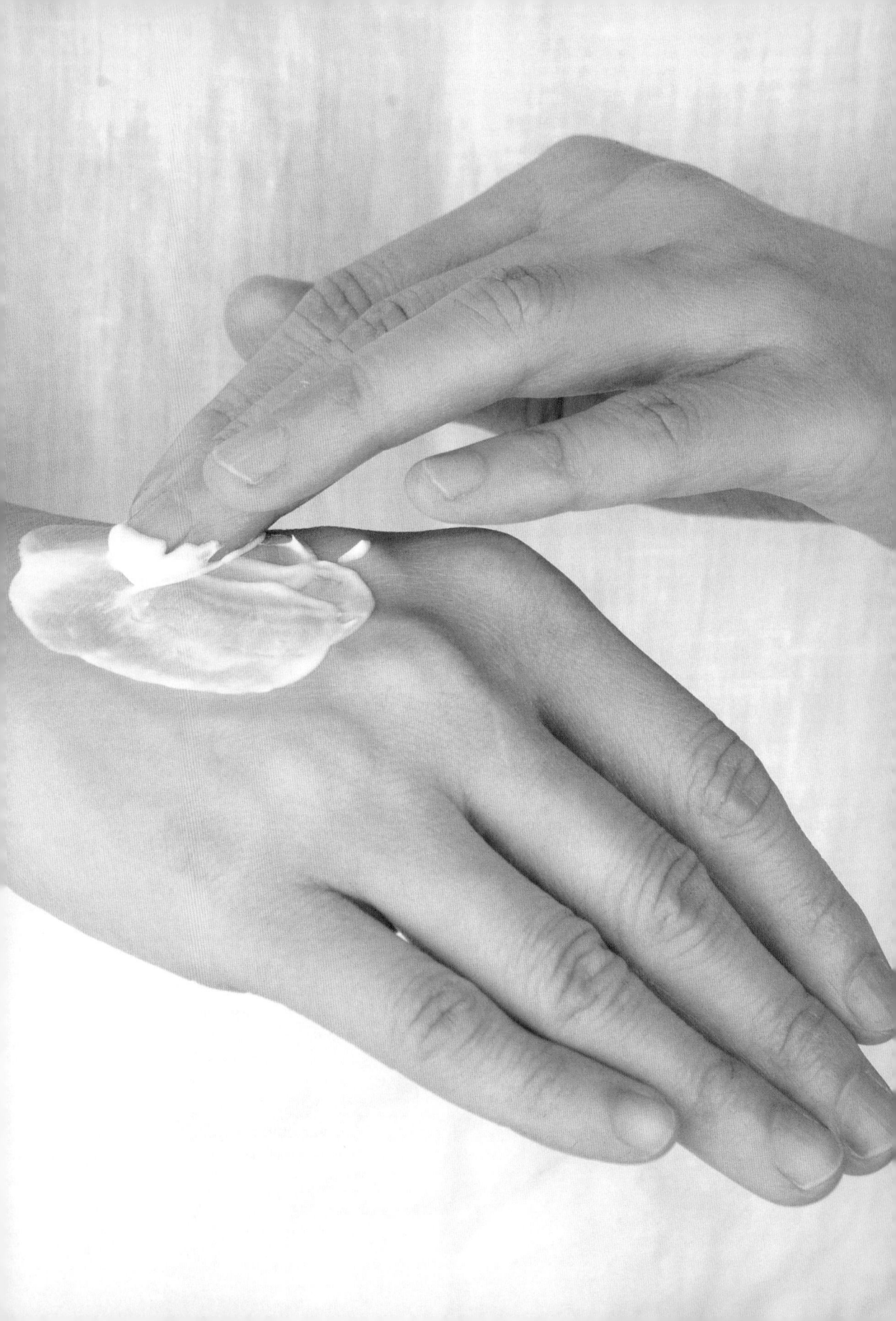

Add at 45°C
  20 drops lavender essential oil
  15 drops frankincense essential oil
  5 drops patchouli essential oil

pH adjustment
  qs citric acid + purified water

Make this hand cream by following the *Method for making an emulsion with emulsifying wax* on page 79.

Hand treatment balm

This is a wonderful treatment for restoring dry, damaged and wrinkled hands. As well as softening the skin, this treatment acts as a barrier preventing water loss from the skin. As a result, any moisture in the skin is forced back into the surface layers of skin cells, hydrating and softening them. For an overnight treatment, apply generously to your hands and put on a pair of cotton gloves and leave on overnight. In the morning, your hands will feel gorgeous.

  35 g shea butter
  10 g castor oil
  5 g rosehip oil
  10 drops lavender essential oil
  5 drops frankincense essential oil

Make this hand balm by following the *Aromatherapy balm method 2* on page 63.

Soft as velvet hand scrub

This hand scrub provides you with velvety soft hands, while the aroma of lavender combined with coconut creates a surprisingly subtle cloud of scent. This scrub also helps remove stains and ingrained dirt.

  15 g coconut milk powder
  5 g lavender flowers
  45 g salt
  30 g sweet almond oil
  5 g coconut oil

1. Sieve the coconut milk powder into a bowl to break down any lumps.
2. Add the lavender flowers and salt and mix well.
3. Add the sweet almond oil and coconut oil and stir well.
4. Store in a jar.
5. Use a teaspoon or so and massage over dampened hands at the basin.
6. Once you have finished massaging your hands, rinse off. You will notice that your hands will feel soft and smooth and a thin layer of oil will remain on your skin to help keep them moisturised. Follow with a moisturising hand cream.

Sandalwood cuticle cream

Cuticle cream is used to soften the cuticles, preventing them from becoming dry and cracked. It also makes them easier to push back.

Oil phase
  25 g shea butter
  12 g plant-derived emulsifying wax
  52 g apricot kernel oil
  1 g antioxidant

Water phase
  102 g purified water
  6 g vegetable glycerin
  2 g preservative

Add at 45°C
  20 drops sandalwood essential oil

pH adjustment
  qs citric acid + purified water

Make this cuticle cream by following the *Method for making an emulsion with emulsifying wax* on page 79.

Nail enhancing oil

50 mL sweet almond oil
16 drops grapefruit essential oil
6 drops rosemary essential oil
3 drops ginger essential oil

Add the essential oils to the sweet almond oil in a glass bottle and shake well.

Massage this blend into the skin at the base of your nails, where your nails begin to grow, and over the nail itself. The massage will stimulate circulation to the nail matrix encouraging better growth, and the oil will reduce nail brittleness.

Foot Care

Narrow, fat, sore, cracked ... Feet are as individual as we are. They take the load for all of us. Treat them well and you will notice how much better the rest of you feels too. Rejuvenate, heal and moisturise your feet with essential oils and plant-based preparations.

Recovery foot and leg massage oil

Use this wonderful massage oil to soothe your aching feet and legs.

100 mL sweet almond oil
22 drops lemon essential oil
13 drops lavender essential oil
8 drops eucalyptus essential oil
7 drops peppermint essential oil

Add the essential oils to the sweet almond oil in a glass bottle and shake well.

Massage a small quantity into your legs and feet or, even better, have somebody else do it for you.

Chill-out foot and leg gel

Soothe and revive your tired, aching legs with this cool gel. Smooth it over your legs whenever you feel like it.

2 g xanthan gum
8 g vegetable glycerin
90 g purified water
1 g preservative
15 drops lavender essential oil
15 drops peppermint essential oil

pH adjustment
qs citric acid + purified water

1. Make this gel by following the *Method for making gel bases* on page 67.
2. Add the essential oils and stir in thoroughly.
3. Store in a container in the refrigerator to add to the gel's cooling sensation.

Smooth recovery foot cream

Keep the skin on your feet smooth with this readily absorbed cream. The essential oils are very soothing and refreshing. Massage it into your feet each morning and evening to keep your feet soft and smooth.

Oil phase
8 g plant-derived emulsifying wax
35 g sweet almond oil
1 g antioxidant

Water phase
148 g purified water
6 g vegetable glycerin
2 g preservative

Add at 45°C
25 drops spearmint essential oil
15 drops lavender essential oil

pH adjustment
qs citric acid + purified water

Make this foot cream by following the *Method for making an emulsion with emulsifying wax* on page 79.

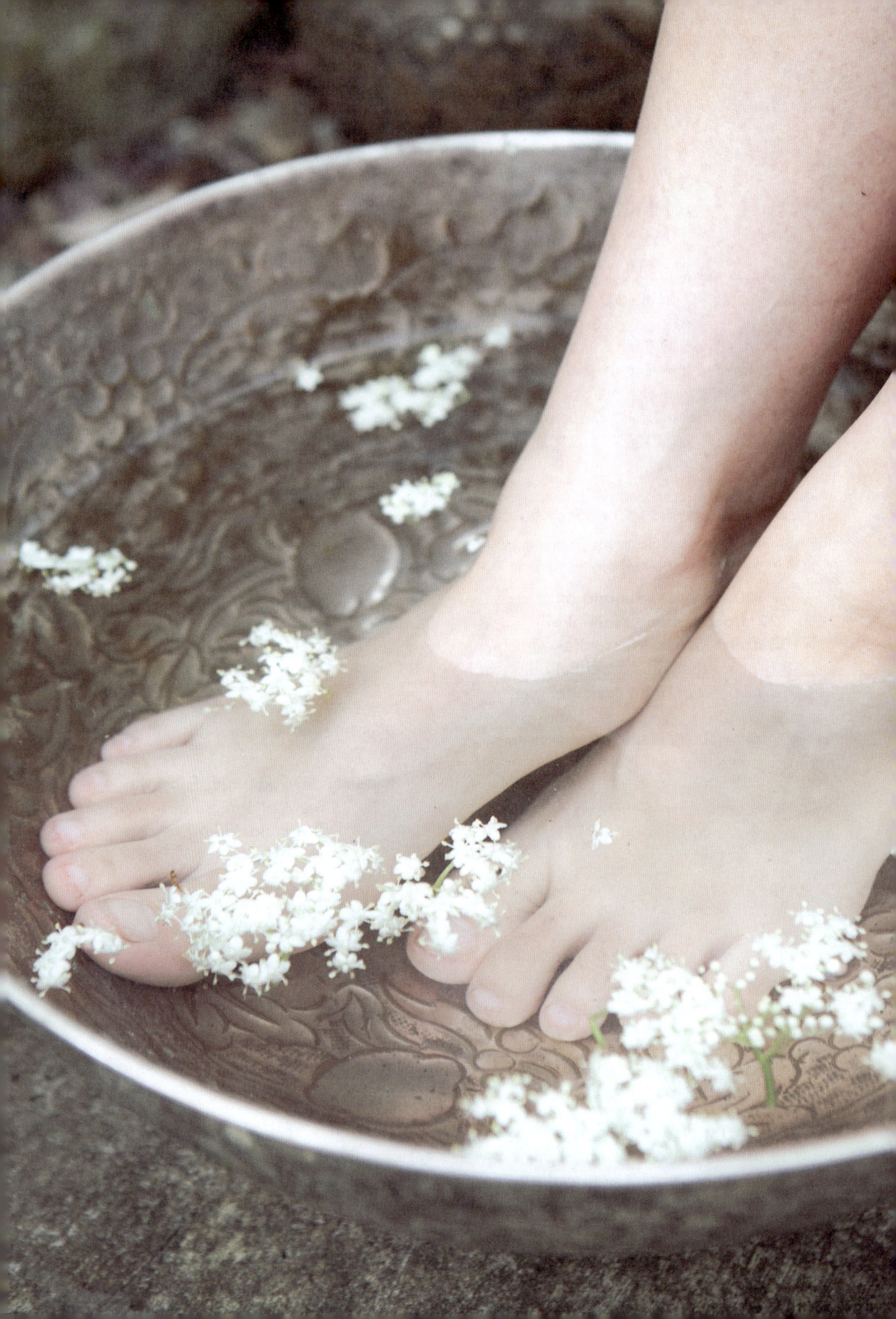

Intense healing foot balm

We all suffer from dry, cracked feet at some time, especially when we neglect taking good care of them. Use this healing foot balm to soften, moisturise and heal those cracks.

Oil phase

15 g shea butter
12 g plant-derived emulsifying wax
34 g macadamia oil
20 g avocado oil
10 g castor oil
1 g antioxidant

Water phase

100 g purified water
6 g vegetable glycerin
2 g preservative

Add at 45°C

25 drops lavender essential oil
25 drops myrrh essential oil

pH adjustment

qs citric acid + purified water

Make this foot balm by following the *Method for making an emulsion with emulsifying wax* on page 79.

Foot Scrubs

Smooth your feet with a granular exfoliant made from ground nuts, grains, seeds or dried pulses.

Mix your granules into a paste using water, milk or yoghurt. Add some honey and cold-pressed vegetable oil to soften the skin.

Salt or sugar crystals mixed with vegetable oil will also remove dry skin from your feet.

Bare feet foot scrub

A smoothing, fresh fragranced foot scrub.

40 g crushed pumice stone
20 g kaolin clay
5 g activated charcoal
5 g poppy seeds
30 g sweet almond oil
45 drops lemon essential oil
15 drops pine essential oil

1. Mix the crushed pumice stone, kaolin, activated charcoal and poppy seeds together in a bowl.

2. Add the essential oils to the sweet almond oil.

3. Add to the dry ingredients, continuing to stir until you form a smooth paste.

4. Add more sweet almond oil if the mixture is too stiff.

5. Store in a jar.

6. Soak your feet first to soften your skin, then massage the foot scrub all over them to remove any rough bits.

Foot Baths

Bath oils, salts or vinegars are blended with essential oils to make therapeutic soaks for your feet.

Soothing foot baths

A wonderful soak for tired, aching, swollen feet and ankles and to moisturise the skin.

Soothing foot bath oil

50 g Castile liquid soap
50 g sweet almond oil
25 drops lavender essential oil
10 drops geranium essential oil
10 drops juniper essential oil
5 drops peppermint essential oil

1. Mix the Castile liquid soap, sweet almond oil and essential oils together.
2. Store in a glass bottle.
3. Shake the mixture well before use.
4. Add 2 teaspoons of the foot bath oil to a basin of warm water and disperse.

Revitalising foot bath salts

A soak to cool and refresh your feet.

200 g Epsom salt
5 g jojoba oil
15 drops lemon essential oil
9 drops lime essential oil
3 drops cypress essential oil
3 drops peppermint essential oil

1. Blend the essential oils with the jojoba oil and mix together with the Epsom salt.
2. Store in a jar.
3. Add 1 tablespoon of the salts to a basin of warm or cool water and dissolve.

Deodorising foot baths

You can combat bad foot odour by choosing to use herbs and essential oils that are both antiseptic and fabulously fragrant. Soak your feet in these foot baths and enjoy the difference.

Funky feet bath soak

An excellent bath for deodorising your feet.

120 g Epsom salt
50 g sodium bicarbonate
25 g citric acid
5 g jojoba oil
10 drops lemongrass essential oil
10 drops petitgrain essential oil
5 drops cypress essential oil
5 drops sage essential oil

1. Mix the sodium bicarbonate, citric acid and Epsom salt together.
2. Blend the essential oils with the jojoba oil and stir this throughout the mixture.
3. Add 1 tablespoon of the bath soak to a basin of water and soak your feet for 10—15 minutes.

Fresh herb vinegar foot soak

A great foot soak to deodorise anybody's smelly feet.

2 tbsp peppermint
2 tbsp rosemary
2 tbsp sage
2 tbsp thyme
1 tbsp lemon peel
1½ cups apple cider vinegar

1. Use fresh herbs to make this foot soak and follow the *Method for making herbal vinegars* on page 54.
2. Add 2 tablespoons to a basin of warm water and soak your feet for 10—15 minutes.

Warming foot baths

Soak your feet in these preparations to stimulate the circulation in your feet and warm them up.

Foot Powders

Foot powders are used to absorb excess moisture and perspiration from your feet and to deodorise them, and may be used as part of a treatment for athlete's foot.

Mustard soak

This is a traditional remedy for warming cold feet.

Add 1 teaspoon of mustard powder to a basin of very warm water and place your feet in there to soak for 10–15 minutes.

Foot deodorant powder

85 g kaolin clay
15 g sodium bicarbonate
22 drops lemon essential oil
14 drops pine essential oil
9 drops geranium essential oil
5 drops patchouli essential oil

Ginger and rosemary foot bath oil

50 mL Castile liquid soap
50 mL sweet almond oil
30 drops ginger essential oil
30 drops rosemary essential oil

1. Mix the Castile liquid soap, sweet almond oil and essential oils together.
2. Store in a glass bottle.
3. Shake the mixture well before use.
4. Add 2 teaspoons of the foot bath oil to a basin of warm water and disperse.

1. Mix together the kaolin and sodium bicarbonate powder in a bowl.
2. Sieve to break down any lumps in the powder.
3. Add the drops of essential oils, ensuring you sprinkle them uniformly over the mixture, then stirring them in.
4. Sieve again a couple of times to ensure any lumps are broken down and the essential oils are evenly distributed throughout the mixture.
5. Store the mixture in a shaker bottle or container such as an icing sugar or parmesan cheese shaker. Alternatively, using a funnel, pour the mixture into a bottle. This way a small amount can be decanted for use each time.

Athlete's foot powder

To assist in the treatment of athlete's foot, keeping feet dry is important, as well as the application of antifungal remedies.

85 g kaolin clay
15 g sodium bicarbonate
20 drops lavender essential oil
15 drops tea tree essential oil
15 drops thyme essential oil

1. Mix together the kaolin and sodium bicarbonate powder in a bowl.
2. Sieve to break down any lumps in the powder.
3. Add the drops of essential oils, ensuring you sprinkle them uniformly over the mixture, then stir them in.
4. Sieve again a couple of times to ensure any lumps are broken down and the essential oils are evenly distributed throughout the mixture.
5. Store the mixture in a shaker bottle or container such as an icing sugar or parmesan cheese shaker. Alternatively, using a funnel, pour the mixture into a bottle. This way a small amount can be decanted for use each time.

Antifungal foot treatment

This lotion is effective in treating tinea due to its antifungal properties and its ability to dry up any moisture, which encourages fungal growth.

50 mL tincture of myrrh
30 drops tea tree essential oil

Add the tea tree oil to the tincture of myrrh in a glass bottle and shake well. Apply the lotion twice a day, especially after your feet have been in water.

Tincture of myrrh can be purchased from herbal medicine suppliers or you can make your own by following the *Method for making herbal tinctures* on page 51.

Special Foot Treatments

Blister treatment

Dab blisters regularly with a couple of drops of lavender essential oil. This will soothe them, help dry them up and heal them quickly.

Baths

Slip off your robe and ease yourself into the tub, lie back, close your eyes and take a deep breath. Let your body become weightless, your arms float to the surface, and your fingers relax and open. This is the perfect time to let your imagination run free. Surrender your fantasies to these creative, beautiful and luxurious bath recipes.

The ritual of bathing is one of the most therapeutic experiences — physically, mentally and spiritually.

Aromatherapy Baths

Essential oils used in bath preparations are incredibly therapeutic. They can relieve aching muscles, revive flagging spirits and be used to create sensual baths for lovers or a sanctuary for those who need time out.

Essential oils can be used in a variety of bath preparations including bath oils, bath bombs, bubble baths, bath salts, soda baths and more.

It is important to dilute or provide a medium of dispersion for essential oils before adding them to your bath as skin irritation may result from sitting directly on essential oils floating on the surface of the water.

Choose from the following essential oils to add to your bath:

- **calming and relaxing** — cedarwood, chamomile, frankincense, geranium, lavender, marjoram, patchouli, sandalwood, vetiver, ylang ylang
- **invigorating and reviving** — eucalyptus, grapefruit, lemon, lemongrass, peppermint, pine, rosemary
- **uplifting** — bergamot, geranium, lime, mandarin, may chang, melissa, neroli, sweet orange, palmarosa, petitgrain, tangerine
- **skin soothing** — chamomile, everlasting, lavender, yarrow
- **aching body relieving** — cajeput, ginger, lavender, marjoram, black pepper, pine, rosemary.

Herbal Baths

Herbs can be used to make bath preparations such as bath oils, bath vinegars, bath infusions, bath decoctions and bath bags. Dried herbs added to bath salts make them look attractive.

Choose from the following herbs to make your herbal bath preparations:

- **calming and relaxing** — chamomile, geranium leaves, hops, lavender, lemon balm, lime flowers, valerian
- **invigorating and reviving** — bay leaves, eucalyptus, grapefruit peel, lemongrass, lemon peel, orange peel, peppermint, pine, thyme
- **aching body relieving** — eucalyptus, ginger root, lavender, mustard powder, rosemary.

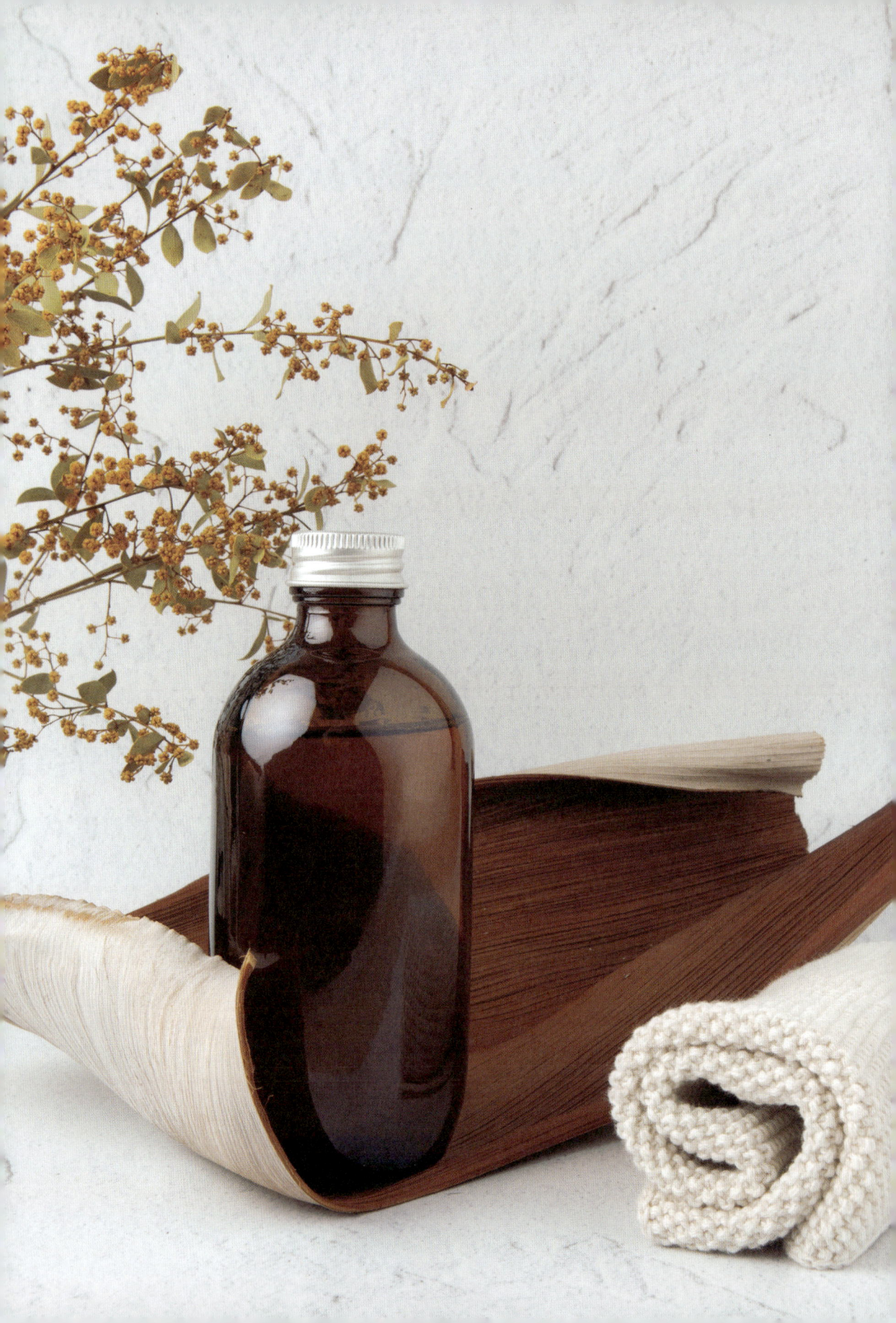

You may like to choose one of these essential oil compositions to add to your bath preparation. The quantities specified here are to be added to each 100 g or mL of base.

Essential oil compositions for baths

Relaxing bath
Relax both body and mind
10 drops sweet orange
7 drops lavender
3 drops sweet marjoram

Anti-stress bath
To calm the nerves and lift your spirits
15 drops sweet orange
5 drops geranium
3 drops clary sage

Sensual bath
A lover's bath
10 drops sandalwood
7 drops bergamot
3 drops ylang ylang

A secret place bath
Revitalising and fortifying
9 drops sandalwood
7 drops bergamot
4 drops frankincense

Zest bath
Totally refreshing
10 drops lemon
6 drops pine
4 drops rosemary

Happy lime bath
Lots of fun
10 drops lime
10 drops sweet orange

Mandarin love bath
Totally delicious
16 drops mandarin
4 drops ylang ylang

Big day out bath
Very relaxing
15 drops lavender
4 drops Roman chamomile
1 drop vetiver

Bath Oils

Bath oils are a wonderful way to moisturise your skin as well as providing a base for adding essential oils to the bathwater. Baths are one of the best ways to enjoy the pure natural fragrances of essential oils and their therapeutic properties.

Dispersing bath oils

The most effective way of using essential oils in the bath is by using a dispersing bath oil. This method ensures the essential oils are dispersed throughout the bathwater. If essential oils are dropped directly into bathwater, without any kind of dispersant, they will float in their concentrated form on top of the bathwater. When you go to sit in the bathwater, the bare skin on your thighs and bottom will come into direct contact with the essential oils and burning and irritation may result. Ensure you have read the safety information on skin irritation and sensitivity on page 38 when selecting essential oils.

A simple dispersing bath oil can be made by combining a vegetable oil with Castile liquid soap. It will disperse essential oils throughout the bathwater and leave your skin feeling soft and moisturised. It does not leave a slippery, oily residue on the bath.

To make your own dispersing bath oils, try the following recipes.

Liquid Castile dispersing bath oil

You may prefer this simple mixture without vegetable oil if you have oily skin.

100 g Castile liquid soap
1–3 g (approx. 20–60 drops) essential oil

1. Choose an essential oil from pages 39–48 or essential oil composition for baths from page 223.
2. Mix the ingredients together and store in a glass bottle.
3. Add 1 tablespoon to your bathwater and swirl to disperse.

Almond Castile dispersing bath oil

This mixture will moisturise your skin.

50 g sweet almond oil
50 g Castile liquid soap
1–3 g (approx. 20–60 drops) essential oil

1. Choose an essential oil from pages 39–48 or essential oil composition for baths from page 223.
2. Mix the ingredients together and store in a glass bottle.
3. Shake well before use, add 1 tablespoon to your bathwater and swirl to disperse.

Floating bath oils

A floating bath oil is the most basic of bath oils and is made from the same ingredients as a body oil. It will float on the surface of the bathwater and leave an emollient film on your skin as you step out of the bath. A floating bath oil will leave a slippery residue on your bath, so it is important to wipe over your bath after using one.

Cold-pressed vegetable oils are recommended for making floating bath oils. They can be used as they are or an aromatherapy bath oil can be made by adding 20–60 drops of essential oil to 100 mL of cold-pressed vegetable oil. Add up to 1 tablespoonful of the bath oil to the bathwater and swirl it throughout the water.

Herbal infused oils can also be used for a fragrant and therapeutic bath. Choose herbs from page 221 and find the *Methods for making herbal infused oils* on page 52. Add up to 1 tablespoonful of the bath oil to the bathwater and swirl it throughout the water.

Bath Vinegars

The addition of apple cider vinegar to the bathwater helps restore your skin's acid mantle and reduces skin irritation. It can be added to the water as it is or you can make a fragrant herbal vinegar. Choose herbs from page 221 and find the *Method for making herbal vinegars* on page 54. Add up to half a cup of the vinegar to the bathwater.

Fragrant botanicals bath vinegar

Gorgeously fragrant, this bath vinegar is made with fresh herbs.

250 mL (1 cup) apple cider vinegar
4 tbsp fresh or dried lavender flowers
2 tbsp fresh or dried rosemary leaves
1 tbsp dried peppermint leaves

Soak the freshly picked herbs from your garden or dried, if you prefer, in vinegar for a couple of weeks before use. Find the for *Method for making herbal vinegars* on page 54.

Soda Baths

Sodium bicarbonate, commonly referred to as bicarbonate of soda or bicarb soda, added to the bath reduces skin irritation. One tablespoon of bicarbonate of soda can be added directly to the bath for this purpose.

Essential oils can be added by mixing 10 drops into 1 teaspoon (5 mL) of vegetable oil before mixing into 100 g of bicarbonate of soda. Stir the mixture well, breaking up any lumps, then store in an airtight container. Dried herbs and flowers can be sprinkled throughout the mixture for a colourful effect.

Bare skin bath

A great bath for irritated or itchy skin.

65 g sodium bicarbonate
15 g oat flour
15 g cocoa butter
5 g apricot kernel oil
9 drops lavender essential oil
3 drops German chamomile essential oil

1. Mix together the sodium bicarbonate and oat flour in a bowl.
2. Sieve to break down any lumps in the powder.
3. Mix the essential oils with the apricot kernel oil.
4. Sprinkle the essential oil and apricot kernel oil blend uniformly over the sodium bicarbonate, then stir in.
5. Sieve again a couple of times to ensure any lumps are broken down and the essential oils are evenly distributed throughout the mixture.
6. Chop the cocoa butter into small, fine pieces.
7. Stir the chopped cocoa butter throughout the mixture.
8. Store the mixture in a jar.
9. Add 2–3 tablespoonfuls to the bathwater and disperse.

Bath Bombs

Sodium bicarbonate mixed with citric acid and thrown into the bathwater creates a wonderful fizzy bath. When the sodium bicarbonate and citric acid dissolve in water, a neutralisation reaction occurs producing carbon dioxide (gas), sodium citrate (salt) and water.

Bath bomb base

Use the *Bath bomb base* recipe to create an exciting range of aromatherapy bath bombs. The addition of corn starch or other starches, such as tapioca flour, arrowroot flour or oat flour, assists in creating a densely packed bath bomb and helps provide a barrier between the sodium bicarbonate and citric acid, slowing down and extending the fizzing time when the bath bomb hits the water.

Vegetable oil assists in moisturising the skin as well as providing a medium into which the essential oils can be diluted. The following recipe creates 500 g of *Bath bomb base*.

240 g sodium bicarbonate
120 g citric acid
120 g corn starch
20 g vegetable oil
2.5–5 g (approx. 50–100 drops)
essential oil or essential oil composition
for baths
spray bottle filled with purified water

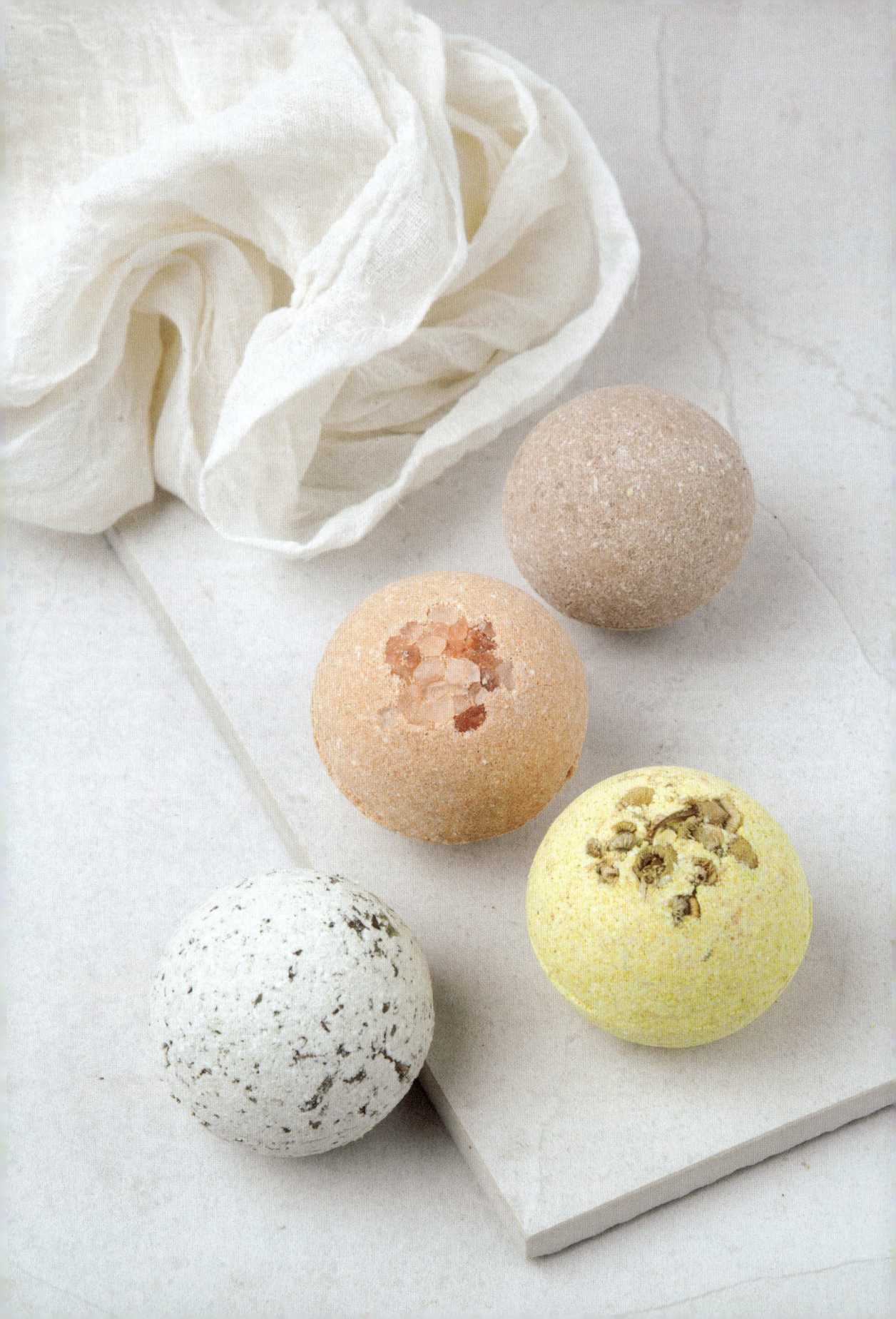

Additional ingredients

The following ingredients can be added to the bath bomb base to benefit your skin, add colour or create texture.

Vegetable oils and butters

Up to approximately 20 g of vegetable oils and butters may be added singly or combined to assist in moisturising the skin as well as providing a medium into which the essential oils can be diluted.

Honey

Up to 20 g of honey may be added for its skin softening and healing properties.

Milk powders

Powdered milk, including coconut and buttermilk, may be added instead of corn starch or a portion of it.

Clays

Up to 20 g of coloured clays may be added to give colour to the bath bombs. The amount added will be determined by the desired colour intensity.

Botanical powders

Up to 20 g of botanical powders may be added depending on the intensity of colour desired, while being mindful of staining or colouring the bath. Botanical powders include acai, beetroot, cacao, matcha, paprika, rose petals, spirulina, turmeric, and other freeze-dried fruit and vegetable powders.

Natural decorations and additives

A small amount of dried herbs and flowers, shredded coconut, Himalayan salt, poppy seeds, rolled oats or brown sugar may be placed into the base of a bath bomb mould before the bath bomb mixture is added or mixed throughout the recipe to provide decoration.

Epsom salt

An additional 125 g of Epsom salt may be added to enhance the muscle-relaxing properties of a bath bomb.

Moulds

The following items may be used as moulds: purpose-made bath bomb moulds, candle moulds, chocolate moulds, muffin trays, small plastic food containers, jelly moulds.

When mixing together large quantities of powders such as sodium bicarbonate and citric acid, it is advisable to wear a dust mask to prevent irritating the mucous membrane of your sinuses and lungs, and to wear glasses or protective eyewear to reduce the potential of irritating your eyes.

Method for making bath bombs

1. Weigh out the ingredients.
2. Mix the dry ingredients together in a large bowl.
3. Sieve the ingredients through a large kitchen sieve to break down any lumps.
4. Mix the essential oil and vegetable oil together.
5. Using a pipette, sprinkle the essential oil and vegetable oil blend uniformly over the mixture, then mix thoroughly.
6. Sieve the mixture several times to ensure any lumps are broken down and the essential oils are evenly distributed throughout the mixture.
7. Mist the mixture with a small amount of water and stir through. Repeat this 4 or 5 times. The mixture needs to be just damp enough so that it holds together when you squeeze it together in your hand (like damp sand). If you add too much water,

the mixture will react before you get it into the bath. On the other hand, if the mixture is not damp enough, the bath bomb will crumble. Humidity will add a certain amount of moisture to the mixture.

8. If using petals or other natural decorations to decorate your bath bombs, sprinkle a few into the mould first so that they will be visible on the surface of the bath bombs. Don't add too many or they will simply fall off.

9. Spoon the mixture into a mould. Press the mixture into the mould as firmly and as tightly as possible.

Using ball-shaped bath bomb moulds

If using purpose-made bath bomb moulds, spoon the mixture into the mould. Press the mixture into it as firmly and as tightly as possible. Overfill the two halves after pressing as much of the mixture into the mould halves as you can. Then press both sides together as firmly as possible. Remove any excess mixture that may be left bulging out of the seam. Gently tap the mould with a spoon from several angles to assist in releasing the bath bomb, then carefully remove it from the mould. Leave the bath bomb to set for at least 8 hours in a dry environment.

Using tray moulds

If using trays or other moulds, spoon the mixture into the tray or mould and press it in with your thumbs to ensure it is compressed as firmly as possible. Leave the bath bombs for 8 hours or overnight to dry. Then place a cutting board over the top of the tray or mould and turn it upside down. Sit the cutting board on a bench and gently tap all over the base of the tray or mould to release the bath bombs. Leave the bath bombs to set for at least 8 hours in a dry environment.

10. Your bath bombs are now ready for you to enjoy.

11. Store your bath bombs in sealed, airtight jars or containers so that they don't absorb moisture from humidity in the air or allow essential oils to evaporate before use.

The following recipes will make 5 large bath bombs or quite a few smaller ones.

Pink cloud bomb
Relaxing.

500 g bath bomb base
10 g beetroot powder
60 drops sweet orange essential oil
30 drops lavender essential oil
10 drops sweet marjoram essential oil

Earth pulse bomb
Revitalising.

500 g bath bomb base
10 g pink clay
10 g pink Himalayan salt
60 drops lemon essential oil
25 drops pine essential oil
15 drops rosemary essential oil

Sprinkle the pink Himalayan salt into the base of the moulds to decorate the top of the bath bombs.

Rose bud bomb
Sensual and luxurious.

500 g bath bomb base
10 g rose petal powder
whole dried rose buds
50 drops geranium essential oil
20 drops ylang ylang essential oil
10 drops patchouli essential oil

Sit 3 rose buds in the base of the moulds to decorate the top of the bath bombs.

Magic mint bomb

Revitalising.

500 g bath bomb base

10 g green Argiletz clay

10 g dried peppermint leaves

30 drops peppermint essential oil

20 drops eucalyptus essential oil

Serene solitude bomb

Calming and uplifting.

500 g bath bomb base

10 g spirulina

dried blue mallow flowers

75 drops sweet orange essential oil

25 drops geranium essential oil

15 drops clary sage essential oil

Sit a few blue mallow flowers in the base of the moulds to decorate the top of the bath bombs.

Zen matcha bomb

Uplifting and refreshing.

500 g bath bomb base

10 g matcha powder

dried elderflowers and rosemary

50 drops lime essential oil

50 drops sweet orange essential oil

Sit a sprinkle of elderflowers and rosemary in the base of the moulds to decorate the top of the bath bombs.

Wholehearted bomb

Sweet and heartening.

500 g bath bomb base

5 g pink Argiletz clay

5 g yellow Argiletz clay

dried blue cornflowers

50 drops sandalwood essential oil

35 drops bergamot essential oil

15 drops ylang ylang essential oil

Sit a few blue cornflowers in the base of the moulds to decorate the top of the bath bombs.

Tranquil glow bomb

Uplifting.

500 g bath bomb base

10 g paprika powder

80 drops mandarin essential oil

20 drops ylang ylang essential oil

Calm under the sun bomb

Relaxing.

500 g bath bomb base

10 g turmeric powder

dried chamomile flowers

75 drops lavender essential oil

20 drops Roman chamomile essential oil

5 drops vetiver essential oil

Sit a few chamomile flowers in the base of the moulds to decorate the top of the bath bombs.

Cosy hug bomb

Comforting and relaxing.

500 g bath bomb base

10 g cacao powder

45 drops sandalwood essential oil

35 drops bergamot essential oil

20 drops frankincense essential oil

Lunar landscape bomb
Relaxing.

500 g bath bomb base
20 g poppy seeds
10 g activated charcoal
100 drops lavender essential oil

Coconut bliss bomb
Tropical delight.

500 g bath bomb base
120 g coconut milk (instead of corn starch)
20 g coconut oil (as the vegetable oil)
25 g coconut sugar
shredded coconut

Sit a sprinkle of shredded coconut in the base of the moulds to decorate the top of the bath bombs.

Unbound nature bomb
An uplifting floral explosion.

500 g bath bomb base
dried lavender flowers
dried rose petals
dried calendula petals
dried peppermint leaves
50 drops lavender essential oil
30 drops geranium essential oil
20 drops ylang ylang essential oil

Sit a sprinkle of the mixture of the botanicals in the base of the moulds to decorate the top of the bath bombs.

TIP

These bath bomb recipes can be used without pressing the mixtures into moulds. Simply make the recipes without adding water and store the powder in a jar. Scoop out a tablespoon or two and add to the bathwater to create a beautiful fizzy bath.

Oat Baths

Oat baths are soothing to the skin and are superb for itchy and irritated skin. It will feel calm and smooth after one of these treats.

Tie a handful of oat bran or rolled oats in a square of cheesecloth or muslin, dip it into your bath and squeeze to release a milky fluid. Massage the bag over your skin to cleanse it.

You can mix the oat bran or rolled oats with other herbs of your choice and with milk powder for a fragrant milky bath. Use these preparations once only before discarding them.

Ahhh skin soother oat bath
A bath treat to soothe red, irritated skin.

In your square of cheesecloth or muslin, tie the following skin-soothing dried herbs and ingredients.

3 tbsp rolled oats
1 tbsp calendula flowers
1 tbsp chamomile flowers
1 tbsp lavender flowers

Botanical bathing bouquet

A dreamy, fragrant bath treat that also moisturises your skin.

In your square of cheesecloth or muslin, tie the following fragrant dried herbs and moisturising ingredients.

3 tbsp rolled oats
2 tbsp crumbled or chopped cocoa butter
1 tbsp lavender flowers
1 tbsp peppermint leaves
1 tbsp rose petals

TIP

If you don't have a bath, soak your precious feet in a foot bath instead. Simply pour a large bowl of warm water or use a bucket and add a tablespoonful or so of your favourite bath preparation. If you have an electric foot spa, please read the instructions regarding the addition of bath products before use.

Bath Salts

Epsom salt, also known as magnesium sulphate, is great to relax in the bath with as it helps relieve tired, sore muscles.

Aromatherapy bath salts can be made by adding up to 1 mL (20 drops) of essential oil to every 100 g of Epsom salt. Dilute the essential oil in a small amount of vegetable oil such as jojoba, sweet almond or apricot kernel first before adding it to the Epsom salt. The vegetable oil assists in moisturising the skin as well as providing a medium into which the essential oils can be diluted. Natural colour and texture can be achieved by sprinkling dried herbs and petals or coloured clays throughout the salts. Half a teaspoon of clay is sufficient to colour

200 g of bath salts. The amount of petals and leaves added to the salts may be determined by their therapeutic effect or by the visual appeal you are wishing to create. They may be added in small amounts or they may be added in larger quantities for maximum effect. Other salts, such as Murray River salt or various local salts, may be added for their visual appeal.

Method for making bath salts

1. Mix together the Epsom salt, any other salt and powdered colourants such as clays, charcoal or botanicals.

2. Mix together the vegetable oil and essential oils and stir into the mixture.

3. Finally, add any petals and dried leaves.

4. Once you have mixed all ingredients together thoroughly, put the mixture into an airtight jar.

5. Add 1—2 tablespoonfuls of bath salts to your bathwater.

Rose petal bath salts
Very pink and pretty.

200 g Epsom salt
½ tsp rose petal powder
1 tsp jojoba oil
6 drops rose otto
2 tbsp dried rose petals

Flourish bath salts
An explosion of colour and petals.

200 g Epsom salt
¼ tsp pink Argiletz clay
1 tsp jojoba oil
20 drops geranium essential oil
1 tbsp dried calendula petals
1 tbsp dried blue cornflower petals
1 tbsp dried rose petals

Soul glow bath salts
A revitalising bath.

100 g Epsom salt
100 g pink Himalayan salt
1 tsp vegetable oil
8 drops lavender essential oil
7 drops geranium essential oil
5 drops peppermint essential oil
1 tbsp blue cornflower petals
1 tbsp lavender flowers

Recharge bath salts
To recharge the spirits.

200 g Epsom salt
1 tsp matcha powder
1 tsp vegetable oil
14 drops lime essential oil
5 drops peppermint essential oil
1 drop lemongrass essential oil

Warm hug bath salts
For when you have been working or playing hard or have sore muscles and joints.

200 g Epsom salt
¼ tsp pink Argiletz clay
¼ tsp turmeric
1 tsp vegetable oil
10 drops ginger essential oil
10 drops lavender essential oil
10 drops rosemary essential oil

Winter warrior bath salts
A warming bath for those feeling the cold or those who have caught a cold.

200 g Epsom salt
¼ tsp turmeric
1 tsp vegetable oil
8 drops eucalyptus essential oil
8 drops ginger essential oil
4 drops black pepper essential oil

Detox bath salts
This combination of essential oils and Epsom salt can be used as part of a detoxification program.

200 g Epsom salt
½ tsp green Argiletz clay
1 tsp vegetable oil
12 drops lemon essential oil
5 drops juniper essential oil
3 drops cypress essential oil

Night sky bath salts
A calming and relaxing bath for the end of the day.

100 g Epsom salt
100 g pink Himalayan salt
½ tsp activated charcoal
1 tsp vegetable oil
10 drops sweet orange essential oil
7 drops lavender essential oil
3 drops sweet marjoram essential oil

Naturopaths often recommend the addition of up to 500 g of plain Epsom salt to a bath for a strong detoxifying effect. This should only be carried out after consultation and recommendation by a qualified naturopath.

Honey Baths

Honey soothes and softens the skin. Dissolve 1 tablespoon of honey in some hot water. Pour this into your bathwater and swirl it throughout the water.

Milk Baths

Milk soothes and softens the skin. Fresh milk can be added directly to the bath.

Milk powder can be used in bath bags, bath salts or bath bombs along with herbs, oats or bran for a fragrant, soothing, milky bath.

Coconut milk added to your bathwater is very soothing to the skin and has a wonderful tropical cocktail fragrance.

Bath Melts

Pop a bath melt into a warm bath as you run the water and its rich emollient ingredients will melt into the water to moisturise your skin. Bath melts are made with cocoa butter, vegetable oils and essential oils, and may include other emollients and botanicals. Moulds such as chocolate moulds or muffin trays may be used to make various shaped bath melts.

Relaxing bath melts

80 g cocoa butter
20 g coconut oil
12 drops mandarin essential oil
5 drops lavender essential oil
3 drops Roman chamomile essential oil
1 tbsp dried chamomile flowers
1 tbsp dried lavender flowers

1. Sprinkle the botanicals into the base of the moulds.
2. Melt the cocoa butter with the coconut oil in a *bain-marie*.
3. Remove from the heat and add the drops of essential oils.
4. Pour into the moulds.
5. Place in the refrigerator or freezer and once set, remove from the moulds.
6. Pop a bath melt into a warm bath as you run the water.
7. In hot weather, store your bath melts in the refrigerator.

Bush spirit bath discs

80 g cocoa butter
20 g coconut oil
10 drops lemon myrtle essential oil
5 drops eucalyptus essential oil
2 tsp dried lemon myrtle powder or pieces

1. Sprinkle the lemon myrtle into the base of the muffin moulds.
2. Melt the cocoa butter with coconut oil in a *bain-marie*.
3. Remove from the heat and add the drops of essential oils.
4. Pour into the muffin tray moulds. Fill them ¼ full to create discs.
5. Place in the refrigerator or freezer and once set, remove from the moulds.
6. Pop a bath melt into a warm bath as you run the water.
7. In hot weather, store your bath melts in the refrigerator.

Aromatherapy Shower Steamers

Aromatherapy shower steamers offer a way to enjoy the benefits of aromatherapy in the shower. They are an alternative to sprinkling essential oils onto the floor of your shower.

Shower steamer ingredients are similar to bath bombs. The main ingredients are sodium bicarbonate, citric acid and essential oil. These ingredients are combined to create a small solid aromatic block.

Place a shower steamer onto the floor of your shower and the sodium bicarbonate and citric acid will gently dissolve and fizz in the water, releasing the essential oil. The heat of the shower encourages the essential oil to diffuse into the air.

Aromatherapy shower steamer base

The shower steamer base can be made in a large batch, then divided into smaller quantities to make various kinds of shower steamers.

TIP

When mixing together large quantities of powders such as sodium bicarbonate and citric acid, it is advisable to wear a dust mask to prevent irritating the mucous membrane of your sinuses and lungs, and to wear glasses or protective eyewear to reduce the potential of irritating your eyes.

The following recipe creates 100 g of *Aromatherapy shower steamer base*.

50 g sodium bicarbonate
25 g citric acid
25 g corn starch
a spray bottle filled with purified water

Method for making shower steamers

1. Weigh out the ingredients.

2. Mix the dry ingredients together in a large bowl.

3. Sieve the ingredients through a large kitchen sieve to break down any lumps.

4. Add the botanical powder or clays used as colourants to the base and stir thoroughly, breaking up any lumps. Sieve again if necessary and stir well.

5. Sprinkle the drops of essential oil uniformly over the mixture, then mix thoroughly.

6. Sieve the mixture several times to ensure any lumps are broken down and the essential oils are evenly distributed throughout the mixture.

7. Mist the mixture with a small amount of water and stir through. Repeat this 4 or 5 times. The mixture needs to be just damp enough so that it holds together when you squeeze it together in your hand (like damp sand). If you add too much water, the mixture will react before you get it into the shower. On the other hand, if the mixture is not damp enough, the shower steamer will crumble. Humidity will add a certain amount of moisture to the mixture.

8. Spoon the mixture into ice cube trays or other moulds and press it in with your thumbs to ensure it is compressed as firmly as possible.

9. Leave the shower steamers for 8 hours or overnight to dry.

10. Remove from the ice cube trays or moulds and allow at least another 8 hours to dry and become firm.

11. Wrap the shower steamers or store them in a sealed, airtight jar or container so that they don't absorb moisture from humidity in the air or allow essential oils to evaporate before use.

12. Place a shower steamer on the floor of your shower and enjoy as you wash.

Nature therapy shower steamer
Revitalising.

100 g shower steamer base
2 g (1 tsp) matcha powder
15 drops blue Mallee eucalyptus essential oil
15 drops lemon myrtle essential oil

Feeling happy shower steamer
Uplifting.

100 g shower steamer base
2 g (1 tsp) pink Argiletz clay
25 drops sweet orange essential oil
5 drops geranium essential oil

Lighten up & let go shower steamer
Calming.

100 g shower steamer base
2 g (1 tsp) turmeric powder
20 drops bergamot essential oil
10 drops lavender essential oil

Snooze time shower steamer
Relaxing.

100 g shower steamer base
2 g (1 tsp) cacao powder
15 drops lavender essential oil
5 drops clary sage essential oil

Mother and Baby Care

Gentle, soothing and safe preparations can be made from natural ingredients to care for babies and mothers-to-be. To ensure essential oils are selected with care, refer to *Pregnancy* on page 38 and *Babies and children* on page 39.

Cocoa butter pregnancy body balm

The balmiest of balms, this cocoa butter body balm is super rich and is suitable for use on very dry skin. It is especially suitable for use during pregnancy to keep your skin soft and supple while it continues to stretch. Use this one to help prevent stretch marks.

60 g cocoa butter
20 g apricot kernel oil
20 g macadamia oil
60 drops tangerine or mandarin essential oil

Make this balm by following the *Aromatherapy balm method 1* on page 63.

Nipple care balm

A protective and healing balm for sore, chafed, cracked nipples. Massage well into the nipples after breastfeeding. Simply stir the calendula infused oil into softened shea butter.

45 mL shea butter
5 mL calendula infused oil

Baby bottom balm

This balm will soothe and protect baby's bottom from nappy rash.

35 g shea butter
10 g zinc oxide powder
5 mL calendula infused oil
3 drops lavender essential oil
2 drops German chamomile essential oil

1. Soften the shea butter in a ceramic or glass mortar and pestle by working the shea butter with the pestle.
2. Stir in the calendula infused oil, essential oils and zinc oxide powder.
3. Continue working the mixture until it is smooth and homogenous.
4. Scoop into a jar.
5. Ensure baby's bottom is completely dry before applying.

Baby wash

A gentle wash to cleanse baby's skin from top to bottom.

90 mL Castile liquid soap
10 mL apricot kernel oil
8 drops lavender essential oil
2 drops German chamomile essential oil

1. Mix the Castile liquid soap, apricot kernel oil and essential oils together.
2. Store in a bottle.
3. Shake the mixture well before use.

Baby massage oil

A soothing and calming massage oil that cares for baby's skin.

100 mL apricot kernel oil
8 drops lavender essential oil
2 drops German chamomile essential oil

1. Add the drops of essential oil to the apricot kernel oil in a glass bottle and shake well.
2. Massage a tiny amount over baby's skin.

Baby powder

75 g corn starch or tapioca flour
15 g oat flour
10 g zinc oxide powder
10 drops lavender essential oil

1. Mix the corn starch or tapioca flour, oat flour and zinc oxide powder together in a bowl.
2. Sieve to break down any lumps in the powder.
3. Add the drops of lavender essential oil, ensuring you sprinkle them uniformly over the mixture, then stir them in.
4. Sieve again a couple of times to ensure any lumps are broken down and the essential oils are evenly distributed throughout the mixture.
5. Store the mixture in a shaker bottle or container such as an icing sugar or parmesan cheese shaker. Alternatively, using a funnel, pour the mixture into a bottle. This way a small amount can be decanted for use each time.

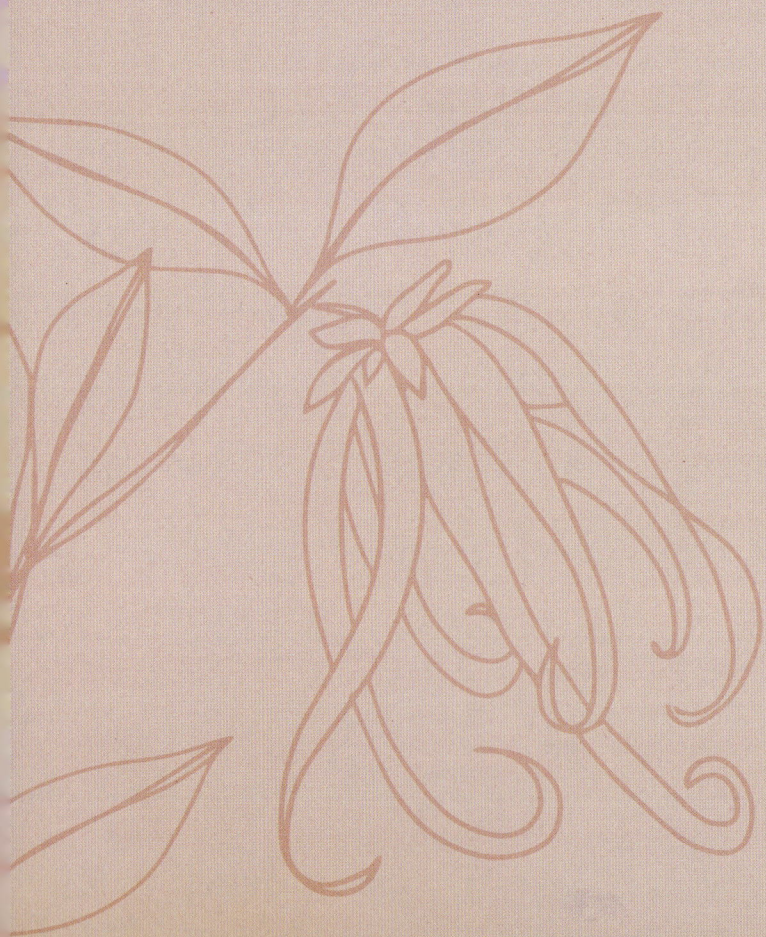

Perfumes

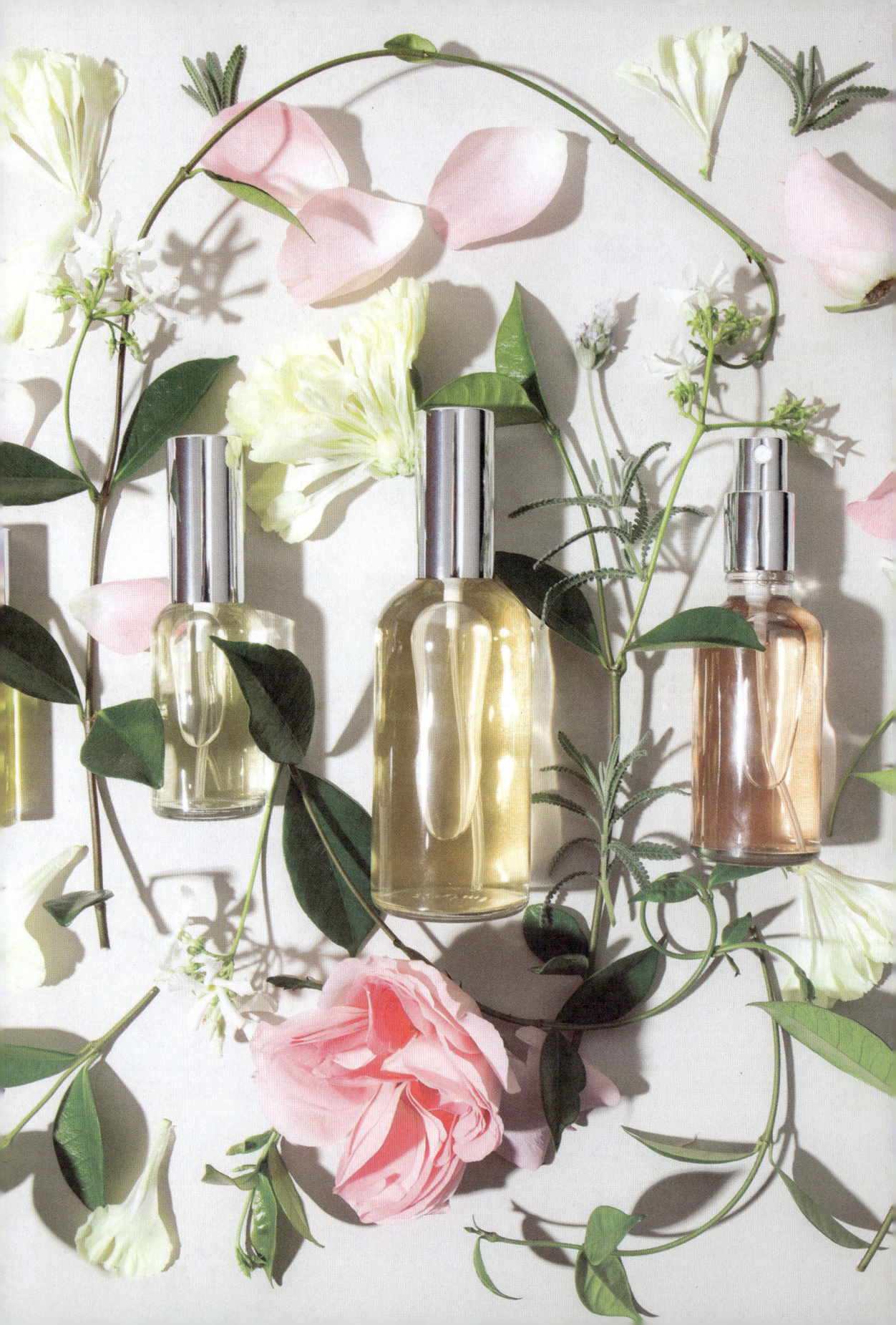

Fragrant Harmony

A natural perfume is a harmonious composition of essential oils — a symphony of top, middle and base notes. Creating a perfume has been described as being like composing music.

As soon as you open a bottle of perfume, you smell the top notes as they quickly escape from the bottle. They are fresh, vibrant, lightweight ingredients that give you the initial impression of a fragrance. After applying the perfume to your skin, the top notes diffuse from your skin for up to half an hour or so, finally giving way to less diffusive middle notes, the heart of the perfume. The middle notes release themselves over several hours, after which all that remains are the base notes. These are the least diffusive notes of all and remain on the skin for most of the day. They are the heavy, woody, resinous notes. They also function as fixatives, ensuring the top notes don't disappear too quickly. Dividing odours into categories of top, middle and base notes provides a means of classifying odours according to their volatility.

Professional perfumers may use hundreds of fragrance ingredients, both natural and synthetic, and take many years to create a unique composition that smells exquisite at all stages as it releases itself from the skin.

When creating a perfume from essential oils, it is important to consider the following:

- Firstly, become familiar with the fragrance of each individual essential oil you have.

- Be aware of the various odour intensities of each essential oil. You will want to use less of an essential oil that has a strong, penetrating odour and more of an oil with a light, fresh or subtle aroma.

- Choose essential oils from each classification of top, middle and base notes to create a perfume that unfolds harmoniously.

- Determine the kind of fragrance you want to achieve — fresh and citrusy, warm and spicy, subtle and woody, sensual and floral, calming and soothing or whatever your heart desires. The essential oils you choose can enhance or balance your mood.

The following proportions give you an indication of the quantity of the essential oil to be used in each note of a perfume blend. However, this will vary according to the notes you wish to have the most impact:

- 45–55% top notes
- 30–40% middle notes
- 15–25% base notes.

The essential oils have been categorised into top, middle and base notes to assist you in your blending. Some essential oils will cross over into another category depending on the other essential oils used in your blend. Thus, these categories are only arbitrary.

Top Notes	Middle Notes		Base Notes
Bergamot	Black pepper	Juniper	Buddha wood
Citronella	Cardamom	Lavender	Cedarwood, Atlas
Grapefruit	Carrot seed	Manuka	Cedarwood,
Lemon	Chamomile, Roman	Marjoram	Virginian
Lemongrass	Cinnamon	Niaouli	Chamomile,
Lemon myrtle	Clary sage	Palmarosa	German
Lemon-scented	Clove bud	Peppermint	Cistus
ironbark	Coriander seed	Petitgrain	Everlasting
Lime	Cypress	Pine	Hinoki wood
Mandarin	Eucalyptus	Rose absolute	Myrrh
May chang	Fennel	Rosemary	Patchouli
Melissa	Fragonia	Sage	Sandalwood
Neroli	Frankincense	Spearmint	Vetiver
Orange, sweet	Geranium	Tea tree	
Rose otto	Ginger	Thyme	
Tangerine	Jasmine	Ylang ylang	

Essential oil concentrations for perfumes

The essential oil compositions for perfumes are balanced blends that may be added to any of the perfume bases to make a parfum, eau de parfum, eau de toilette, eau de cologne, body mist, perfume oil or perfume balm. Of these, parfum has the highest concentration of essential oils, with the concentration falling until it is lowest in a body mist. You would use only a small quantity of parfum to fragrance your body, whereas you would use a body mist quite liberally.

Personal Fragrance	Essential Oil	Alcohol/Water
Parfum/extrait	15–30%	Alcohol 90% Water 10%
Eau de parfum	8–15%	Alcohol 85% Water 15%
Eau de toilette	4–8%	Alcohol 80% Water 20%
Eau de cologne/aftershave	3–5%	Alcohol 70% Water 30%
Body mist	1–3%	Alcohol 60% Water 40% or Essential oil solubiliser 2–6% Water 94–98%
Perfume oil/balm	10–30%	Base oil or balm base

You may like to choose one of these essential oil compositions to add to a base to create an aromatherapy perfume before taking the next step of trusting your nose and your knowledge to make your own perfume composition.

The total quantity of essential oils in each composition is equivalent to adding approximately 1% to 100 mL of perfume base. This makes it easy to calculate the quantity of essential oil you will need to add to a perfume base to make your desired strength of perfume. If, for example, you would like to make 100 mL of eau de parfum, multiply the quantity of drops by 10 to give you just under a 10% dilution.

Essential oil compositions for perfumes

Composition 1
Spicy and oriental
5 drops sweet orange
4 drops bergamot
3 drops cinnamon
2 drops lavender
3 drops Atlas cedarwood
3 drops patchouli

Composition 2
Rich floral
6 drops rose absolute
6 drops geranium
3 drops frankincense
5 drops sandalwood

Composition 3
Green, herbaceous and lively
8 drops lemon
4 drops lemongrass
3 drops petitgrain
3 drops rosemary
1 drop ginger
1 drop vetiver

Composition 4
Green and cool
5 drops lavender
5 drops spearmint
4 drops geranium
2 drops fennel
4 drops sandalwood

Composition 5
Warm and woody
6 drops mandarin
3 drops grapefruit
2 drops palmarosa
7 drops sandalwood
2 drops myrrh

Composition 6
Floriental
4 drops bergamot
3 drops lime
4 drops jasmine
2 drops clove bud
2 drops ylang ylang
3 drops Atlas cedarwood
2 drops patchouli

Composition 7
Traditional eau de cologne
4 drops bergamot
4 drops lemon
4 drops sweet orange
3 drops neroli
2 drops rosemary
2 drops lavender
1 drop petitgrain

Creating Perfumes

Creating a pure and natural perfume from essential oils satisfies both your nose and your soul. To make a perfume, you will require a selection of essential oils as well as base ingredients that act as carriers.

Perfume Bases

There are several perfume base ingredients into which you can blend your essential oils. These include water, alcohol and oil. The type of base determines how much essential oil can be added to the perfume, how it diffuses into the air and the way in which it is used on the body. Water-based perfumes are able to incorporate the least amount of essential oil and are used as body mists, whereas alcohol-based and oil-based perfumes and balms can incorporate higher amounts of essential oils, making them more concentrated with less being applied to the body. Alcohol-based perfumes are more diffusive, creating a cloud of fragrance around you, whereas oil-based or balm-based perfumes are less diffusive and may remain on the skin longer.

Water

Distilled water is the water of choice. If this is not readily available to you, bottled spring or filtered water will suffice. Waters of distillation such as lavender water, rosewater or neroli water may also be used where their fragrance complements the essential oils chosen. Essential oils do not readily disperse throughout water. If you add essential oils to water alone, you need to shake your container each time you use your perfume. An essential oil solubiliser will ensure the essential oils remain solubilised in the water.

Alcohol

Alcohol is used as a perfume base for essential oils and assists in their gentle diffusion into the air around your body.

Perfume grade ethanol is the alcohol of choice. It is a fine grade alcohol made by the fermentation of starches, for example, sugar. Its smell does not compete with the aroma of the essential oils added to it. Generally, perfume grade ethanol is 95% pure ethanol mixed with water and denaturant. It is often denatured to prevent its internal consumption.

As perfume grade ethanol is not available for purchase without an alcohol licence, some aromatherapy companies provide a perfume base that has had benzoin gum steeped in it, for example, which also acts as a fixative for the perfume, helping the oils remain on the skin longer.

Oil

Jojoba oil is the base oil of choice in making a perfume oil or oil-based perfume. It is relatively odourless and is very stable over a long period of time. Your next choice would be sweet almond oil or apricot kernel oil. They are not as stable as jojoba oil in the long term, but they are suitable if you are making small quantities that you intend to use within 6 months.

Balm

Essential oils may be added to a balm, which you can store in a small pot. Make a perfume balm, also known as a solid perfume, by following the *Methods for making aromatherapy balms* on page 63.

Making Your Perfume

This recipe is suitable for making an eau de toilette. Modify the quantities of ingredients according to the table on page 242 to make other perfume concentrations.

80 g perfume ethanol
20 g purified water
5 g (approx. 100 drops) essential oils

1. Blend the essential oils.
2. Mix the essential oils with an equivalent quantity of perfume ethanol.
3. Mix the water and remaining perfume ethanol together.
4. Slowly add the essential oil and ethanol mixture to the water and ethanol mixture, stirring as you go. This will assist in avoiding or reducing cloudiness.
5. Store in a closed glass bottle for at least a week in a cool place to allow for any sedimentation that may occur to drop out.
6. Filter the perfume through filter paper such as coffee filter paper.
7. Store in a sealed glass bottle to allow your perfume to develop to its full maturity for at least 3 months. Keep it in a cool place out of the light.
8. Your perfume is now ready for use.

This is a traditional method of making perfumes. It requires time and patience. However, if you choose, your perfume may be used at any time after you have blended it.

Aftershave

Follow the same procedure as above. However, at step 3, add some glycerin to the ethanol and water. The glycerin will help reduce the drying effects the ethanol may have on the skin. Add approximately 3–5 g of essential oil to each 100 g of aftershave.

The body mist method below can be an alternative for making a gentle aftershave.

Body mists

1. Blend the essential oils.
2. Add essential oil solubiliser to the essential oil blend and mix well.
3. Add the water to the essential oil and solubiliser blend, and stir well.
4. Pour into a spray bottle.

Perfume oils

1. Blend the essential oils.
2. Add the base oil to the essential oil blend and mix well.
3. Pour into a dropper bottle or rollerball bottle.
4. Allow a day or two for the blend to mature if desired.

Perfume balms/solid perfumes

1. Blend the essential oils.
2. Add the essential oil blend to a balm base by following the *Methods for making aromatherapy balms* on page 63.
3. Store in a small glass jar or perfume pot.

Fresh from the Garden Perfumes

Eau de colognes, body mists and aftershaves can be made from the fragrant herbs and flowers in your garden. They are simple to make and truly worth the effort.

Try any of these fragrant ingredients or others that you may have in your garden. Harvest herbs and flowers in the warmer months and at the time of day when their scent is strongest.

Flowers

frangipani, honeysuckle, jasmine, lavender, roses

Pick the flowers in the early evening, being careful not to bruise or damage the flowers.

Allow any moisture to evaporate from them for around an hour before macerating them in the perfume base for 24 hours. Replace with a fresh round of flowers several times to reach the intensity of perfume you desire.

Herbs

eucalyptus, geranium, lemon balm, lemongrass, lemon myrtle, lemon verbena, peppermint, rosemary, sage, thyme

Ensure the leaves are dry then chop them up before macerating them in the perfume base for 24 hours. Replace with a fresh round of herbs a couple of times to reach the intensity of perfume you desire.

Citrus

grapefruit, lemon, lime, mandarin, orange rinds

Remove the rinds from the fruit and remove any moisture that may be on them. Chop them into pieces before macerating them in the perfume base for 24 hours. Replace with a fresh round of rinds a couple of times to reach the intensity of perfume you desire.

Spices

cinnamon, clove, coriander seeds

Crush the dried spices before macerating them in the perfume base for 24 hours. Replace with a fresh round of spices a couple of times to reach the intensity of perfume you desire.

Ingredients

**your chosen fragrant plant material
perfume ethanol
or
vodka**

To make your fresh from the garden eau de cologne, body mist or aftershave, follow this maceration method.

Maceration method for making perfumes

1. Place the prepared plant material into a glass jar, filling it no more than two-thirds full.
2. Pour enough perfume ethanol or vodka into the jar, ensuring the ingredients are properly covered with a small excess.
3. Close the lid and macerate (steep) the ingredients for 24 hours.
4. Strain the mixture through a strainer lined with muslin.
5. Discard the spent plant material.
6. To intensify the perfume, repeat the process several times with fresh plant material and the same alcohol.
7. Once you have reached the intensity of perfume you desire, strain the final mixture through a dampened coffee filter, then pour it into a bottle, storing it away from heat and light.

8. Allow to mature from a week to a fortnight before using.

Perfume cocktail

This recipe is easy to make and smells light, fresh, herbaceous and summery. It contains ingredients you would want to make a cocktail with.

1 handful fresh lavender leaves and flowers
1 handful fresh mint
1 handful fresh rosemary
rind of 3 lemons
approximately 500 mL vodka

Make this perfume by following the *Maceration method for making perfumes* on page 246.

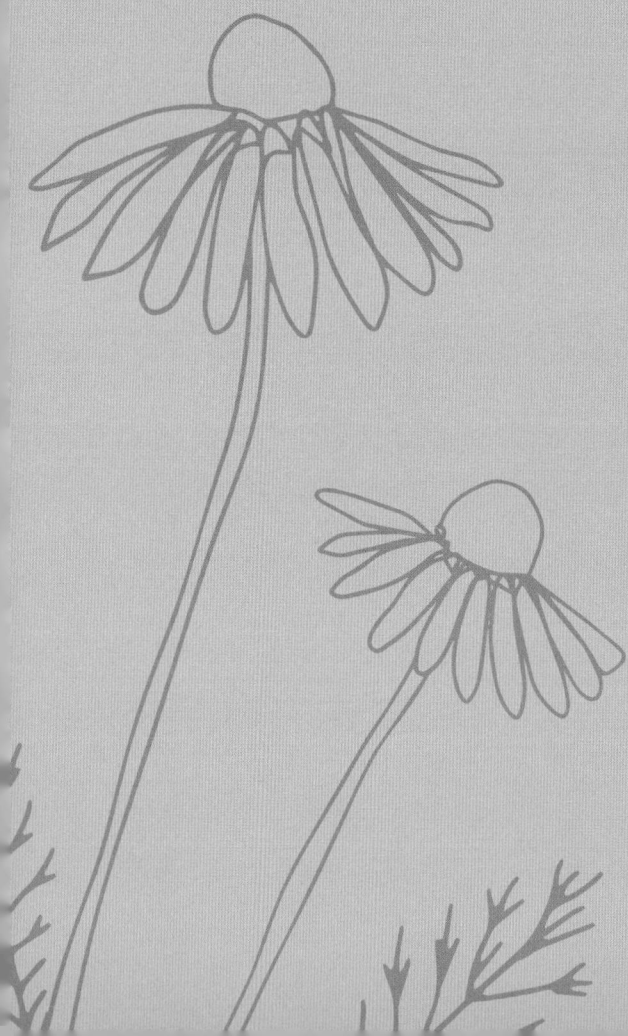

Hair

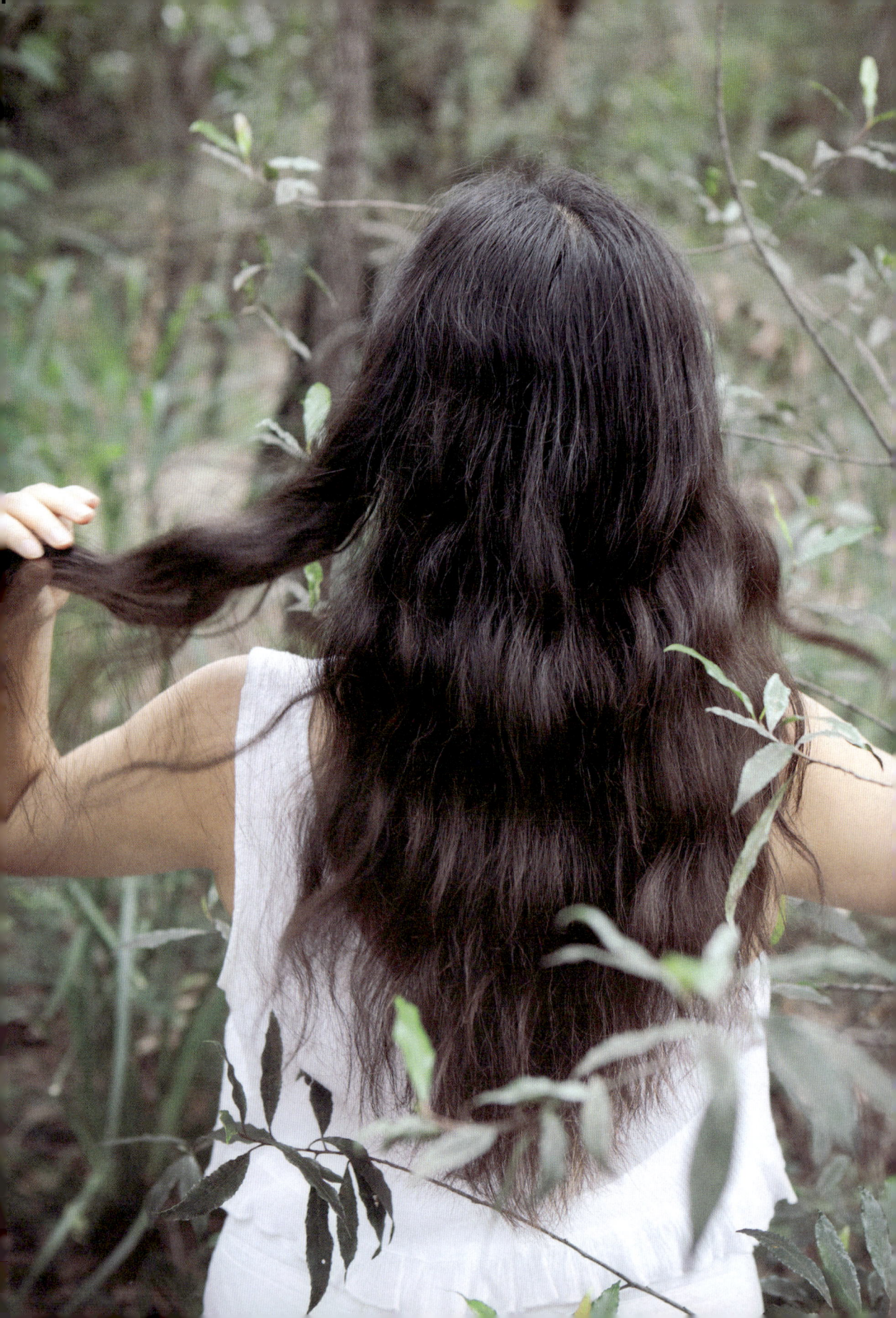

Hair and Scalp Care Ingredients

Understanding the active ingredients that are used to make your hair and scalp preparations will allow you to create many new preparations and adapt the ones given here to suit your own needs.

Essential Oils for Hair and Scalp

Essential oils have many properties that benefit the hair and scalp. They are most beneficial therapeutically when massaged into the scalp, where they improve the health of the scalp and subsequently the health of the hair. Do not choose essential oils according to hair colour as they do not affect hair colour.

- **Ginger, pine** and **rosemary** stimulate the circulation in the scalp, which in turn improves blood flow to the hair papillae and follicles where hair growth takes place. Use these oils when poor hair growth is a concern.

- **Sandalwood** improves dry scalp conditions.

- **Bergamot, cedarwood, cypress, geranium, grapefruit, lemon** and **patchouli** help balance excessively oily scalp and hair.

- **Chamomile** and **lavender**, due to their anti-inflammatory properties, may be used on inflamed, irritated scalps and are gentle enough to use on babies' scalps as well.

- **Atlas cedarwood, lavender, patchouli, peppermint, rosemary, tea tree** and **thyme** will help clear dandruff conditions.

- **Geranium, lavender, rosemary** and **ylang ylang** may be used on most hair and scalp types.

The essential oils above or the essential oil compositions on the next page may be added to hair and scalp preparations in the following quantities:

- **Shampoos** — add 1 mL (approx. 20 drops) of an essential oil or essential oil composition to 100 mL of shampoo base.

- **Hair and scalp treatment oils** — add up to 0.5 mL (approx. 50 drops) of an essential oil or essential oil composition to each 100 mL of cold-pressed vegetable oil.

- **Hair conditioning preparations** — add 1 mL (approx. 20 drops) of an essential oil or essential oil composition to each 100 mL of conditioner base.

- **Hair vinegars and rinses** — add 5 drops of an essential oil or essential oil composition to each 500 mL of the herbal infusion and herbal vinegar rinse recipes on page 253.

Essential oil compositions for hair and scalp

Oily hair composition
Balances oiliness
10 drops lemon
5 drops geranium
3 drops lavender
2 drops cypress

Dry hair composition
Gentle on dry hair
10 drops sandalwood
7 drops lavender
3 drops ylang ylang

All hair types composition
A general hair and scalp tonic
8 drops geranium
8 drops lavender
4 drops rosemary

Inflamed, irritated scalp conditions composition
Anti-inflammatory and soothing
7 drops lavender
5 drops sandalwood
3 drops German chamomile

Baby's hair composition
Gentle and soothing
4 drops lavender
1 drop German chamomile

Dandruff and itchy scalp composition
Relieves dry, flaky scalp
10 drops Atlas cedarwood
6 drops patchouli
4 drops rosemary

Psoriasis of the scalp composition
Helps relieve this scalp condition
8 drops bergamot
7 drops lavender
3 drops juniper
2 drops German chamomile

Hair loss composition
Stimulates scalp circulation
8 drops peppermint
7 drops rosemary
6 drops ginger

Herbs for Hair and Scalp

Herbal extracts, including infusions, vinegars and oils, are wonderful preparations to use to improve the condition of your hair and scalp.

- **Horsetail**, **lavender**, **rosemary** and **sage** can be used to improve the condition of all hair and scalp types.

- **Aloe vera**, **chamomile**, **comfrey**, **marshmallow root** and **soapwort** are gentle and suitable for use on dry hair and scalps.

- **Nettle**, **peppermint**, **thyme** and **yarrow** are suitable for use on oily hair and scalps.

- **Calendula**, **chamomile** and **lavender** are gentle and suitable for use on baby, fine hair and sensitive scalps.

- **Lavender**, **nettle**, **parsley**, **peppermint**, **rosemary**, **sage** and **thyme** can help improve dandruff.

- **Calendula**, **chamomile**, **comfrey**, **lavender**, **liquorice root**, **marshmallow root** and **soapwort** are soothing on inflamed and irritated scalps.

- **Bay**, **ginger**, **nettle**, **peppermint** and **rosemary** help improve circulation in the scalp and assist healthy hair growth.

Herbal infusions

Herbal infusions may be used as final hair rinses to add shine to your hair and to improve the health of your scalp. Make a herbal infusion by following the *Method for making herbal infusions* on page 49.

After shampooing and conditioning your hair, pour the infusion over your scalp and throughout your hair. There is no need to rinse it out; it leaves a subtle fragrance in your hair, depending on the herb.

Herbal infusions may also be mixed in your hand with your shampoo just before shampooing your hair.

Herbal infusions can be used to add subtle coloured highlights to your hair. For more information, see the section on herbal hair colours on page 273.

Use herbal infusions fresh or store them in the refrigerator for up to 2 days to prevent the proliferation of microbes.

Herbal vinegars

Herbal vinegars may be used to improve the condition of your scalp and help to reduce dandruff. They not only re-establish the acid pH of your scalp and hair, but also include the therapeutic properties of the herbs. Herbal vinegars may be used regularly after shampooing and conditioning.

Follow the *Method for making herbal vinegars* on page 54.

Add 20 mL (1 tbsp) of your herbal vinegar to 250–500 mL of water and massage it into your scalp and pour throughout your hair. You may want to follow with a quick rinse of warm water or herbal infusion.

Herbal oils

Herbal oils condition your hair and treat your scalp. They can also be beautifully fragrant depending on the herbs you choose to infuse into your base oil. Follow the *Method for making a cold-infused oil* on page 52. Your herbal oils may be used in your shampoos and conditioners, especially if your hair is dry. However, they are best used as they are, as treatments for your hair and scalp. Essential oils may also be incorporated into your herbal oil preparations.

Infused Oils

Infused oils such as carrot and calendula are beneficial for scalp problems.

- **Carrot infused oil** is beneficial for alleviating dry, flaky scalp conditions.
- **Calendula infused oil** is beneficial for alleviating irritated scalp conditions.

Infused oils may be applied to your scalp directly or blended with cold-pressed vegetable oils. Essential oils may be combined with the infused oils for a scalp treatment.

Cold-pressed Vegetable Oils

Cold-pressed vegetable oils have been used traditionally to smooth and protect the hair, improving its shine and lustre. They are also used as scalp treatments to improve the condition of the scalp.

- **Coconut oil** is traditionally used as a hair and scalp treatment in the Pacific Islands.

- **Olive oil** is traditionally used in the Mediterranean region.
- **Jojoba oil** is traditionally used by First Nations People in the south-west USA and western Mexico.
- **Sweet almond and apricot kernel oil** are also suitable hair and scalp oils.

Fruits and Vegetables

Grapefruit and lemon

Grapefruit and lemon juice that has been strained and diluted may be used in preparations for oily hair.

Avocado

Avocado is rich in conditioning oil. Ripe avocado flesh mashed into a smooth creamy paste makes a wonderful hair conditioner.

Henna

Henna is a natural hair colourant. It is a herb that coats the hair shaft, giving it a lustrous shine. It is available in a variety of shades of red/orange colours.

Shampoos

Clean your hair with a plant-derived shampoo and give yourself a stimulating scalp massage. This will leave you and your hair feeling clean and refreshed.

Plant-derived shampoo bases are readily available and simplify the process of making shampoos. However, complex shampoos are possible if you undertake further studies to understand the chemistry of surfactants.

Using a Shampoo Base

A gentle unscented shampoo base that is pH balanced and made from plant-based surfactants can be simply and effectively customised to provide a shampoo for your hair type.

Normal to oily aromatherapy shampoo

100 mL shampoo base
20 drops essential oil

1. Choose an essential oil or essential oil composition for your hair from pages 251–252.
2. Add the essential oils to the shampoo base and shake or stir thoroughly.
3. Store in a bottle or container.

Normal to dry aromatherapy shampoo

80 mL shampoo base
10 mL argan oil
10 mL macadamia oil
20 drops essential oil

1. Choose an essential oil or essential oil composition for your hair from pages 251–252.
2. Mix the essential oils, macadamia oil and argan oil (or your choice of vegetable oil) together.
3. Stir this mixture into the shampoo base.
4. Store in a bottle or container.
5. Shake the bottle each time before use.

Herbal shampoo

90 mL shampoo base
10 mL herbal tincture

1. Choose the appropriate herbs for your hair and scalp from page 252 and follow the *Method for making herbal tinctures* on page 51.
2. Add the tincture to the shampoo base and shake or stir thoroughly. If your hair is dry, add 10 mL of cold-pressed vegetable oil or herbal infused oil to the mixture.
3. Store in a bottle or container.
4. Shake the bottle each time before use.

Green clay shampoo

An effective shampoo for oily hair.

100 mL shampoo base
25 g green Argiletz clay
20 drops essential oil

1. Choose an essential oil or essential oil composition for oily hair from page 252.
2. Stir all ingredients together thoroughly.
3. Store in a bottle or container.
4. Shake well before use if you see the ingredients have separated.
5. Use as you would a normal shampoo by massaging into wet hair and scalp, then rinsing thoroughly and conditioning.

Shampoo Bars

Shampoo bars are a concentrated water-free alternative to liquid shampoos. They are long lasting and don't require packaging. Their size and absence of water makes them convenient for travel too.

A gentle, anionic surfactant, sodium cocoyl isethionate, is the main ingredient. It is a powder that is combined with a liquid surfactant to form a paste, then pressed into a mould to form a solid bar. Other ingredients include hair conditioning agents to ensure the hair maintains its moisture, condition and shine. Conditioning agents include behentrimonium methosulphate & cetearyl alcohol, vegetable oils, vegetable butters and d-panthenol (pro-vitamin B5). In regard to the behentrimonium methosulphate & cetearyl alcohol used in the recipe in this book, BTMS 25 has been selected. This ingredient is made up of 25% behentrimonium methosulphate and 75% cetearyl alcohol.

To use a shampoo bar, wet your hair thoroughly. Create a lather on your shampoo bar and massage it throughout your hair. Encourage further lathering by massaging your hair and scalp with your finger tips and adding more water if necessary. Rinse well and follow with a conditioner. The following shampoo bar recipe is suitable for normal to dry hair.

Equipment

- dust mask
- digital scales
- saucepan
- metal trivet
- heat-resistant jug
- stovetop or hot plate
- 2 metal stirring spoons
- mixing bowl
- silicon mould

Ingredients

62 g sodium cocoyl isethionate powder
20 g cocamidopropyl betaine
5 g BTMS 25
(behentrimonium methosulphate & cetearyl alcohol)
10 g cocoa butter
2 g d-panthenol
1 g pink Argiletz clay
1 g (approx. 20 drops) essential oil

Method for making a shampoo bar

1. Choose an essential oil or essential oil composition for your hair type from pages 251–252.
2. Wearing a dust mask, add the sodium cocoyl isethionate and pink clay into a mixing bowl. Take particular care with the sodium cocoyl isethionate as it is a fine powder and the particles become airborne very easily, making it easy to inhale.

3. Carefully stir the sodium cocoyl isethionate and pink clay together so that the pink clay is evenly mixed throughout the sodium cocoyl isethionate.

4. Add the drops of essential oil to this mixture.

5. Into the heat-resistant jug, add the d-panthenol, BTMS 25 and cocoa butter and heat in a *bain-marie* until melted.

6. Add the cocamidopropyl betaine to the melted panthenol, BTMS 25 and cocoa butter in the *bain-marie*.

7. Stir together until the liquid is smooth and milky/creamy. The solid ingredients may seize up momentarily when you add the cocamidopropyl betaine before they melt again, forming a milky/creamy liquid.

8. Add this mixture into the sodium cocoyl isethionate and pink clay in the mixing bowl.

9. Stir together with a mixing spoon. At first the mixture will be a powder, then form crumbs. Eventually, with continued stirring, it will form a dough.

10. Fill the mixture into a silicon mould, such as a muffin mould, pressing it in carefully and smoothing over the surface. Alternatively, it could be hand-formed into a ball or disc without using a mould.

11. Place in the refrigerator or freezer to solidify.

12. When the shampoo bar has set, carefully remove it from the mould.

13. Leave it to air dry for a day or two before using.

14. Store it in a dry place in between hair washes.

Shampoo Alternatives

Soapwort hair cleanser

This is an excellent hair cleanser for sensitive or problem scalps as well as for fine or damaged hair. Soapwort root is rich in saponins which, when released through simmering, produce a mild foam that will gently cleanse your hair and scalp.

20 g soapwort root
500 mL water

1. Make a soapwort root decoction following the *Method for making herbal decoctions* on page 51.

2. Pour into a bottle or container and shake well to create a gentle foam.

3. Massage into damp hair and rinse thoroughly. Your hair will feel soft and clean.

4. Store any remaining liquid in the refrigerator and use it within a couple of days.

Moroccan clay hair cleanser

This is a simple cleansing preparation for most hair types and may be used as an alternative to regular shampoo. Double this mixture or increase proportionally if you have long hair.

75 mL herbal infusion or purified water
20 g rhassoul clay
5 mL (1 tsp) apple cider vinegar

1. Choose the appropriate herbs for your hair and scalp from page 252 and follow the *Method for making herbal infusions* on page 49 or simply use purified water.

2. Add the herbal infusion or purified water and apple cider vinegar to the clay and mix into a smooth slurry.

3. Pour the mixture into a bottle so that you can apply the mixture easily to your scalp and hair.

4. Wet your hair and scalp, then wring out the excess water.

5. Carefully apply small quantities of the mixture to your scalp and massage it in well. Then apply more of the mixture to the rest of your hair, especially the oily parts, and spread through well. Be careful not to get the mixture on your face or in your eyes as the apple cider vinegar can be irritating.

6. Leave on for 2—5 minutes before rinsing. Give your scalp a massage during this time. Do not allow the mixture to dry.

7. Rinse the mixture thoroughly from your hair and condition as normal.

Pure pulse shampoo

This is another traditional hair cleansing method. It is made from finely milled dried pulses. You may choose to grind them yourself or alternatively you can purchase them as flour. Chickpeas and lentils are both traditionally used ingredients. They absorb any dirt and grime from the hair, which is then rinsed away.

50 g chickpea or lentil flour
400 mL herbal infusion or purified water

1. Place the flour into a saucepan.

2. Choose the appropriate herbs for your hair and scalp from page 252 and follow the *Method for making herbal infusions* on page 49 or simply use water.

3. Slowly add the herbal infusion or purified water and mix into a smooth paste.

4. Gently heat the mixture for about 15 minutes.

5. Stir the mixture constantly to ensure it does not stick to the bottom of the saucepan.

6. Remove from the heat and pour into a bowl to cool down. It will thicken up over this time.

7. Apply to your scalp and hair, starting at the roots and massaging in well.

8. After a couple of minutes, rinse your hair thoroughly and follow with a conditioner.

Simple dry shampoo

This is not exactly a shampoo but is used in between shampooing to absorb excess oil from the hair, leaving it looking cleaner. It also leaves your hair smelling wonderfully aromatic. Use it whenever you don't want to or can't shampoo your hair with water.

25 g corn starch or arrowroot flour
25 g kaolin clay
0.5 g (approx. 10 drops) essential oil

1. Mix the corn starch or arrowroot and kaolin together in a bowl.

2. Sieve to break down any lumps.

3. Add the drops of essential oil, ensuring you sprinkle them uniformly over the mixture, then stir them in.

4. Sieve again a couple of times to ensure any lumps are broken down and the essential oils are evenly distributed throughout the mixture.

5. Store the mixture in a shaker bottle or container such as an icing sugar or parmesan cheese shaker. Alternatively, using a funnel, pour the mixture into a bottle. This way a small amount can be decanted for use each time.

6. Massage small quantities into your hair close to your scalp, then spread and massage the mixture throughout your hair.

7. Use a brush to distribute the mixture throughout your hair and to remove any excess.

8. Remove the rest of the excess by tipping your head upside down and continuing to brush.

See page 97 for more recipes for dry shampoos, including different colours.

Oily hair toner

Whenever your scalp is particularly oily, apply pure witch hazel water or lavender water to a cotton wool ball or pad and wipe throughout your hair and over your scalp to remove the excess oil.

Using Castile Liquid Soap as Shampoo

Some people find Castile liquid soap a simple and effective alternative to shampoo to clean their hair. However, it is not suitable for everyone.

There are a few important considerations to keep in mind when deciding whether or not it is suitable for your hair.

- Castile liquid soap is highly alkaline, i.e. around pH 9–11 while your scalp is pH 4.5–5.5. It is recommended that you follow it with a vinegar rinse, which is acidic. The soap removes grime and lifts the cuticles on the hair shaft, while the acidity of the vinegar encourages the cuticles to lie flat again. Dry, itchy scalp problems may also develop if the pH is not re-established.
- It will leave your hair dry and tangled if you don't follow it with a vinegar rinse.
- Do not get it in your eyes as it will sting. If you do, rinse immediately. You will need to do the same with the vinegar rinse as it is acidic and will also sting your eyes.

- If you have hard water, high in minerals such as calcium and magnesium, the Castile liquid soap will not rinse properly from your hair and may build up on your hair.
- Not all Castile liquid soaps are the same. Some will foam up more than others and rinse better from your hair, while others may leave your hair feeling greasy and dull.
- You may need to use the Castile liquid soap and vinegar rinse method several times before your hair completely adjusts to being washed this way.
- If your hair is very dry, you may need to work a few drops of vegetable oil or hair oil blend through your hair while it is still damp at the end of the process of washing and rinsing.

What to prepare

Castile liquid soap shampoo
- 1 tbsp (20 mL) Castile liquid soap
- 100 mL warm purified water (tap water is not recommended, especially if it is high in minerals, as the salts precipitate as scum)
- bottle (any bottle that has a narrow opening so that you can squeeze the mixture from it and distribute it throughout your hair)

Apple cider vinegar rinse
- 1 tbsp (20 mL) apple cider vinegar
- 500 mL warm purified water
- bottle (any bottle that has a narrow opening)

Rinsing water
- a jug or large bottle filled with warm purified water

Method for using Castile liquid soap as a shampoo

1. Add the Castile liquid soap hair shampoo ingredients to one bottle and shake well.

2. Add the apple cider vinegar rinse ingredients to another bottle and shake well.

3. Fill your jug or large bottle with warm purified water.

4. Wet your hair with a little of the purified water from the jug.

5. Squeeze the Castile liquid soap hair shampoo mixture over your hair and lather. Make sure you massage your scalp.

6. Rinse well with purified water from the jug and squeeze out any excess water.

7. Squeeze the apple cider vinegar rinse over your hair and massage throughout your hair and scalp. Leave on for a minute or two.

8. Rinse well with purified water from the jug.

9. Dry as normal.

10. If your hair is very dry, squeeze out any excess water from your hair and drop a few drops of vegetable oil or hair oil blend onto the tips of your fingers and spread well throughout your hair and dry as normal.

Conditioners

While shampoos remove dirt and grime, they also lift the cuticle scales on the hair shaft and remove the hair's natural oil. Conditioning ensures that the cuticle scales are, once again, smoothed down and the hair is hydrated. This is particularly important for dry, dehydrated, damaged or brittle hair.

Amazing avocado conditioner

A softening conditioner for fine, dry hair. This recipe makes enough for one application.

½ ripe avocado
5 mL (1 tsp) avocado oil
1 egg yolk

1. Mash the avocado flesh into a smooth paste.
2. Blend in the avocado oil and egg yolk.
3. After shampooing, spread the conditioner throughout your hair and leave it on for a few minutes before rinsing.
4. Rinse thoroughly.

Ultra-rich hair conditioner

Slather this conditioner on your hair if it is dry and damaged. This recipe makes enough for one application.

2 egg yolks
10 mL (2 tsp) apple cider vinegar
10 mL (2 tsp) cold-pressed vegetable oil
(coconut, olive or jojoba oil)
10 mL (2 tsp) honey
5 mL (1 tsp) liquid lecithin

1. Mix all of the ingredients.

2. After shampooing, spread the conditioner throughout your hair and leave it on for a few minutes before rinsing.
3. Rinse thoroughly.

Hair moisturiser

This is more of a hair moisturiser for normal to dry hair. However, it is used the same way as you use a conditioner. It leaves the hair feeling soft and smooth.

<u>Oil phase</u>
10 g plant-derived emulsifying wax
35 g jojoba oil

<u>Water phase</u>
148 g purified water
5 g vegetable glycerin
2 g preservative

<u>Add at 45°C</u>
2 g (approx. 40 drops) essential oil

<u>pH adjustment</u>
qs citric acid + purified water

1. Choose an essential oil or essential oil composition for your hair from pages 251–252.
2. Make this hair moisturiser by following the *Method for making an emulsion with emulsifying wax* on page 79.
3. Store in a container and use after each shampoo.
4. Spread the hair moisturiser throughout your hair and leave it on for a few minutes.
5. Rinse thoroughly.

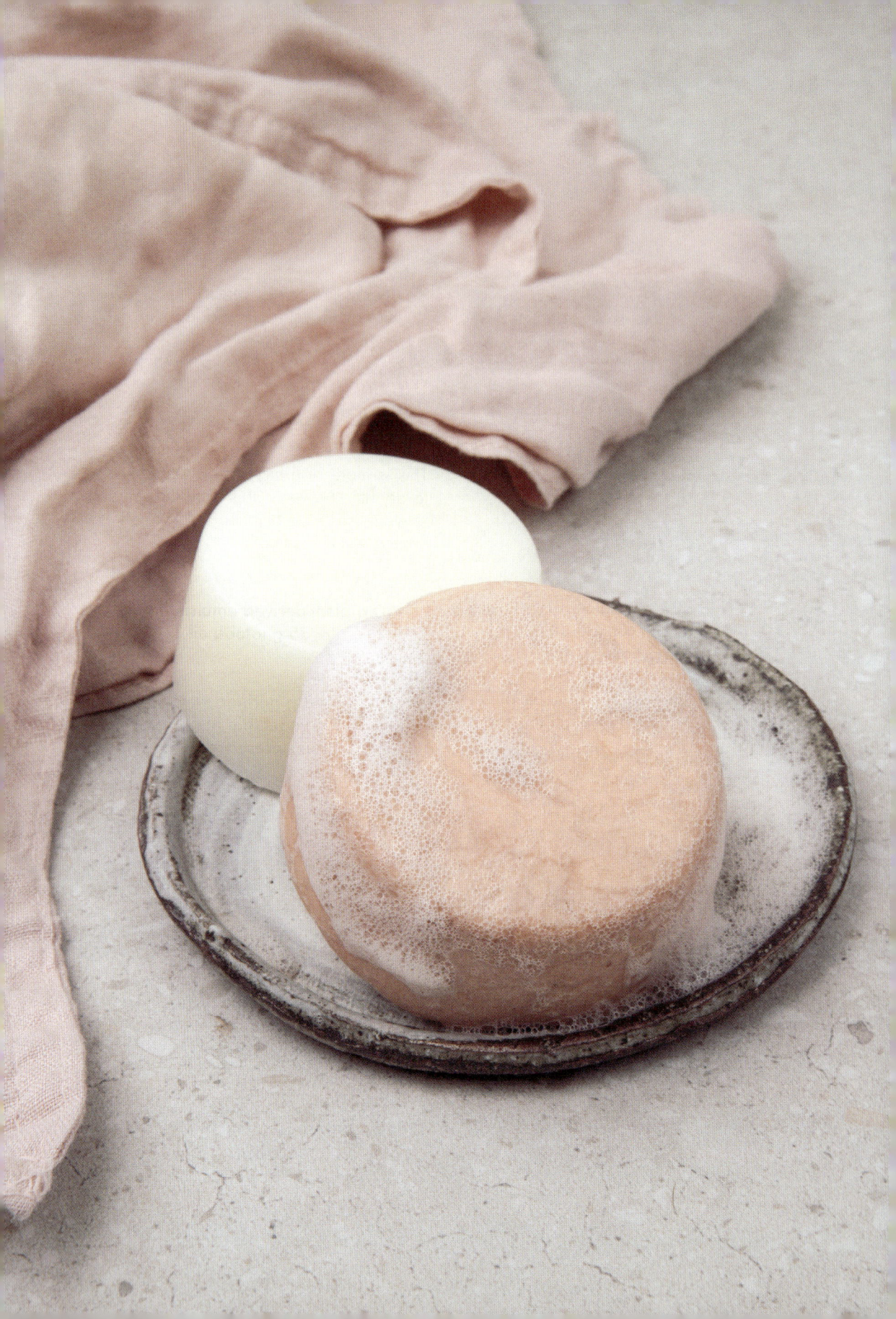

Conditioner Bars

Conditioner bars are a concentrated water-free alternative to liquid conditioners. They are long lasting and don't require packaging. Their size and absence of water makes them convenient for travel too.

A cationic conditioning agent is the main ingredient. It smooths the hair cuticle along the hair shaft via a positive charge. This recipe utilises behentrimonium methosulphate in combination with cetearyl alcohol. It is available as a solid wax and creates a hard conditioner bar. Behentrimonium methosulphate is a quaternary ammonium compound synthesised from canola oil. It is combined with cetearyl alcohol to further harden the bar and smooth the hair. In regard to the behentrimonium methosulphate & cetearyl alcohol used in the recipe in this book, BTMS 25 has been selected. This ingredient is made up of 25% behentrimonium methosulphate and 75% cetearyl alcohol.

Vegetable oils and butters are included to smooth, protect and add shine to the hair, while d-panthenol (pro-vitamin B5) moisturises the hair.

To use, wash your hair then smooth the conditioner bar down the length of your hair, concentrating on the ends. If you have long hair, use a wide-tooth comb to distribute throughout your hair and to remove any tangles. Rinse well. The following conditioner bar recipe is suitable for normal to dry hair.

Equipment

- digital scales
- measuring glass or beaker
- saucepan
- heat-resistant jug
- metal trivet
- stovetop or hot plate
- metal stirring spoon
- silicon mould

Ingredients

80 g BTMS 25
(behentrimonium methosulphate &
cetearyl alcohol)
9.5 g cocoa butter
5 g jojoba oil
3 g shea butter
0.5 g tocopherol
2 g d-panthenol
1g (approx. 20 drops) essential oil

Method for making a conditioner bar

1. Choose an essential oil or essential oil composition for your hair type from pages 251–252.
2. Weigh out the ingredients.
3. Melt all the ingredients except for the d-panthenol and essential oils together in a *bain-marie*.
4. Once they have fully melted, add the panthenol and stir well until fully incorporated.
5. Remove from the heat, add the essential oils and stir in well.
6. Pour the mixture into a silicon mould, such as a muffin mould.
7. Place in the refrigerator to solidify.
8. When the conditioner bar has set, carefully remove it from the mould.
9. Store it in a dry place in between hair washes.

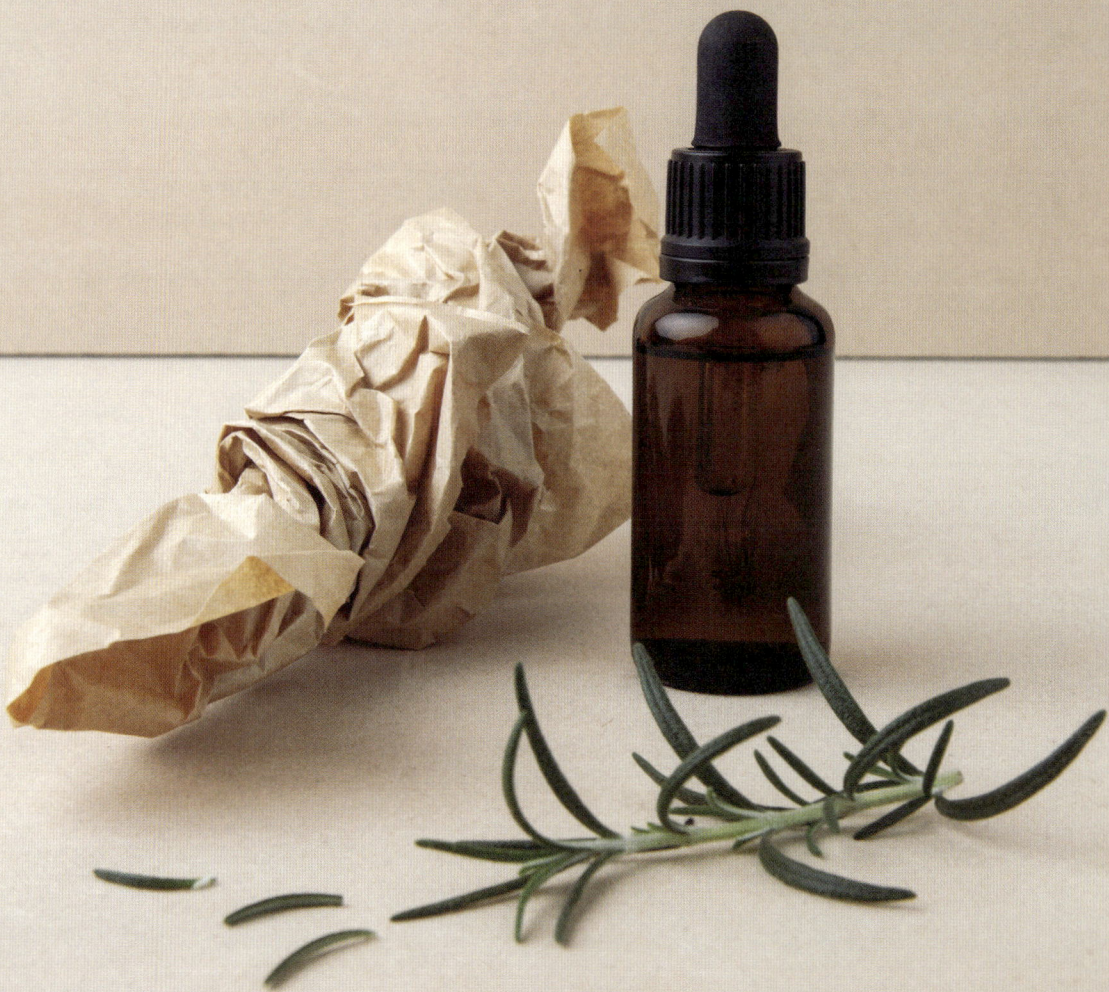

Hair and Scalp Treatments

Improve the health of your hair and scalp by choosing to use a treatment on a regular basis.

Hair and Scalp Treatment Oils

Treatment oils are particularly beneficial for treating dry and damaged hair, as well as scalp problems such as dandruff and dry, flaky scalp, inflamed and irritated scalp, psoriasis of the scalp and hair loss. They can also improve circulation in the scalp.

Dandruff treatment oil

An aromatherapy oil for relieving itchy scalp and dry flakes of dandruff.

50 mL jojoba oil
5 drops Atlas cedarwood essential oil
5 drops patchouli essential oil
5 drops rosemary essential oil

1. Add the drops of essential oils to the jojoba oil in a glass bottle and shake well.
2. Using an eyedropper, distribute just enough of the treatment oil over your scalp to cover it, and massage it in.
3. Leave on for at least half an hour before shampooing and conditioning.
4. Follow with a herbal vinegar rinse for dandruff or rinse with diluted apple cider vinegar. Add 1 tablespoon (20 mL) of vinegar to 500 mL warm water and pour over your scalp.

5. Use this treatment each time you wash your hair until the condition improves, then reduce it to once a week, then to once a fortnight.

Healthy hair growth treatment oil

Use this aromatherapy oil to encourage circulation to the hair follicle and to encourage hair growth.

50 mL jojoba oil
5 drops ginger essential oil
5 drops peppermint essential oil
5 drops rosemary essential oil

1. Add the drops of essential oils to the jojoba oil in a glass bottle and shake well.
2. Using an eyedropper, distribute just enough of the treatment oil over your scalp to cover it and massage it in.
3. Perform a gently stimulating massage on the scalp for a few minutes.
4. Leave on for at least half an hour before shampooing and conditioning.
5. Use this treatment once or twice a week.

Cradle cap treatment oil

Sweet almond oil, apricot kernel oil and evening primrose oil, either combined or applied individually, may be massaged into your baby's scalp to help soften the build-up of cradle cap. A drop of German chamomile essential oil may be added to 50 mL of the base oil to soothe the scalp. This can be stored in a bottle and a small quantity applied with an eyedropper and massaged into baby's scalp.

Following the massage, shampoo with a mild shampoo and gently lift the scales by massaging baby's scalp with a soft baby brush.

Heavy duty hair conditioning treatment oil

A rich treatment oil for dry, damaged hair.

50 mL coconut oil
10 drops essential oil

1. Choose an essential oil or the dry hair essential oil composition from pages 251–252.
2. Add the drops of essential oil to the coconut oil, mix well and store in a glass jar.
3. Using an eyedropper or the tips of your fingers, distribute the treatment oil over your scalp and massage it in. Then smooth more oil along the length of your hair. If your hair is dry and damaged on the ends only, use this treatment on the ends only.
4. Perform a gently stimulating massage on the scalp for a few minutes.
5. Leave on for at least half an hour before shampooing and conditioning.
6. Use this treatment once a week.

Fine hair conditioning treatment oil

A lighter treatment oil for normal to dry and fine hair.

30 mL jojoba oil
20 mL argan oil
20 drops essential oil

1. Choose an essential oil or essential oil composition for your hair from pages 251–252.

2. Add the drops of essential oil to the jojoba oil in a glass bottle and shake well.
3. Using an eyedropper, distribute the treatment oil over your scalp and massage it in. Then, smooth more oil along the length of your hair. If your hair is dry on the ends only or you have an oily scalp, use this treatment on the ends only.
4. Perform a gently stimulating massage on the scalp for a few minutes.
5. Leave on for at least half an hour before shampooing and conditioning.
6. Use this treatment once a week.

Hair Conditioning Treatments

We subject our hair to many damaging elements, which strip the hair of its natural oil and moisture, making it dry and brittle and prone to split ends.

Hair conditioning treatments lubricate and protect our hair, improving its shine and lustre. They replace or supplement the natural oil, which normally flows from the sebaceous glands of our scalp down the shaft of each hair, helping to smooth the cuticle scales of the hair shaft.

Henna conditioning treatment

This conditioning treatment utilises the hair conditioning properties of the herb *Cassia obovata*, which is commonly referred to as clear or neutral henna. This conditioning treatment can be used every 2–4 weeks.

100 g neutral/clear henna powder
500 mL boiling water
20 mL cold-pressed vegetable oil
(coconut, olive or jojoba oil)
1 egg yolk (optional)

If your hair is blonde, grey or has been bleached, to confirm the colour of your hair will not be affected, mix a small amount of the henna powder with hot water and apply to a discrete section of your hair, leave on for an hour before rinsing. Do this the day before you plan to use this conditioning treatment as sometimes the colour can continue to develop after removal.

1. To make the conditioning treatment, mix the neutral/clear henna powder, boiling water and cold-pressed oil together in a bowl.
2. Once the mixture has cooled a little, mix in the egg yolk.
3. Spread the treatment throughout your hair and wrap it in an old plastic bag or shower cap.
4. Leave on for at least half an hour.
5. Rinse thoroughly, shampoo and condition.

Lecithin conditioning treatment

An ultra-rich conditioning treatment for dry, damaged hair.

5 g liquid lecithin
25 g cold-pressed vegetable oil (coconut, olive or jojoba oil)
20 g cocoa butter
1 g (approx. 20 drops) essential oil

1. Choose an essential oil or the dry hair essential oil composition from pages 251–252.
2. Melt all ingredients together in a *bain-marie*.
3. Once melted, pour the mixture into a container and use it as required.
4. Spread the treatment throughout your hair.
5. Leave on for at least half an hour before shampooing and conditioning.

6. Apply shampoo to the hair first, then add water to lather and rinse.
7. Use this treatment once a week.

Head Lice Treatments

Head lice are small insects that live and breed in human hair and feed by sucking blood from the scalp. They are spread through direct head-to-head contact and sometimes by direct contact with items that have been in contact with the head, such as hats, brushes and pillowcases. Clean hair does not prevent their infestation. Their eggs (nits) hatch in 7 to 10 days and they can live for up to 35 days on the scalp.

Head lice oil

A concentrated aromatherapy blend that can be used to eliminate head lice.

15 drops tea tree essential oil
50 mL jojoba oil
or
5 drops eucalyptus essential oil
5 drops lavender essential oil
5 drops tea tree essential oil
50 mL jojoba oil

1. Add the drops of essential oil to the jojoba oil in a glass bottle and shake well.
2. Spread the treatment oil throughout the hair and comb through well.
3. Leave on for at least half an hour.
4. Then, section the hair and using a nit/head lice comb, comb the hair from the scalp through to the ends of the hair, working methodically to make sure you have combed through all of the hair.
5. Each time you run the comb through the hair, wipe it on a tissue or paper towel to ensure the head lice have been removed.

6. Shampoo and condition the hair.

7. Spray the hair with *Head lice spray* (recipe below).

8. Thoroughly scrub and clean the comb.

9. You may need to carry out this process every couple of days for 2 weeks to ensure all eggs and hatched lice have been removed entirely.

Head lice spray

10 drops tea tree essential oil
50 mL purified water
or
4 drops eucalyptus essential oil
4 drops lavender essential oil
4 drops tea tree essential oil
50 mL purified water

1. Add the drops of essential oil to the water in a spray bottle.

2. Shake the bottle each time before spraying through the hair.

3. Spray the hair each day as a preventative if there is an outbreak of head lice occurring.

Styling

Slick your hair back and keep it in place with a natural hair spray or give it volume and style with a natural hair gel. Keep in mind that these natural styling products will not have the same strong holding properties as commercial products.

Hair spray

A gentle hair spray for holding those stray hairs into place. This hair spray is not a strong hold hair styling spray, rather it holds hairs in place and reduces frizzy hair and fly-aways.

20 g sugar
80 g purified water

1. Dissolve the sugar into the water in a jug.
2. Pour into a spray bottle.
3. Lightly mist over your hair.
4. Store in the refrigerator and use within 2 or 3 days of making.

Hair gel

Slick your hair into place with this one. This natural gel contains no alcohol or synthetic polymers.

85 g purified water
4 g xanthan gum
12 g vegetable glycerin
1 g preservative
0.5 g (approx. 10 drops) essential oil

pH adjustment
qs citric acid + purified water

1. Choose an essential oil or essential oil composition for your hair from pages 251–252.
2. Make this hair gel by following the *Method for making gel bases* on page 67.
3. Add your choice of essential oils and mix thoroughly.
4. Store your hair gel in a suitable container in the refrigerator.

Curl and wave hair balm

This balm will help keep hair in place, add gloss, and is great for enhancing curls and waves and reducing frizz. The first recipe contains beeswax while the second recipe is vegan.

50 g castor oil
5 g coconut oil
20 g shea butter
10 g cocoa butter
15 g beeswax
1 g (approx. 20 drops) essential oil
or
50 g castor oil
5 g coconut oil
30 g shea butter
5 g cocoa butter
10 g candelilla wax
1 g (approx. 20 drops) essential oil

1. Choose an essential oil or essential oil composition for your hair from pages 251–252.
2. Melt the cocoa butter and beeswax or candelilla wax in a *bain-marie*.
3. Once they have fully melted, add the shea butter, coconut oil and castor oil.

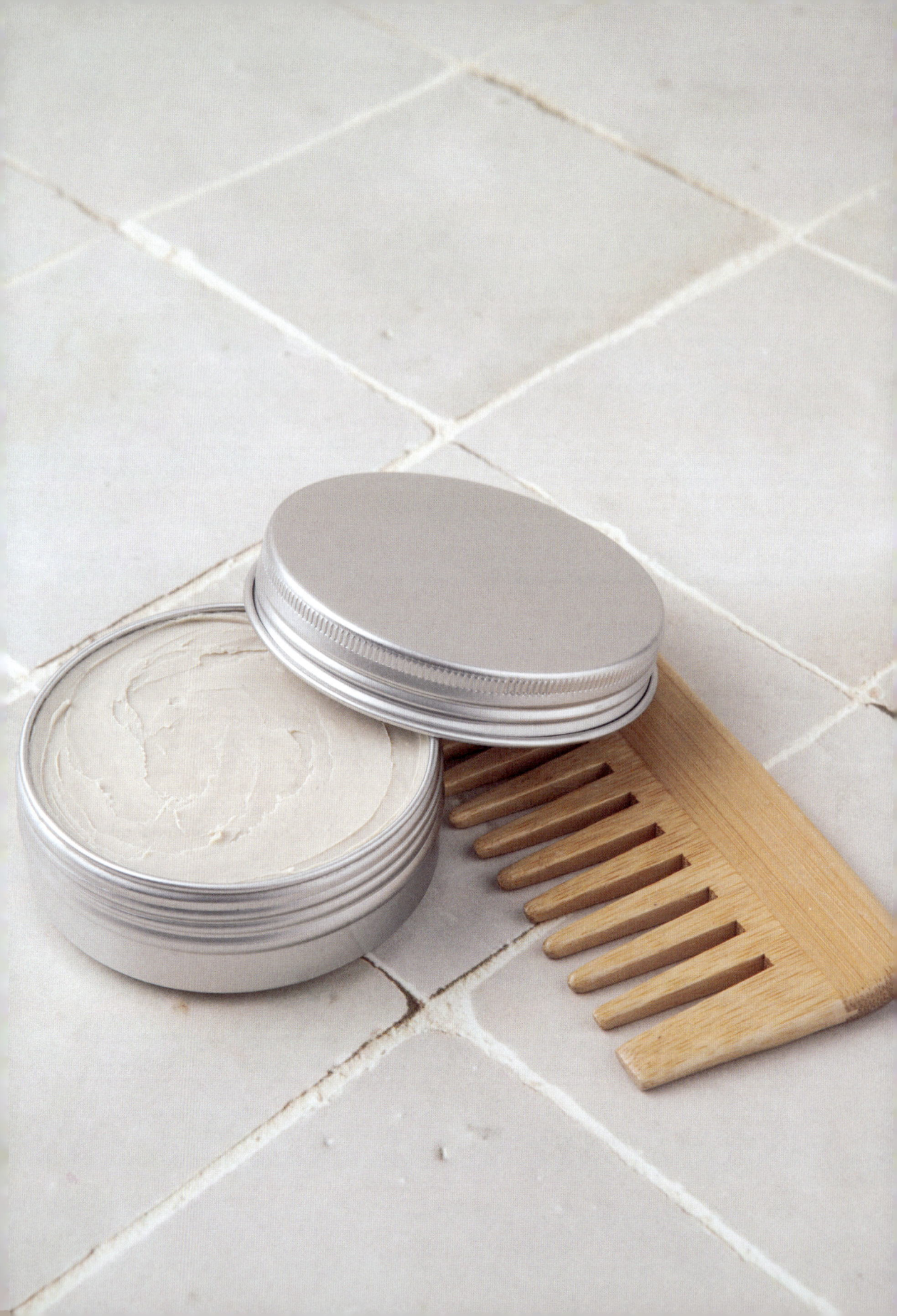

4. Ensure all ingredients have melted and remove from the heat.

5. Once the mixture cools a little, add the essential oils.

6. Pour into a clean jar to store.

7. Allow to cool to room temperature before adding lids. The jar of balm can be put in the freezer for 2 hours to speed up solidification time, but allow to come back to room temperature before adding lids.

8. Using a tiny amount on the tips of your fingers, spread the hair balm through your hair and style accordingly.

Glossy hair balm

A simple balm for adding gloss to thick, dry hair. The first recipe contains beeswax while the second recipe is vegan.

80 g cold-pressed vegetable oil (coconut, olive or jojoba oil)
10 g beeswax
10 g cocoa butter
1 g (approx. 20 drops) essential oil
or
85 g cold-pressed vegetable oil (coconut, olive or jojoba oil)
10 g cocoa butter
5 g candelilla wax
1 g (approx. 20 drops) essential oil

1. Choose an essential oil or essential oil composition for your hair from pages 251–252.

2. Heat the cocoa butter, beeswax or candelilla wax and vegetable oil in a *bain-marie* until the ingredients have all melted.

3. Once the mixture cools a little, add the essential oils.

4. Pour into a jar to store.

5. Allow to cool to room temperature before adding lids. The jar of balm can be put in the freezer for 2 hours to speed up solidification time, but allow to come back to room temperature before adding lids.

6. Using a tiny amount on the tips of your fingers, spread the hair balm over your hair. Then, using the palms of your hands, smooth it throughout your hair. You may choose to use it on dry ends only.

Clay hair styling balm

This balm will help texturise hair with a somewhat matte finish. The first recipe contains beeswax while the second recipe is vegan.

20 g castor oil
5 g coconut oil
15 g shea butter
5 g cocoa butter
15 g beeswax
40 g kaolin clay
1 g (approx. 20 drops) essential oil
or
20 g castor oil
5 g coconut oil
20 g shea butter
5 g cocoa butter
10 g candelilla wax
40 g kaolin clay
1 g (approx. 20 drops) essential oil

1. Choose an essential oil or essential oil composition for your hair from pages 251–252.

2. Melt the cocoa butter and beeswax or candelilla wax in a *bain-marie*.

3. Once they have fully melted, add the shea butter, coconut oil and castor oil.

4. Ensure all ingredients have melted and remove from the heat.

5. Once the mixture cools a little, add the essential oils.

6. Stir in the kaolin and continue stirring until the mixture is smooth.

7. Scoop into a jar to store.

8. Allow to cool to room temperature before adding lids. The jars of balm can be put in the freezer for 2 hours to speed up solidification time, but allow to come back to room temperature before adding lids.

9. Using a tiny amount on the tips of your fingers, spread the hair balm through your hair and style accordingly.

Hair smoothing serum

A lightweight serum to smooth your hair and help tame fly-aways. Rub a small amount between your palms and smooth over your hair.

Oil phase
10 g plant-derived emulsifying wax
25 g jojoba oil

Water phase
158 g purified water
5 g vegetable glycerin
2 g preservative

Add at 45°C
1 g (approx. 20 drops) essential oil

pH adjustment
qs citric acid + purified water

1. Choose an essential oil or essential oil composition for your hair from pages 251–252.

2. Make this serum by following the *Method for making an emulsion with emulsifying wax* on page 79.

Colours

You can enhance your own natural hair colour by using herbs or change it dramatically by using henna, a plant which is used traditionally as a hair dye.

Herbal Hair Colours

Herbal hair colours are generally subtle, require several and regular applications and encourage healthy, shiny hair.

Choose from the following list of herbs to enhance your natural hair colour:

- golden highlights — calendula petals, turmeric, rhubarb root
- fair highlights — chamomile flowers, lemon juice
- brown — espresso coffee, sage, strong black tea, walnut husks.

1. Make a strong decoction of your chosen herb or herbs and include 1 teaspoon of apple cider vinegar. Follow the *Method for making herbal decoctions* on page 51.
2. Simmer until the colour is strong.
3. Strain the herbs from the water.
4. Massage the warm decoction thoroughly throughout clean hair.
5. Cover your hair and leave it on for at least 1 hour.
6. Rinse with lukewarm water.

Henna

The use of henna and other herbs as hair colouring agents and conditioners has a long history. Henna is an excellent conditioner for the hair. It protects the ends from splitting and gives a glorious shine. It colours the hair, giving various colours and shades depending on the henna used and the original colour of your hair.

Henna was used extensively in ancient Egypt; Cleopatra and Nefertiti are reputed to have enhanced their beauty with it. Many women and men throughout the world continue to use it today, not only to dye their hair, but to colour their fingernails and to decorate their hands and bodies with intricate henna tattoos. Henna has also been shown to have antiseptic properties, hence its traditional use on the soles of the feet as a form of protection.

It is made from the pulverised leaves of the henna plant (*Lawsonia* species), which is widely distributed throughout the tropics. In 1709, botanist and traveller Dr Lawson isolated the active compound in henna, lawsone, which is responsible for both its colouring and conditioning properties.

Henna varies a great deal in its lawsone content and thus its quality. Hot regions of the world yield the best henna, which include countries such as Egypt, Iran, Pakistan and India. However, there are variations of quality produced within each of these countries. Poor quality henna is cheap and coarse, with little or no colouring ability due to the absence of lawsone. The consistency of poor quality henna, when mixed with water, is very gritty and not smooth. It is difficult to apply. Good quality henna, even though still messy to apply, mixes with water into a smooth mud consistency and is much easier to apply.

Pure henna ranges in colour from red to orange. Various herbs and spices are mixed with the pulverised henna powder to produce other colour variations. Indigo (*Indigo tinctoria*) and woad (*Isatis tinctoria*) are used to produce a darker or black henna. Clear henna or neutral henna is used as a conditioning treatment without colouring the hair, but may give grey or blonde hair a yellow tinge. It is not actually from the henna plant but from the herb *Cassia obovata*.

Considerations and precautions

- Because the colouring outcome is more difficult to predict with henna than synthetic colours, it is essential to do a strand test first to help gauge the final colour outcome. Mix approximately a teaspoon of the henna powder with a small amount of boiling water into a paste. Apply the henna to a small section of your hair, wrap in foil and, after the recommended period of time (1–4 hours), rinse your hair and check the colour. This will help you decide whether it is appropriate for you.

- The ultimate colour of your hair depends on your original hair colour and this will vary from person to person.

- With each application of henna, the colour becomes richer and deeper.

- On darker hair, henna will produce red highlights.

- On bleached hair, the red-based hennas will take very strongly and the colour will be very bright.

- Henna does not take as well to grey hair and several applications may be required

to build up initial depth of colour. As grey hair is lighter in colour, the red-based colours will initially tend to be lighter and brighter.

- The use of henna is not recommended if you intend to have your hair permed or use another hair colour in the near future. Henna does not allow the perming solution to penetrate the hair shaft properly.

- Henna may be used over coloured hair as long as it has been several months since the colour was applied. A strand test must be carried out to check the colour interaction.

- In general, henna is relatively permanent. It will fade gradually over time; however, it will never completely fade from the hair and will need to grow out or be cut off. Alternatively, another colour may be applied over the top.

Applying henna to the hair

To make your henna hair colour you will require the following.

Equipment

- rubber gloves
- ceramic, glass or metal bowl
- mixing spoon
- paper to cover the floor and table
- old towel
- old clothes to wear
- plastic grocery bag or designated shower cap
- hairdryer (optional)

Ingredients

- henna (100 g will cover shoulder-length hair)
- boiling water

- vinegar or lemon juice
- vegetable oil (optional)
- egg (optional)

Method for applying henna

1. Set aside several hours to apply henna to your hair and to allow the colour to develop. Read a good book, watch a good movie or two, or do the housework while you're waiting for the colour to develop.

2. Cover your table and the floor around you with newspaper (or better still, do it in the backyard), prepare your utensils, and put on your old clothes.

3. Apply vegetable oil to the skin around your hairline to prevent it staining.

4. Mix the henna powder with enough boiling water to give it the consistency of a cake batter. (Water may be replaced with wine, beetroot juice, tea or strong coffee to vary the shade of the henna. You can replace the water completely with these liquids, but the liquid should be hot). Add a good dash of apple cider vinegar or lemon juice to the mixture to create an acidic environment that will enhance colour development.

5. Mix an egg into the mixture (optional) so that it sticks to the hair better and gives it extra conditioning properties.

6. If your hair is particularly dry, add a tablespoon of cold-pressed vegetable oil to the mixture.

7. Apply the mixture with a tint brush or gloved fingers to clean dry hair. Apply to small sections at a time. Work from the underneath layers to the top layers, smoothing the henna mixture from the roots to the ends. Clip your hair up and release a layer of hair at a time until completed.

8. Make sure your hair is evenly coated. Leave the mixture on your hair to develop. Warmth assists colour development. Cover your hair with plastic (such as an old plastic grocery bag or a shower cap) to keep the mixture warm, and wrap in an old towel. If you're in a cold climate, a warm hairdryer on a low setting may be used to warm it up every so often.

9. Leave the henna on from 1 to 4 hours, depending on the depth of colour you desire.

10. Rinse the henna thoroughly from your hair. This could take a while if your hair is long. Then shampoo and condition.

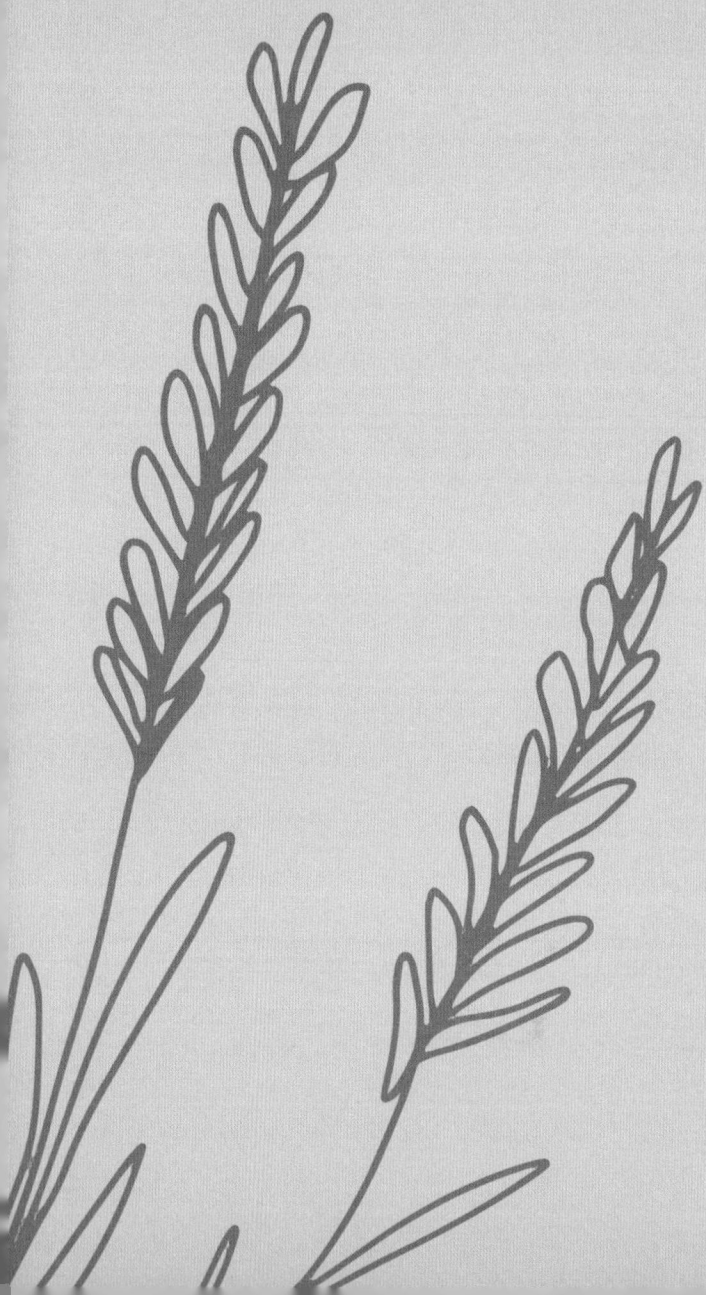

Home

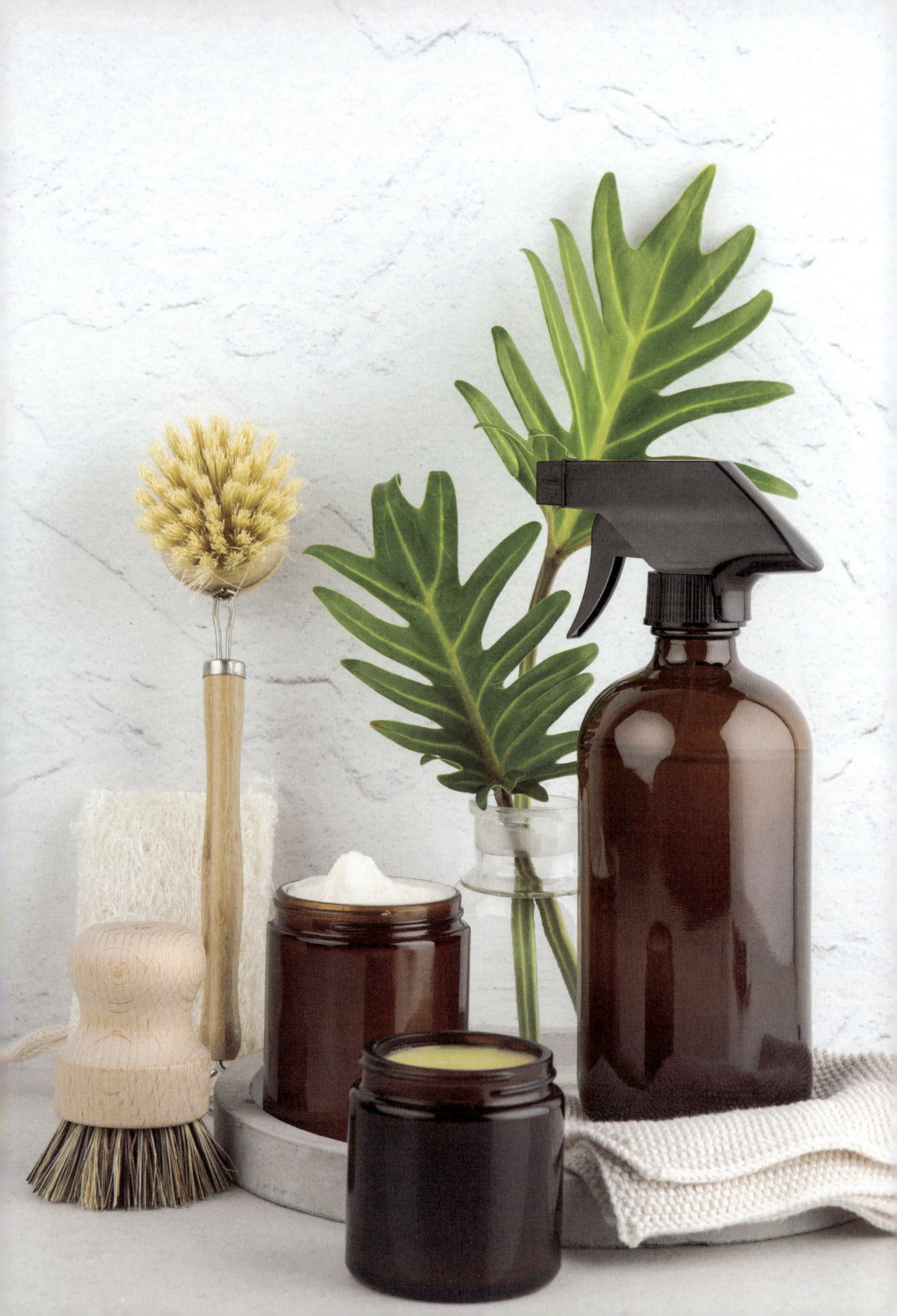

Cleaning your home naturally reduces waste and environmental pollution. It eliminates the use of allergenic and harmful ingredients and allows you to create cleaning products that are cost-effective.

Considerations and precautions

- Household surfaces vary, so test a little of the product in a discreet place first and check for scratches, discolouration or damage to the surface. Observe the surface for any changes that may occur over time.
- Do not use undiluted essential oils on paint, varnish or plastic surfaces as they will damage these surfaces.
- Follow safety precautions on all ingredients including essential oils, and keep out of reach of children.
- Always label your products with their purpose, ingredients and date made.

Basic Cleaning Ingredients

You will require a few basic ingredients to make your own household cleaning products:

Green cleaning essential oils: to disinfect, repel insects and create a fresh-smelling home.

- **Antibacterial** — bergamot, cinnamon bark, blue Mallee eucalyptus, lavender, lemon, lemongrass, lemon myrtle, lime, pine, rosemary, sage, tea tree
- **Antifungal** — lemon-scented eucalyptus, kunzea, lavender, lemon myrtle, tea tree
- **Anti-mould** — cinnamon bark, clove bud, lemon
- **Dissolve grease** — blue Mallee eucalyptus, grapefruit, lemon, lemongrass, lime, sweet orange
- **Insect repellent** — cajeput, Virginian cedarwood, citronella, blue Mallee eucalyptus, lemon-scented eucalyptus, peppermint eucalyptus, geranium, lemon myrtle, niaouli, peppermint, spike lavender, tea tree, lemon scented tea tree
- **Deodorising** — bergamot, blue Mallee eucalyptus, lemon-scented eucalyptus, lavender, lemon, lemongrass, lemon myrtle, peppermint, pine, lemon-scented tea tree

Sodium bicarbonate (bicarb soda): acts as a gentle non-scratching abrasive. It absorbs odours and acts as a mild disinfectant.

Sodium carbonate (washing soda): removes oil and grease, disinfects, softens water and removes stains. It may irritate the skin, so wear rubber gloves when handling it.

White vinegar: dissolves grease, deodorises and acts as a mild disinfectant. Great for cleaning glass and shiny surfaces. Do not use vinegar on anything made of stone, including marble, granite, travertine and terrazzo.

Castile liquid soap: makes an excellent cleaner.

Green Cleaners

Surface cleaning paste

Use this paste to clean sinks, basins, tiles, stovetops, benchtops and toilets.

245 g sodium bicarbonate
55 g Castile liquid soap
2 g (approx. 40 drops) essential oil

1. Choose a *Green cleaning* essential oil from page 279.
2. Mix the essential oil into the Castile liquid soap.
3. Stir this mixture into the sodium bicarbonate until you form a smooth paste.
4. Store in a wide-mouthed glass jar.
5. To use, rub the mixture over the surface with a damp cloth, then wipe off with a clean damp cloth.

Surface cleaning spray

Use this spray to clean sinks, basins, tiles, stovetops, benchtops and toilets. Not suitable for wooden surfaces.

460 g warm purified water
20 g sodium carbonate (washing soda)
20 g Castile liquid soap
2.5 g (approx. 50 drops) essential oil

1. Choose a *Green cleaning* essential oil from page 279.
2. In a glass jug, dissolve the sodium carbonate into the warm water.
3. In a separate glass jug, mix the essential oil into the Castile liquid soap.

4. Stir the dissolved sodium carbonate/warm water mix into the essential oil/Castile liquid soap mix.
5. Decant into a spray bottle.
6. To use, spray onto the surface you wish to clean and wipe over with a damp cloth.

Window, glass and mirror cleaning spray

160 g white vinegar
340 g purified water
1 g (approx. 20 drops) essential oil

1. Choose a *Green cleaning* essential oil from page 279.
2. Pour the white vinegar, water and essential oil into a spray bottle and shake well.
3. Spray onto a clean dry cloth and wipe over the glass surfaces you wish to clean.

Furniture polish

A beautifully aromatic polish to condition and add shine to your wooden furniture.

20 g beeswax
80 g jojoba oil or olive oil
1.5 g (approx. 30 drops) wood essential oil (such as Atlas cedarwood or hinoki wood)

1. Choose a wood essential oil.
2. Melt the beeswax and jojoba or olive oil in a heat-resistant jug in a *bain-marie*.

3. Once the beeswax has melted, remove the jug from the heat and add the essential oil before the mixture starts to set.

4. Pour into a wide-mouthed glass jar to store.

5. Allow to cool to room temperature before adding lids. The jar of furniture polish can be put in the freezer for 2 hours to speed up solidification time, but allow to come back to room temperature before adding lids.

6. Apply a small amount to a cloth, lightly smooth over your furniture and massage in.

Simple wooden furniture polish oil

100 mL olive oil or jojoba oil
20 drops wood essential oil
(such as Atlas cedarwood or hinoki wood)

1. Add the essential oil to the olive oil or jojoba oil in a glass bottle and shake well.

2. Using a slightly damp cloth, add a few drops of the furniture polish oil to the cloth and wipe over the furniture.

Cockroach deterrent surface spray

80 g perfume ethanol
20 g purified water
20 drops eucalyptus essential oil
16 drops lemon myrtle essential oil
16 drops peppermint essential oil
8 drops clove bud essential oil

1. Add the essential oils to the ethanol and stir well.

2. Slowly add and stir in the water.

3. Pour into a spray bottle.

4. Spray into cupboards inhabited by cockroaches and refresh as often as needed. Do not use on painted or varnished surfaces.

5. Peppermint essential oil can also be put onto cotton wool balls and placed in strategic positions to help repel cockroaches.

Home Fragrance

Scented Wardrobe

Add a few drops of your favourite essential oil to a strip of cotton or linen and tie in a bow to the neck of a coat hanger. Avoid direct contact with other fabric. This will scent your wardrobe and will gently infuse into your clothes.

Moth deterrent

As above, add a few drops of essential oil from the *Insect repellent* list under the *Green cleaning essential oils* on page 279 to a strip of cotton or linen and tie it to a coat hanger and hang it in your wardrobe. Refresh regularly.

Pot Pourri

Pot pourri is a simple and attractive way to fragrance a space. Dried flowers, herbs and spices can be mixed together in an attractive jar or bowl and sprinkled with essential oils. The following recipes will make a enough to fill a small bowl

Spice bowl pot pourri

2 tbsp star anise
1 tbsp cardamom pods
6 dried orange pieces
5 cinnamon sticks
1 tbsp clove buds
10 drops orange essential oil
4 drops cinnamon essential oil
2 drops clove essential oil

1. Add the drops of essential oil to the dried botanicals and stir in.
2. Display in a glass or ceramic bowl or jar and refresh the essential oils when necessary.

Flower petals pot pourri

1 tbsp lavender flowers
4 tbsp rose buds or petals
1 tbsp jasmine flowers
1 tbsp calendula flowers
10 drops lavender
6 drops geranium
4 drops ylang ylang

1. Add the drops of essential oil to the dried botanicals and stir in.
2. Display in a glass or ceramic bowl or jar and refresh the essential oils when necessary.

Herb garden pot pourri

2 tbsp crushed lemon myrtle leaves
2 tbsp crushed lemon verbena leaves
2 tbsp cut pieces of lemongrass
1 tbsp rosemary
12 drops lemon myrtle essential oil
4 drops rosemary essential oil

1. Add the drops of essential oil to the dried botanicals and stir in.
2. Display in a glass or ceramic bowl or jar and refresh the essential oils when necessary.

Room Sprays

Create a clean, fresh-smelling environment or a place of calm by making your own aromatherapy room spray. Choose one of the essential oil compositions for room sprays to add to a room spray base.

Simple aromatherapy room spray

100 mL purified water
40–60 drops essential oil

1. Choose an essential oil or an essential oil composition for room sprays from those below.
2. Add the water and essential oils to a spray bottle and shake each time before you spray. Avoid spraying directly on fabrics.

Aromatherapy room spray

This room spray recipe ensures the essential oils are properly dispersed throughout the mixture without the need for shaking each time it is used. The use of perfume alcohol also allows for the mist to dry quickly if it lands on any surfaces.

80 mL perfume ethanol
20 mL purified water
40–60 drops essential oil

1. Choose an essential oil or an essential oil composition for room sprays from those below.
2. Add the essential oils to the perfume ethanol and stir well.
3. Slowly add and stir in the water.
4. Pour into a spray bottle and mist around the room. Avoid spraying directly on fabrics.

You may like to choose one of these essential oil compositions to add to your room spray base. The quantities specified here are to be added to each 100 g or mL of base.

Essential oil compositions for room sprays

Garden fresh composition
Perfect for freshening up the kitchen
20 drops lemon myrtle
20 drops sweet orange
6 drops rosemary
2 drops sage

Insect repellent composition
Helps clear the room of flies and mosquitoes
30 drops citronella
20 drops lavender
5 drops blue Mallee eucalyptus
5 drops peppermint

Tranquil space composition
Creates a space of tranquillity
18 drops sandalwood
15 drops petitgrain
8 drops geranium

Evening rest composition
Turn off for the day
24 drops lavender
14 drops geranium
3 drops sweet marjoram

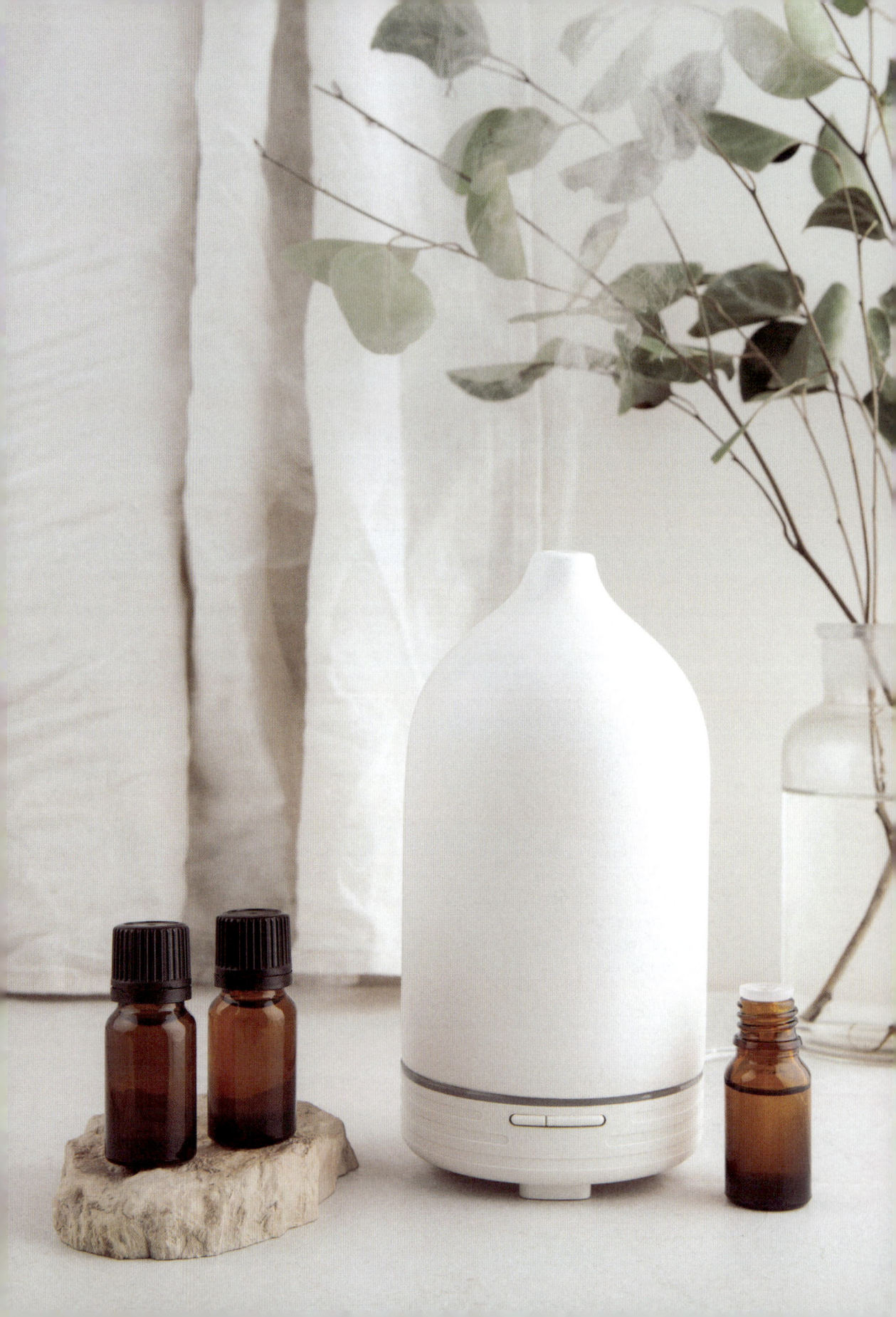

Aromatherapy Diffuser Blends

Create an atmosphere of calm positivity, or purify the air. Choose one of these essential oil compositions to add to your aromatherapy diffuser or oil burner.

Essential oil compositions for aromatherapy diffusers

Peaceful composition
3 drops mandarin
1 drop geranium
1 drop Roman chamomile

Serene composition
3 drops ylang ylang
1 drop clary sage
1 drop vetiver

Restful composition
4 drops bergamot
2 drops geranium
1 drop clary sage

Sleep well composition
4 drops sweet orange
3 drops lavender
1 drop sweet marjoram

Elevate composition
3 drops lemon
1 drop geranium
1 drop juniper

Refreshed spirit composition
2 drops grapefruit
1 drop geranium
1 drop patchouli
1 drop petitgrain

Awaken composition
3 drops lemongrass
2 drops pine
1 drop Atlas cedarwood

Vitality composition
5 drops lemon
3 drops juniper
2 drops peppermint
1 drop cypress

Heartfelt composition
2 drops geranium
2 drops jasmine absolute
1 drop ylang ylang

Purify composition
3 drops manuka
2 drops lavender
2 drops tea tree

Insect away composition
5 drops citronella
4 drops lavender
2 drops blue Mallee eucalyptus
2 drops peppermint

Breathe deeply composition
2 drops blue Mallee eucalyptus
2 drops peppermint
2 drops pine

Useful Information

Guide to Herbs and Essential Oils for Skin Care

Skin Type or Condition	Essential Oils	Herbs
All skin types	Roman chamomile, jasmine, lavender, neroli, rose	Aloe vera, calendula, chamomile, comfrey, lavender, soapwort
Oily	Bergamot, Atlas cedarwood, clary sage, cypress, geranium, grapefruit, juniper, lemon, lime, mandarin, sweet orange, petitgrain, tangerine, ylang ylang	Aloe vera, lavender, witch hazel, yarrow
Combination	Geranium, lavender, palmarosa, ylang ylang	Aloe vera, elderflowers
Dry	Neroli, palmarosa, rose, sandalwood, ylang ylang	Aloe vera, comfrey, marshmallow root, rose, slippery elm
Mature	Carrot seed, cistus, everlasting, frankincense, jasmine, lavender, myrrh, patchouli, rose, sandalwood, blue tansy, vetiver	Ginseng, gotu kola, green tea, rose
Dehydrated	Palmarosa, rose, sandalwood	Aloe vera, comfrey, marshmallow root, rose, slippery elm
Sensitive	German chamomile, everlasting, jasmine, lavender, neroli, rose otto, sandalwood, blue tansy, yarrow	Aloe vera, calendula, chamomile, comfrey, gotu kola, green tea, liquorice, marshmallow root, soapwort
Devitalised	Grapefruit, lemon, peppermint, rosemary, vetiver	Lemongrass, nettle, rosemary

Skin Type or Condition	Essential Oils	Herbs
Acne	Bergamot, Atlas cedarwood, chamomile (German and Roman), cistus, clary sage, cypress, eucalyptus, everlasting, fragonia, geranium, grapefruit, juniper, lavender, lemon, lime, mandarin, manuka, may chang, myrrh, palmarosa, patchouli, petitgrain, pine, rosalina, sage, sandalwood, tangerine, blue tansy, tea tree, thyme, yarrow	Aloe vera, calendula, comfrey leaves, gotu kola, lemon balm, lemongrass, sage, thyme, yarrow
Boils	Myrrh, tea tree, thyme	Fenugreek, marshmallow root, myrrh, slippery elm
Broken capillaries	Carrot seed, German chamomile, cypress, geranium, lemon, neroli, rose otto	Gotu kola
Bruises	Black pepper, lavender, spike lavender	Arnica, comfrey, hypericum, witch hazel
Burns	German chamomile, everlasting, lavender	Aloe vera, calendula, chamomile
Herpes simplex (cold sores)	Bergamot, cistus, melissa, myrrh, palmarosa, tea tree, thyme	Lemon balm, myrrh
Cracked skin	Myrrh, patchouli, sandalwood	Aloe vera, calendula, comfrey, marshmallow root
Dermatitis/ eczema	Carrot seed, German chamomile, cistus, everlasting, kunzea, lavender, myrrh, palmarosa, patchouli, sandalwood, blue tansy, yarrow	Aloe vera, calendula, chamomile, chickweed, comfrey, liquorice root, marshmallow root
Tinea	Myrrh, tea tree, thyme	Calendula, myrrh
Pruritis, urticaria (itching, rashes)	German chamomile, lavender, peppermint, tea tree	Aloe vera, calendula, chamomile, chickweed, lavender, liquorice root, marshmallow root, peppermint

Skin Type or Condition	Essential Oils	Herbs
Psoriasis	Bergamot, carrot seed, German chamomile, everlasting, juniper, lavender, sandalwood, blue tansy, yarrow	Aloe vera, calendula, chamomile, chickweed, comfrey, liquorice root, marshmallow root
Scarring	German chamomile, everlasting, frankincense, lavender, myrrh, patchouli	Aloe vera, calendula, comfrey, gotu kola
Verruca (warts)	Cinnamon bark and leaf, lemon, tea tree, thyme	Thuja
Wounds, cuts, sores	Bergamot, chamomile (German and Roman), everlasting, frankincense, geranium, lavender, manuka, myrrh, palmarosa, patchouli, rose, sage, sandalwood, blue tansy, tea tree, thyme, yarrow, vetiver	Aloe vera, calendula, comfrey, fenugreek, myrrh, thyme, yarrow
Mosquito bites	Lavender, peppermint, tea tree	Aloe vera, calendula, chamomile, peppermint

Skin Uses	Essential Oils	Herbs
Insect repellent	Atlas cedarwood, Virginian cedarwood, citronella, eucalyptus, geranium, lavender, lemongrass, peppermint, pine, rosemary, spike lavender, tea tree	Lavender, pennyroyal
Deodorant	Bergamot, clary sage, cypress, eucalyptus, frankincense, geranium, juniper, lavender, patchouli, petitgrain, pine, sandalwood, tea tree, ylang ylang	Lemon balm, lemongrass, peppermint, rosemary, sage, thyme

Guide to Herbs and Essential Oils for Hair Care

Hair Type or Scalp Condition	Essential Oils	Herbs
All hair types	Roman chamomile, geranium, lavender, rosemary, ylang ylang	Henna, horsetail, lavender, rosemary, sage
Dry scalp and hair	Sandalwood	Aloe vera, chamomile, comfrey, marshmallow root, soapwort
Oily scalp and hair	Bergamot, Atlas cedarwood, Virginian cedarwood, clary sage, cypress, geranium, grapefruit, juniper, lemon, lime, patchouli, petitgrain	Nettle, peppermint, thyme, yarrow
Baby and fine hair	Chamomile (German and Roman), lavender	Calendula, chamomile, lavender
Dandruff	Atlas cedarwood, Virginian cedarwood, clary sage, spike lavender, patchouli, peppermint, rosalina, rosemary, sage, tea tree, thyme	Lavender, nettle, parsley, peppermint, rosemary, sage, thyme
Inflamed, irritated scalps (eczema and psoriasis)	German chamomile, lavender, patchouli, sandalwood	Calendula, chamomile, comfrey, lavender, liquorice root, marshmallow root, soapwort
Hair loss	Ginger, peppermint, pine, rosemary	Bay, ginger, nettle, peppermint, rosemary
Lice	Cinnamon leaf, geranium, tea tree, thyme	

Ingredient Suppliers

Ingredients can be found easily, either locally
or online and in:

- your garden
- farmers markets
- green grocers
- bulk food stores
- health food stores
- supermarkets
- pharmacies
- aromatherapy shops and suppliers
- herb shops and suppliers
- cosmetic ingredient suppliers
- soap ingredient suppliers.

Guide to Green Terms

Animal testing

The cruel tests to which animals are exposed and the reality of their life in testing laboratories in the name of beauty are abhorred by many seeking a healthier life for themselves and the planet. Increasingly, cruelty-free skin care and cosmetics, which mean a final product and its ingredients have not been tested on animals, are conscientiously sought after.

While cosmetic testing bans in the European Union, India, South Korea, New Zealand, Australia and several US states are an important step to ending the practice of product testing on animals once and for all, certain legislative loopholes still exist. For this reason, cruelty-free certification programs continue to operate, including the following.

Cruelty Free International is a US-based organisation that certifies products that have not been tested on animals and do not contain ingredients tested on animals, under its Leaping Bunny program.
For more information, visit:
https://www.crueltyfreeinternational.org/

PETA is a US-based organisation that certifies products that have not been tested on animals and do not contain ingredients tested on animals, under its Beauty Without Bunnies program.
For more information, visit:
https://www.peta.org/

Choose Cruelty Free is an Australian organisation that certifies products that have not been tested on animals and do not contain ingredients tested on animals. It has recently teamed up with Cruelty Free International.
For more information, visit:
https://choosecrueltyfree.org.au

Certified Organic and Natural

The ultimate objectives of organic certification are to safeguard the welfare of the environment and people and to ensure clear and transparent information is available so that sustainable choices can be made.

Organic practices aim to work with the environment towards a better future. Focusing on organic, sustainable farming practices, soil health, land regeneration and biodiversity protection, organic farmers take into consideration any potential impact on native flora or fauna on their land. The Australian Certified Organic Standard prohibits the use of synthetic agricultural chemicals including pesticides, fungicides and herbicides; therefore, organic farmers who certify to this standard adhere to these strict rules and help to protect local eco-systems.

In Australia, the term 'organic' is not regulated as it is in the United States, Japan and China. This means that, in Australia, a product can be called 'organic' without providing the consumer with any proof that it is actually organic. Unfortunately, the term 'organic' can be used on a product anywhere, anytime without any legal consequences.

On the other hand, formal organic certification of products is the producer's guarantee to you that along the entire supply chain, a Certified Organic product has been produced in line with the strict national and industry Organic and Biodynamic Standards.

If a product claims to be Certified Organic, and a consumer questions its validity, the vendor must by law (Australian Competition and Consumer Act) be able to show the certificate of registration that confirms the product's integrity or provide their certification number. The processor's certification number can be entered on the certifier's website for verification.

For a product to be labelled Certified Organic, it must go through a rigorous certification process at every part of the supply chain to ensure it meets organic standard requirements — from the farm and the sourcing of the ingredients, to manufacturing and processing, all the way through to the final product sold to consumers.

Every Certified Organic farm, food manufacturer, processor, wholesaler and retailer that handles or modifies the product in any way must comply and agree to a thorough inspection at least once a year (as well as spot checks from time to time). They must have robust systems in place and paperwork to prove that standards are being met.

Once organic farms and companies are certified and pass initial compliance, they are issued with a certificate. The awarded status can be 'Organic' or 'In Conversion' (which indicates they are in the process of converting to organic), and includes a list of land, products, ingredients or processes that have been certified. This certificate acts like a passport to prove the organic status of their

goods. After having their labels approved by the certification body, they are permitted to use the certification bodies' logo (like the ACO bud logo) with their own certification number.

There are six reputable Australian organic logos, and many others from around the world. The six certifying bodies in Australia are ACO (Australian Certified Organic), NCO (NASAA Certified Organic), OFC (Organic Food Chain), BDRI (Bio-Dynamic Research Institute), AUS-QUAL and SXC (Southern Cross Certified Australia). The USA and EU have achieved some consistency in their markets — so you may also see the USDA or EU organic logos, especially on imported products.

In Australia, the most recognised and most trusted organic logo is the ACO bud logo. If you're ever unsure if a product is certified, or if there is a logo you don't recognise, always be sure to check with the retailer or manufacturer.

The key international certified organic standard for cosmetics is the COSMOS-standard. The founding members include the Soil Association (UK), Ecocert and Cosmebio (France), BDIH (Germany) and ICEA (Italy). Australian Certified Organic manages the COSMOS-standard in Australia, including auditing.

Certified organic cosmetics are designed to preserve the essential characteristics and benefits of ingredients and to minimise environmental impacts.

The COSMOS-standard is guided by four core principles:

- promoting the use of products from organic agriculture, and respecting biodiversity

- using natural resources responsibly, and respecting the environment
- using processing and manufacturing that are clean and respectful of human health and the environment
- integrating and developing the concept of 'Green Chemistry'.

All ingredients used in certified organic beauty and skin care products are natural and effective and not tested on animals. They are free from synthetic colouring agents, fragrances, ethoxylated ingredients, parabens, phthalates, silicones, paraffin, nano-particles or petroleum. GMOs (genetically modified organisms) are not permitted.

COSMOS Natural certification is applied to products that comply with the COSMOS-standard in all respects but do not meet the required minimum organic percentages as specified in the COSMOS-standard. COSMOS Natural products do not have to contain any organic ingredients — although in practice many do. All ingredients, whether certified organic or not, must be approved by COSMOS.

Certified COSMOS Natural products contain 95–100% ingredients of natural origin (water is counted as natural).

Certified COSMOS Organic products contain 95–100% ingredients of natural origin. 95–100% of the plant-based ingredients must be from certified organic farming, and the portion of ingredients from organic farming must represent 20–100% of the total product, with the exception of wash-off products, which is 10–100%.

COSMOS Natural is most suitable for products containing a lot of ingredients that cannot be organically grown, such as water

(body sprays), salt (bath salts) or clay (face masks).

The benefits of COSMOS Organic or COSMOS Natural products include higher levels of antioxidants, sustainably sourced ingredients, biodegradable ingredients, minimal packaging, transparency in manufacturing processes, and protection of wildlife and biodiversity.

COSMOS standards have a holistic approach encompassing and going beyond singular claims such as clean beauty, green chemistry, zero waste and not tested on animals.

The full COSMOS Organic and Natural Standard can be read here: https://www.cosmos-standard.org

For further information on organic certification in Australia, visit: https://www.budorganic.com.au/what-are-organic-standards/

Clean beauty and 'free from' claims

The term 'clean beauty' is not regulated nor does it have a set of standards, with each business defining its own set of standards depending on what it leaves in or out of its products. Largely, clean beauty is concerned with a 'free from' list of ingredients that are deemed potentially harmful to health and wellbeing.

The following example reveals how it is often little more than a marketing tool. One company may list 'free from' the preservative phenoxyethanol, while another company that uses this ingredient will leave it off their free from list.

Fairtrade

The FAIRTRADE Mark was established specifically to support the most disadvantaged producers in developing countries by using trade as a tool for sustainable development. Farmers and producers in developing countries often have little infrastructural support, social security systems or other safety nets if they cannot get a fair price for their products.

The Fairtrade scheme ensures producers have an equal say in how it is run and are included in all decision-making.

For farmers and workers, Fairtrade means:

- prices that aim to cover the average costs of producing their crop sustainably — a vital safety net when market prices drop
- the Fairtrade Premium — an extra sum of money paid on top of the selling price to invest in business or community projects of their choice
- decent working conditions and a ban on discrimination, forced labour and child labour
- access to advance credit ahead of harvest time
- being able to plan more for the future, with more security and stronger relationships with buyers.

For further information on Fairtrade, visit: https://www.fairtrade.net/

Green chemistry

The principles of green chemistry in the production of cosmetic ingredients and products aim to reduce environmental harm and eliminate hazards to human health and wellbeing while producing safe and effective products.

Green chemistry applies across the life cycle of a chemical product, including its design, manufacture, use and ultimate disposal. Green chemistry is also known as sustainable chemistry.

The Twelve Principles of Green Chemistry, originally published by Paul Anastas and John Warner in *Green Chemistry: Theory and Practice* (Oxford University Press, New York, 1998) include:

1. prevention of waste, rather than cleaning it up
2. maximise atom economy
3. design less hazardous chemical syntheses for workers and the environment
4. design safer chemicals and products for end use applications
5. use safer solvents or eliminate them entirely
6. increase energy efficiency
7. use renewable feedstocks
8. avoid chemical derivatives in the reaction process
9. use catalysts rather than stoichiometric reagents
10. design products to biodegrade after use
11. analyse reactions in real time to prevent polluting by-products
12. minimise the potential for accidents.

Production of key cosmetic ingredients, such as polymers and surfactants, involves chemical processing. There are a number of manufacturers that produce these ingredients based on green chemistry principles.

Palm free

Going palm free is one recommendation being made in an effort to reduce the environmental degradation and human rights issues surrounding the production and consumption of palm oil.

Palm oil is extracted from the flesh of the fruit of *Elaeis guineensis*, while palm kernel oil is extracted from its kernel. Palm yields higher amounts of oil than any other oil crop and can do so for up to 30 years. It grows easily in the tropics, is highly profitable for farmers and is the cheapest vegetable oil available.

Palm oil and its derivatives are used in food, cleaning products, cosmetics, hair care, personal care items, soaps and candles. With petrochemicals and animal fats previously used to make these products, palm oil was seen as a more ethical and environmentally friendly choice.

Another palm product is palm kernel cake used as feed for livestock including cattle and poultry. However, the manufacture of biofuel uses the most palm oil. Due to the versatility and a growing human population, demand for palm oil continues to rise.

Indonesia and Malaysia are the largest producers of palm oil in the world, with large areas of tropical forests and other ecosystems continually being cleared to make room for more oil palm plantations. Aside from the benefits palm oil has brought to producers and consumers, it has affected local communities, destroyed natural habitats for endangered species, including orangutans, elephants and tigers, and become a critical factor in climate change.

In 2004, the Roundtable on Sustainable Palm Oil (RSPO) was established with the objective of promoting the growth and use of sustainable palm oil products through global standards and multi-stakeholder governance.

The RSPO developed a set of environmental and social criteria that companies must comply with in order to produce Certified Sustainable Palm Oil. When properly applied, these criteria can help to minimise the negative impact of palm oil cultivation on the environment and communities in palm oil producing regions.

Many companies in the West purchase Certified Sustainable Palm Oil; however, demand for and willingness to pay a premium for it throughout the world is limited. Furthermore, the RSPO has been criticised by various environmental NGOs and studies that show adherence to the scheme shows no difference in environmental, social and economic sustainability than non-certified plantations. Issues include the ongoing impact on the orangutan population, destruction of tropical forests and tracts of peat swamp forest in Malaysia, and the clearing of pristine forests in Indonesia when there are large areas of grassland available. Labourers have also protested against abuses on RSPO certified plantations.

However, simply replacing palm oil with other crops that yield less oil and require more land would be moving the environmental impact elsewhere.

Other places that produce palm oil include South America and Africa. While circumstances vary from country to country, there are concerns similar problems that are being faced in Malaysia and Indonesia are now occurring in these places.

The issues surrounding palm oil are challenging. As with the production of all commodities, a wholistic approach is required, with better agricultural and environmental planning from government ministries and social pressure for sustainable production along with a reduction in consumption.

For further information on palm oil visit:

Orangutan Alliance — certified palm oil free https://orangutanalliance.org

Roundtable on Sustainable Palm Oil https://rspo.org/

https://theconversation.com/how-palm-oil-became-the-worlds-most-hated-most-used-fat-source-161165

https://www.theguardian.com/news/2019/feb/19/palm-oil-ingredient-biscuits-shampoo-environmental

Veganism

Veganism, which excludes the consumption and use of animal products, has been a way of life for many people throughout the ages, whether for religious, spiritual, philosophical or health reasons.

The first official vegan organisation to be established was The Vegan Society in 1944 in the United Kingdom. According to The Vegan Society:

> Veganism is a philosophy and way of living which seeks to exclude — as far as is possible and practicable — all forms of exploitation of, and cruelty to, animals for food, clothing or any other purpose; and by extension, promotes the development and use of animal-free alternatives for the benefit of animals, humans and the environment. In dietary terms it denotes the practice of dispensing with all products derived wholly or partly from animals.

Since that time, vegan organisations have been established across the globe, educating and providing information on leading a vegan lifestyle and advocating on behalf of animal rights.

They have established certifications and logos to assist consumers in purchasing products that are vegan. The certification procedure differs from one organisation to another, where some certifications are granted on simple declaration whereas others carry out in-depth controls and audits in the field. Boundaries of what is acceptable may vary according to their politics and history.

For further information on veganism and vegan certification visit:

Expertise Vegan Europe (EVE Vegan) created by Vegan France — Europe https://www.certification-vegan.org/

Sello Vegano certification by Vegetarianos Hoy — Latin America https://www.certificacionvegana.org/

The Vegan Society — UK https://www.vegansociety.com/

Vegan Belarus certification by the Vegan community of Belarus https://vegan.by/

VEGANOK — Italy https://www.veganok.com/

Certified Vegan by Vegan Action — US https://vegan.org/

Vegan Australia certification by Vegan Australia https://www.veganaustralia.org.au/

Certified Vegan NZVS certification by NZ Vegetarian Society http://www.vegetarian.org.nz/

Zero waste

Zero waste goes beyond recycling with a vision to move from a linear economy to a circular economy. Zero waste principles aim to conserve resources and prevent waste through responsible production, consumption, re-use and recovery of all products, packaging and materials, without burning them, and without discharges to land, water or air that threaten the environment or human health. It encompasses the actions of reducing and re-using with least reliance on current methods of disposing then recycling.

The role of design is to ensure long-lasting, easily maintainable and repairable products. Every 'waste' output of one process is considered and becomes an input for another, such that the utility of the material is maximised.

Plastic is of particular concern as it is less easily recycled. Unlike glass and metal, which can be melted down and recycled indefinitely, plastic's molecular stability downgrades over time. It can only be recycled 2 or 3 times before it's unusable. After that, it becomes rubbish and will break down into microplastics.

For further information on zero waste, visit: https://zerowasteeurope.eu/about/principles-zw-europe/

Glossary

Absorption and adsorption

Absorption refers to molecules being taken into a substance, whereas adsorption refers to molecules adhering to the surface of a substance.

Acid mantle

The thin, slightly acidic layer of sebum and other secretions present on the surface of the skin having mild antimicrobial properties.

AHAs and BHAs

AHAs (alpha hydroxy acids) and BHAs (beta hydroxy acids) are acids that are used as exfoliants. AHAs are derived from fruit and sugar cane and can also assist with skin moisturisation. Commonly used AHAs include lactic acid, glycolic acid, malic acid, tartaric acid and citric acid. BHAs, such as salicylic acid, which is exfoliating only, can be found in willow bark extract.

Allergy · irritation · sensitisation

An adverse reaction to an ingredient or skin care product may result in itching, stinging, redness, burning and swelling, or may involve an allergic reaction with an intense immune response.

Irritation is normally less severe and shorter in duration and is confined to the area where a product is applied. Irritation may occur immediately or may suddenly occur after repeated use, in combination with other products or with change in climate.

Allergic reactions, which can require immediate medical care, last for days and spread beyond the area of product application. Reactions may be immediate or delayed.

Skin irritation, once gone, may allow for the re-introduction of the ingredient or skin care product to the skin in some way. However, a person who is allergic to an ingredient or skin care product may never use it again without eliciting a reaction.

Ingredients such as fragrances, preservatives and some chemical sunscreens are known to cause adverse skin reactions.

Anti-inflammatory

Reduces inflammation (redness, swelling and pain).

Antioxidant

Antioxidants slow down, prevent or block the damaging effects of free radical activity. The skin has its own antioxidant defence system to protect it from free radical damage; however, when free radical activity is greater than the skin's capacity to deal with it, cellular damage occurs. This protective capacity also diminishes with age. Damaged skin cells manifest as aging skin with wrinkles, dry and dull skin, dark circles under the eyes, decreased elasticity and hyperpigmentation.

The addition of antioxidants to skin care products supplements the skin's own antioxidant defence system. Antioxidants assist the skin in dealing with free radical activity produced by sunlight (UV and infrared rays), air pollution (vehicle exhaust fumes and industrial pollution) and other environmental factors.

Natural antioxidant ingredients include green tea, Kakadu plum, beta-carotene and tocopherols (vitamin E).

The addition of antioxidants such as mixed tocopherols and rosemary oleoresin to skin care products also improves stability and reduces the rancidity of ingredients such as vegetable oils.

Antiseptic · antibacterial · antifungal · disinfectant

Antiseptics, disinfectants and antibacterials are all antimicrobial substances.

Antiseptics work by preventing or inhibiting the growth of bacteria, fungi and viruses on the skin.

Disinfectants, on the other hand, are stronger than antiseptics and kill bacteria, fungi and viruses. They are used on hard surfaces such as countertops and door handles.

Antibacterial substances are also used on the skin, but are only effective against bacteria.

Astringent

An ingredient or product that causes the contraction of skin and body tissues.

Bain-marie

Bain-marie is a French term for a double boiler or a water bath. It is used to heat ingredients gently and reduce the risk of over-heating or burning the ingredients. A simple *bain-marie* used to make the recipes in this book consists of a saucepan and heat-resistant glass jug. The saucepan is first filled to about halfway with water, then a metal trivet is placed on the bottom of the saucepan. The glass jug is then sat on the trivet in the saucepan. The saucepan is then heated on a hot plate.

Deodorant · antiperspirant

Deodorants mask the odour produced by the action of our bacteria on perspiration, whereas antiperspirants inhibit or prevent perspiration by blocking sweat glands.

Dispersion

Dispersion refers to the particles of one material dispersed into the continuous phase of another material. It often refers to powders such as minerals, pigments and clays dispersed in a liquid.

Emollient

Emollients are fatty or oily substances with a lubricating action that make the skin feel soft, smooth and more pliable. They include lipids such as vegetable oils, fats, butters and waxes. Emollients reduce moisture loss from the skin. They are used in face and body oils, ointments and balms, creams and lotions.

Exfoliant

An exfoliant is a mechanical or chemical agent that is applied to the skin to remove dead skin cells from the surface of the skin. Chemical exfoliants (often referred to as peels) include natural acids such as AHAs and BHAs, while natural mechanical exfoliants (scrubs) include granules such as ground seeds and nuts.

Fixative

A substance that helps slow the rate of evaporation of components of perfume formulations. It helps the perfume last longer on the skin. Extracts from resins, such as benzoin and myrrh, can act as fixatives.

Humectant

A substance that attracts and holds moisture. Humectants assist in keeping the skin hydrated and are most often used in moisturising creams and lotions. They can be added to products to counteract the drying effects of other ingredients such as alcohol. Humectants also improve the aesthetic qualities of products and can reduce a product's susceptibility to drying out. Glycerin is an example of a humectant.

INCI

INCI is the abbreviation for International Nomenclature of Cosmetic Ingredients. It is a uniform system for identifying the ingredients found in cosmetics using conventional scientific names, Latin and English names. It is a regulatory requirement in many countries to have cosmetic ingredients listed on their packaging using their INCI names. This provides a certain level of transparency, allowing consumers to know what they are buying and to identify potential allergens.

Lipid

Lipids include vegetable oils, fats, butters and waxes. They are not soluble in water. They provide a protective barrier on the skin and reduce moisture loss, thus keeping the skin soft and supple.

pH

pH is a measure of how acidic or alkaline (basic) an aqueous solution is. pH denotes 'potential (or power) of hydrogen'. It refers to the level of acidity or alkalinity of a given aqueous solution on a logarithmic scale of 1 to 14. The concentration of hydrogen determines the level of acidity (higher concentration of hydrogen ions) or alkalinity (higher concentration of hydroxide ions). A pH of 7 is considered neutral, while the pH of acidic substances is below 7 and that of alkaline substances is above 7. Pure water is neutral with a pH of 7. The pH of healthy skin ranges around 5 or just below. The skin has the ability to equalise its pH when mildly disrupted. However, the use of highly acidic or alkaline products can make the skin take longer to equalise its pH, and during this time make it vulnerable to sensitivity, redness, breakouts, eczema and hence progressive skin damage. The skin's healthy microflora may also be disrupted if highly acidic or alkaline products are used regularly. The pH of a healthy scalp is 5.5 or below, while the pH of hair is around 3.67.

Solubiliser

In aromatherapy preparations, a solubiliser is a surfactant that helps make essential oils soluble in water. A solubiliser is used in formulations such as face and body sprays, room sprays, toners, micellar waters and gels. Solubilisers are also used in products such as body washes and shampoos to improve clarity and reduce any separation of essential oils.

Solvent

A liquid in which another substance can be dissolved, suspended or extracted. Water, vegetable oil and ethanol are well-known natural solvents.

Surfactant

A shortened term for 'surface active agent'. A substance with the ability to reduce the surface tension at the interface between two unlike surfaces. Soaps, detergents, foaming agents, emulsifiers, solubilisers and dispersants are examples of surfactants. Surfactants are used in products such as shampoos, creams and mists to name a few.

Starting material used in the manufacture of surfactants may include coconut oil, palm oil, sugar and petro-chemicals.

Viscosity

Viscosity is a measure of a fluid's resistance to flow. Informally, it is often referred to as the 'thickness' of a liquid.

Vitamins

Vitamins are organic compounds that our bodies use, in very small amounts, for a variety of metabolic processes. The inclusion of vitamins in skin care products may stimulate collagen synthesis, act as antioxidants or be anti-inflammatory depending on the vitamin.

Bibliography and Further Reading

Advanced Professional Skin Care, Peter T Pugliese, APSC Publishing, Bernville, 1991.

For information on the anatomy and physiology of the skin and the pathology and diagnosis of skin disorders. It also covers treatment of the skin as it relates to beauty therapists.

Aromadermatology: Aromatherapy in the Treatment and Care of Common Skin Conditions, Janetta Bensouilah and Philippa Buck, Radcliffe Publishing, Oxford, 2006.

Accessible information especially suited to therapists using aromatherapy to treat skin conditions. Key topics covered include skin structure and function, essential oils and their effects on the skin, essential oil safety issues in relation to the skin, discussion of a range of skin conditions and the practical application of essential oils in their treatment. Underpinned by sound reference to dermatology and current scientific studies.

Aromatherapy Soap Making, Elizabeth Wright, Print Wright, Gladstone, 1996.

This book contains easy to follow recipes on how to make your own vegetable soaps using natural ingredients. An excellent book for those of you who have never made soap before, and would like to make your own soap from scratch.

Australian Native Plants — Cultivation and Uses in the Health and Food Industries, edited by Yasmina Sultanbawa and Fazal Sultanbawa, CRC Press, Boca Raton, 2016.

Provides a comprehensive view of native food crops grown commercially in Australia that possess nutritional and health properties. It examines their antioxidant and antimicrobial bioactive compounds and properties, with discussions on their cosmetic applications.

A–Z of Natural Cosmetic Formulation, Gail Francombe with Tina Svetek, Goodness & Wonder, Coppell, 2029.

A guide to the most commonly used terminology, theories, methods and protocols in natural cosmetic formulation, with further information on natural ingredients used in skin care formulations. A great first book for those who want to get serious about the business of formulating natural cosmetics.

Bodycraft, Nerys Purchon, Hodder and Stoughton, Sydney, 1993.

This book contains many recipes for natural skin and hair care preparations. It also briefly discusses aromatherapy, nutrition and taking time out.

Clays and Health: Properties and Therapeutic Uses, Michel Rautureau, Cleso de Sousa Figueiredo Gomes, Nicole Liewig, Mehrnaz Katouzian-Safadi, Springer International Publishing, Cham, 2017.

Examines the research that has been carried out on clays and their effects on human health, including the long history of clays used as pharmaceutical and therapeutic agents, the origins of clays, their structural properties and modes of action.

The Complete Guide to Aromatherapy — second edition, Salvatore Battaglia, The International Centre of Holistic Aromatherapy, Brisbane, 2003.

A comprehensive book on the subject of aromatherapy and its various applications, whether for personal use, product formulation or professional health care. It includes quality control of essential oils, essential oil safety, essential oil chemistry, pharmacological studies on essential oils, olfaction and the psychological effects of essential oils, subtle aromatherapy, the role of aromatherapy in primary health care, comprehensive monographs of over 80 essential oils, detailed studies of conditions for each body system, the role of aromatherapy in day spa treatments and more.

The Complete Guide to Aromatherapy — third edition, vol. 1 — Foundations & Materia Medica, Salvatore Battaglia, Black Pepper Creative, Brisbane, 2018.

Provides a framework for the practice of holistic aromatherapy. It includes monographs for 110 essential oils including botany and origins, organoleptic profile, chemical composition, history and traditional uses, a comprehensive view of pharmacological and clinical studies, actions and indications, blending tips, and advice on safety.

The Complete Soapmaker, Norma Coney, Sterling Publishing, New York, 1996.

Contains many beautiful photographs and recipes for soaps. An excellent book for those of you wanting to expand your soap-making horizons.

Greeniology 2020: Greener Living Today, And In The Future, Tanya Ha, Melbourne University Press, Melbourne, 2011.

A guide to sustainable living with many practical tips and recipes, including green cleaning recipes.

The Herbal Medicine-Maker's Handbook: A Home Manual, James Green, Crossing Press, New York, 2000.

A great book providing practical details on how to make a wide range of herbal preparations for health and wellbeing.

How Clay Works: Science and Applications of Clays and Clay-like Minerals in Health and Beauty, Galina St George, Pure Nature Cures School of Mineral and Spa Therapies, Middletown, 2019.

Describes various types of clays and clay-like minerals, their properties, and how the properties of different clay types can be used for a range of skin types and health issues.

It's So Natural, Allan Hayes, Bay Books, Pymble, 1993.

A compilation of environmentally friendly recipes and remedies for health, home and garden.

Jackie French's Natural Solutions, Jackie French, Australian Consolidated Press, Sydney, 1999.

A book of homemade solutions using natural ingredients for health, beauty, home and garden, including green cleaning recipes.

Jeanne Rose's Herbal Body Book: The Herbal Way to Natural Beauty and Health for Men and Women, Jeanne Rose, North Atlantic Books, Berkeley, 2000.

A kitchen cosmetics book containing information on making many preparations using a wide array of common and interesting ingredients.

Make Your Own Cosmetics, Neal's Yard Remedies, Aurum Press, London, 1997.

Contains many simple recipes made from readily available ingredients, which you can prepare at home. It also contains an excellent section discussing ingredients found in many commercially available products.

Milady Skin Care and Cosmetic Ingredients Dictionary — fourth edition, M Varinia Michalun and Joseph C Dinardo, Milady, New York, 2015.

This book discusses many of the ingredients, including natural, which are contained in today's cosmetics. It also discusses the anatomy and physiology of the skin as well as skin care.

Index

EO = essential oil

A
Acne 48, 119, 289
Active ingredient 33, 251
Adzuki beans 9, 155
Aftershave 56, 242, 245
Alcohol 22, 51, 73, 242, 244
Algae 9, 27
Allergic reaction 300
Almond meal 9, 96, 156, 157, 186
Almond oil, sweet 10, 60, 191
Aloe vera 14, 67, 208
Alpha hydroxy acid (AHA) 155, 300
Anisic acid 73
Annatto 169
Antimicrobial 73, 301
Antioxidant 74, 300
Apple 7, 151, 156
Apple cider vinegar 27, 54, 129, 130
Apricot kernel oil 10, 60, 191
Argan oil 11, 140
Argiletz (see Clay) 20, 150
Arnica 61
Arnica infused oil 28
Aromatherapy 35
Arrowroot 10, 23, 97, 258
Athlete's foot (see Tinea) 289
Atlas cedarwood EO 40, 243, 252
Avocado 7, 254, 261
Avocado oil 11, 104, 106, 139, 189

B
Baby 37, 236, 291
    bottom balm 236
    massage oil 237
    powder 237
    wash 236
Bain-marie 53

Balm 59
    aromatherapy 63, 193
    beauty 111
    body 111, 193
    cleansing 112, 123
    hair 113, 269
    hand 111, 213
    healing 112
    herbal 61
    lip 111, 143
    perfume 112, 245
Banana 7, 151, 156, 186
Base products 32
    balm 59
    body wash 181
    cream 77
    gel 65
    lotion 77
    ointment 59
    shampoo 255
Bath 221
    aromatherapy 221
    bomb 225
    herbal 221
    honey 232
    infusion 92
    melt 233
    milk 233
    oat 230
    oil 106, 223
    salt 231
    soda 225
    vinegar 109, 224
Beer 24
Beeswax 23, 60, 86, 141, 193, 280
Beetroot 7
Behentrimonium methosulphate 23, 256, 263
Benzoic acid 73
Benzoin tincture 23
Benzyl alcohol 73
Bergamot EO 39, 196, 223, 243

Bicarbonate of soda (see Sodium bicarbonate) 27, 159, 197, 225
Black pepper EO 39, 221, 242
Blemish gel 137
Blister 220
Blueberry 7
Blue Mallee eucalyptus EO 47, 202, 279
Blue tansy EO 45
Blush 161
Body
    balm 111, 193
    lotion 77, 189
    mask 95, 187
    mist 242, 245
    moisturiser 189
    oil 104, 191
    powder 210
    scrub 96, 99, 100, 183
    wash 101, 181
Body bar
    exfoliating 185
    massage 195
    moisturising 195
Boils 289
Borax 24
Bran 9
Brewer's yeast 24
Broken capillaries 48, 289
Buddha wood EO 47, 242

C
Cabbage leaves 57
Cacao 11, 24, 161,169, 227
Cajeput EO 39, 202, 221, 279
Calendula 14, 61, 91, 170
Calendula infused oil 28, 112, 134, 139, 211
Candelilla wax 11, 60, 193, 199, 269
Cantaloupe (see Rockmelon) 9
Cardamom EO 40, 242
Carnauba wax 11, 60

Carrot infused oil 28, 111, 134, 169, 189
Carrot seed EO 40
Castile soap 24, 101, 181, 259
Castor oil 11, 111, 213, 269
Caustic potash 24, 26, 168
Caustic soda 24, 26, 168
Cedarwood, Atlas EO 40, 107, 202, 251
Cedarwood, Virginian EO 40, 201,202
Cetearyl alcohol 23, 71, 256, 263
Cetearyl glucoside & cetearyl alcohol 71
Cetearyl olivate & sorbitan olivate 71, 72
Chamomile 16, 57, 91, 92, 273
Chamomile, German EO 40, 48, 140, 211, 236
Chamomile, Roman EO 40, 123,193, 233
Chamomile water 29
Champagne 24
Charcoal, activated 24, 95, 159, 163
Chickpea 10, 258
Chickweed 16, 61
Chlorophyll 27, 169
Cinnamon 16, 99, 169, 282
Cinnamon EO 40, 242, 279
Cistus EO 40, 242
Citric acid 24, 74, 225
Citronella EO 40, 202, 279, 283
Clary sage EO 41, 106, 196, 223
Clay 19
    Argiletz 20, 150
    Australian 21, 95, 100, 157
    bentonite 21, 197
    Brazilian 22
    French green montmorillonite 22
    green Argiletz 21, 150, 157
    kaolin 22, 95, 199
    Mediterranean 22
    pink Argiletz 21, 156, 178
    red Argiletz 21, 95, 150, 163
    rhassoul (ghassoul) 22, 186, 257
    white Argiletz 21
    yellow Argiletz 21, 95, 150
Clay mask 20, 95, 150, 187

Cleaning 280
Cleanser 101, 103, 112, 121
Cleansing
    balm 112, 123
    cream 124
    foaming 101, 125
    lotion 124
    milk 125
    oil 103, 123
Clove bud EO 41, 101, 279
Cocamidopropyl betaine 25, 256
Cockroach spray 281
Cocoa 11, 24
Cocoa butter 11, 60, 134, 185, 195, 233, 236
Coconut 7, 95, 96, 177
Coconut oil 12, 195, 253, 266
Coffee 25, 96, 99, 185
Cold cream 124
Cold sore 144
Cologne (see Eau de cologne) 242, 243
Colourant 163, 169, 231, 254
Colour cosmetic 161
Combination skin 48, 117, 136, 157
Comedogenic 13
Comfrey 16, 57, 61, 91, 152
Compress 29, 37, 57, 145
Conditioner 251, 253, 254, 261
    bar 263
Coriander EO 41, 242
Corn starch 10, 200, 210, 237, 258
Couperose 120, 140
Cradle cap 265
Cream
    body 189
    face 134
    moisturising 134, 189
Cream, dairy 25
Cucumber 8, 131, 152, 209
Cuticle cream 213
Cypress EO 41, 97, 101, 140, 197, 251

D
Dandruff 107, 252, 265, 291
Decoction, herbal 49
Dehydrated skin 48, 91, 95, 118, 139

Dehydroacetic acid 73
Deodorant
    block 199
    paste 197
    powder 97, 200
    spray 200
    vinegar 109, 200
Dermatitis 61, 119, 134
Devitalised skin 48, 120
Diffuser essential oil blends 285
Dilution, essential oil 36
Dry shampoo 97, 258
Dry skin 48, 86, 103, 106, 117, 123, 134, 139, 189, 193, 195

E
Eau de cologne 242
Eau de parfum 242
Eau de toilette 242
Eczema 61, 119, 134
Elderflowers 16, 91
Elixir
    face 104, 139
    body 104, 192
Emollient 10, 121, 133, 169, 301
Emulsifier 71, 121, 133
Emulsifying wax 25, 71, 72
Emulsion 69
Epsom salt 25, 231
Equipment 1
Essential fatty acids 10
Essential oil dilution 36
Essential oils 39
Essential oil solubiliser 25, 131, 244, 245, 302
Ethanol 22, 73, 244
Ethyl lactate 73
Eucalyptus, blue Mallee EO 47, 202, 279, 283
Eucalyptus, lemon-scented EO 47, 202
Eucalyptus, peppermint EO 47, 100, 279
Evening primrose oil 12, 134, 139, 265
Everlasting EO 41, 48, 104, 112, 134, 140, 192
Exfoliants
    body 96, 99, 183
    enzymatic 155
    face 96, 99, 155

fruit acid (*see* AHA) 155, 300
gommage 155
granular 155
paste 96, 156
Exfoliating body bars 185
Extrait 242
Eyebrow powder 163
Eye colour 163
Eye cream 147
Eye gel 147

F
Face powder 161
Facial treatment oil 104, 139
Facial wash 101, 126
Fake tan 208
Fats 10, 169
Fatty alcohol 23
Fennel 16
Floral water 29, 129
Flours 10, 93, 97, 161, 210
Foaming cleansers 101, 125
Fomentation 57
Foot
    balm 217
    bath 217
    cream 215
    gel 215
    massage oil 215
    powder 219
    scrub 96, 100, 217
    treatment 220
Fragonia EO 47, 242
Frankincense EO 41, 48, 104,
    112, 134, 139, 192
Fruit acid 155, 300
Fruits 7
Furniture polish 280

G
Galen 124
Gel 65
    base 65
    blemish 67, 137
    eye 67, 147
    face 67, 136
    hair 67, 269
    linseed 68
    mask 67, 149
    moisturiser 67, 136

Geranium EO 41, 48, 136, 140,
    196
German chamomile EO 40, 48,
    140, 211, 236
Ginseng 16
Glass cleaner 280
Glycerin 25, 69, 73, 133, 245
Glycerol (*see* Glycerin) 25, 69,
    73, 133, 245
Glyceryl caprylate 73, 74
Glyceryl stearate 71
Glyceryl stearate citrate 71
Glyceryl stearate SE 71
Gotu kola 16, 91, 95
Grains 9
Grapefruit EO 41, 48, 185, 242
Grapes 8, 151
Green tea 18, 91, 99, 183
Guar gum 25, 65, 67, 149

H
Hair 251
    balm 113, 269
    colour 273
    conditioner 261
    gel 67, 269
    loss 265
    oil 107, 265
    removal 205
    rinse 92, 253
    shampoo 255
    spray 269
    styling 113, 269
Hand 211
    cream 211
    scrub 96, 100, 213
    treatment balm 111, 213
    wash 101, 181
Head lice 267
Hemp flour 9, 157
Hemp seed oil 12
Henna 254, 273
Herbal
    balm 61
    bath 92, 221
    decoction 49
    extract 49
    infusion 49
    infused oil 52
    ointment 61
    tincture 51

vinegar 54
Herbs 14
High blood pressure 38
Hinoki wood EO 42, 242, 280
Home cleaning 280
Honey 26, 130, 141, 143, 156,
    232
Humectants 133, 302
Hydrophilic 71
Hydrosol (*see* Floral water) 29,
    129
Hygiene 2
Hypericum infused oil 29

I
Infused oil 28, 52
Insect repellent 202
    balm 202
    cream 202
    oil 202
    spray 202
Ironbark, lemon-scented EO 47,
    242

J
Jasmine absolute 42, 48, 106,
    243
Jojoba oil 12, 123, 136, 244
Juniper EO 42, 48, 140, 150

K
Kakadu plum 8, 95, 157, 301
Kaolin 20, 21, 22, 151, 161
Kelp 9, 95, 152, 187
Kunzea EO 47, 140, 279

L
Lanolin 26
L-ascorbic acid 26, 186
Lavender 16, 91, 92, 282
Lavender EO 42, 48, 135, 139,
    196, 221, 223, 237
Lavender, spike EO 42, 202
Lavender water 29, 244
Lecithin 26, 71, 82, 136
Lemon 8, 205, 246, 254
Lemon balm 17, 221, 246
Lemon EO 42, 48, 140, 279
Lemongrass 17, 221, 282
Lemongrass EO 42, 170, 243,
    279

Lemon myrtle 17, 185, 233, 282
Lemon myrtle EO 47, 100, 141
    283
Lemon-scented eucalyptus EO 47,
    202, 279
Lentils 9, 155, 258
Lettuce 8
Lice 267
Lime 8, 246
Lime EO 42, 100, 126, 143, 183
Linseeds 26, 57, 65, 68
Lip balm 111, 141
Lipophilic 71
Lip scrub 99, 143
Liquorice 17, 252
Loofah 26
Lotion 77
    body 189
    face 136
Lye 24, 26, 168

M
Macadamia oil 12, 139, 140, 141,
    192, 193
Madder root 169
Magnesium sulphate 25, 231
Mandarin EO 42, 136, 141, 236
Manuka EO 43, 101, 197, 285
Marjoram, sweet EO 43, 196,
    223, 285
Marshmallow 17, 152
Mask
    body 95, 187
    face 95, 149
Massage balm 193
Massage oil
    aromatherapy 191
    herbal infused 191
Matcha 18, 95, 99, 157, 227
Mature skin 48, 95, 96, 104, 112,
    118, 134, 139, 152, 153, 156
May chang EO 43, 170, 221
Melissa EO 43, 144
Milk 26
Mist
    body 245
    face 131
Moisturiser 133, 189
Myrrh 17, 95, 130, 144, 220
Myrrh EO 43, 141, 217, 243

N
Nails 214
Nappy rash 236
Neem 17, 95, 159
Neroli EO 43, 48, 123, 139
Neroli water 29, 150, 244
Nettle 17, 92, 252
Niaouli EO 43, 202, 279
Nipple balm 236
Normal skin 48, 117, 125, 135
Nuts 9

O
Oats 8, 9, 152, 230
Occlusive 133
Oil
    body 104, 191
    face 104, 139
    massage 191
Oil-in-water emulsion 69
Oil phase 69
Oily skin 48, 101, 117, 136, 140
Ointment 59
Olive oil 12, 124, 169, 211, 254
Orange 8, 183, 246, 282
Orange, sweet EO 43, 196, 223,
    243
Orange flower water (see Neroli
    water) 29, 150, 244

P
Palmarosa EO 43, 48, 243
Panthenol 26, 256, 263
Papaya (see Paw paw) 8, 151, 156
Paprika 169, 227, 229
Parfum 242
Parsley 17, 152
Passionfruit 8, 151
Patchouli EO 44, 48, 139, 196,
    201, 243
Paw paw 8, 151, 156
Peach 8, 151
Pear 8, 151
Pectin 65
Peppermint 17, 224, 229, 231
Peppermint EO 44, 141, 159, 215
Peppermint eucalyptus EO 47,
    100, 279
Perfume 241
Perfume balm 112, 245
Perfume oil 242, 244, 245

Petitgrain EO 44, 48, 97, 243
pH 302
    strip 74
    meter 74
Phenethyl alcohol 73
Photosensitivity 38
Pineapple 8, 151, 155
Pine EO 44, 182, 221, 279
Pomegranate 9, 96
Potash 26, 168
Potassium hydroxide 24, 26, 168
Potassium sorbate 73, 74
Potato 9, 10, 187
Pot pourri 282
Poultice 57
Powder
    body 210
    face 161
Precautions 38
Pregnancy 38, 236
Pregnancy balm 236
Preservative 72, 121, 133
Psoriasis 119, 134, 252
Pulses 9
Pumice 26, 96, 217

Q
Quandong 9, 183
QS, quantum sufficit 2

R
Rice flour 9, 96, 156, 157
Rockmelon 9
Roman chamomile EO 40, 123,
    193, 233
Room spray 283
Rosacea 120
Rosalina EO 47, 183, 193
Rose 17, 91, 92, 95, 99, 156, 161
Rose absolute 44, 192, 243
Rosehip oil 13, 134, 139, 153
Rosemary 18, 191, 252, 282
Rosemary EO 44, 196, 251, 252,
    265
Rosemary oleoresin 75
Rose otto 44, 48, 136, 139
Rosewater 31, 134, 147, 153

S
Sage 18, 91, 92, 108, 252
Sage EO 44, 107, 113, 279

Salicylic acid 73
Salt 27, 99, 183
Salt solution 125, 181
Sandalwood EO 45, 48, 139, 243
Sandalwood powder 27, 96
Sanitisation 2
Saponification 167
Scales 1
Scalp oil 107, 265
Scalp treatment 107, 265
Scar treatment 139, 192
Scrub
    body 96, 99, 100, 183
    face 96, 99, 156
    foot 96, 100, 217
    granular 155
    hand 96, 100
    salt 100, 183
    sugar 99, 183
Seaweed 9, 100, 152, 187
Seeds 9
Semolina 9
Sensitisation 3, 39, 300
Sensitive skin 3, 39, 48, 119, 124, 134, 135, 140, 152, 156, 186, 187, 199
Serum 104, 139, 272
Shampoo 255
    bar 256
    dry powder 97, 258
Shaving cream 126
Shaving gel 127
Shea butter 13, 60, 112, 134, 135, 143, 195, 211, 213, 236
Shower steamer 233
Skin cleanser (see Cleanser) 121
Skin condition 118
Skin freshener 91, 129
Skin irritation 39, 300
Skin type 117
Slippery elm 18, 57
Soap 165
    ball 177
    cold-process 172
    ingredients 168
    making 168
    mould 170
    recipes 174
    shave 178

    tracing 173
Soapwort 18, 126, 181, 257
Sodium anisate 73
Sodium benzoate 73, 74
Sodium bicarbonate 27, 159, 197, 225
Sodium cocoyl isethionate 27, 256
Sodium hydroxide 24, 26, 167
Sodium levulinate 73
Solid body bars 195
Solubiliser (see Essential oil solubiliser) 25, 131, 245, 302
Sorbic acid 73
Soyabean oil 13
Spirulina 27, 169, 227
Strawberry 9, 95, 156
Sugar 27, 99, 143, 183, 269
Sugaring 205
Sunburn 208
Surface cleaning paste 280
Surface cleaning spray 280
Surfactant 121, 302
Sweet orange EO 43, 196, 223, 243
Sweet marjoram EO 43, 196, 223, 283, 285

T
Tahini 151
Tangerine EO 42, 221, 236
Tansy, blue EO 45
Tapioca starch 10, 161, 210, 237
Tea 208, 209
Tea, green 18, 91, 99, 183
Tea tree EO 48, 137, 140, 144, 267, 279
Teeth powder 159
Thalassotherapy 9
Thermometers 1
Thyme 18, 91, 252
Thyme EO 45, 144, 220, 251
Tincture, herbal 51
Tinea 220
Tocopherol 75
Tomato 9, 96
Toothpaste 160
Toner 91, 108, 129
Turmeric 18, 169, 183, 227

U
Utensils 1

V
Vanilla 141, 177
Vegetable oil 10
Vegetables 7
Vetiver EO 45, 48, 140, 243
Vinegar 27
    bath 109
    deodorant 109, 200
    hair 108, 253
    herbal 54
    scalp 108, 253
    toner 108, 129
Vitamin C (see L-ascorbic acid) 26, 186
Vitamin E (see Tocopherol) 74
Vodka 23, 51, 246, 247

W
Wash
    body 101, 181
    face 101, 125
Water-in-oil emulsion 71
Watermelon 9, 151
Water phase 69
Wattle seeds 9, 96, 157
Waxes 10, 11, 23
Wheatgerm oil 13, 139, 140, 189
Window cleaner 280
Wine, red 27
Witch hazel water 31

X
Xanthan gum 28, 65, 81, 149

Y
Yarrow 18, 61, 91, 252
Yarrow EO 45, 192
Ylang ylang EO 45, 48, 135, 139, 196, 223, 243, 285
Yoghurt 28, 150, 151

Z
Zinc oxide 28, 236, 237